Frederick William Pavy

A Treatise on Food and Dietetics

Physiologically and Therapeutically Considered

Frederick William Pavy

A Treatise on Food and Dietetics
Physiologically and Therapeutically Considered

ISBN/EAN: 9783744644839

Printed in Europe, USA, Canada, Australia, Japan

Cover: Foto ©Andreas Hilbeck / pixelio.de

More available books at **www.hansebooks.com**

A TREATISE

ON

FOOD AND DIETETICS

PHYSIOLOGICALLY AND THERAPEUTICALLY CONSIDERED

BY

F. W. PAVY, M.D., F.R.S.,

FELLOW OF THE ROYAL COLLEGE OF PHYSICIANS; PHYSICIAN TO, AND LECTURER ON PHYSIOLOGY AT, GUY'S HOSPITAL.

SECOND EDITION

NEW YORK
WILLIAM WOOD & COMPANY
27 GREAT JONES STREET
1881

INSCRIBED

By the Author

TO

THE RIGHT HONORABLE

LYON PLAYFAIR, M.P., C.B., F.R.S.,

AS A MARK OF

APPRECIATION OF HIS SCIENTIFIC

LABORS IN RELATION TO FOOD,

AND

IN ADMIRATION OF

THE SERVICES HE IS NOW RENDERING

IN HIS POLITICAL CAREER.

PREFACE TO THE SECOND EDITION.

A LARGE impression having become exhausted in less than a year, I feel myself warranted in concluding that I was not mistaken in judging that a work of the kind produced was wanted, and at the same time am emboldened to cherish the idea that the labor bestowed has not proved fruitless in usefulness to others.

The favorable reception accorded to the first edition has served alike as a source of gratification to me and a stimulus to renewed exertions to render the work worthy of approbation. Without presuming to think that there does not still exist much room for improvement, I hope that something in that direction has been effected by the revision which has been carried out. Wherever it has appeared to be required, the wording has been altered to render the meaning clearer; various modifications (in part suggested by the valued hints of reviewers) have been introduced; and a considerable amount of new matter added—notably, attention may be directed to the preliminary part of the section on Wine as having undergone extensive amplification.

I am glad to avail myself of the opportunity here afforded of expressing my thanks to those who, since the appearance of this work, have supplied me with information drawn from scattered sources upon the subject of Food.

35 GROSVENOR STREET,
GROSVENOR SQUARE, LONDON,
June 1, 1875.

PREFACE TO THE FIRST EDITION.

In the Preface to the second edition of my work on "Digestion: its Disorders, and their Treatment," I mentioned that I had originally intended to add a section on Food to the contents of that volume, but that for the reasons given I afterward determined to publish a separate treatise on the subject. Thus originated the present work, which, with the progress of time, and a large consumption of midnight oil, has grown to dimensions far exceeding those I had at first contemplated.

From the fact that the subject of Food is one of deep concern, both to the healthy and the sick—that the information which has been obtained during the last few years has completely revolutionized some of the cardinal scientific notions formerly entertained—and that no modern systematic treatise of the kind here presented exists in the English language, I have been encouraged to think that the task I have undertaken may not be deemed superfluous. Whatever the results obtained, I have steadily striven, sparing no pains for the purpose, to render the work produced instructive and useful.

On account of the change recently introduced in chemical notation, I have given both old and new formulæ, placing the latter within square brackets after the former.

35 GROSVENOR STREET,
GROSVENOR SQUARE, LONDON,
March, 1874.

CONTENTS.

A TREATISE

ON

FOOD AND DIETETICS.

INTRODUCTORY REMARKS ON THE DYNAMIC RELATIONS OF FOOD.

THE discoveries and inductions of the present age have thrown a new light on the physiology of food.

Around us we have to deal with Matter and Force—the one a substantive entity, the other appreciable only as a principle of action. It has long been known that matter (as cognizable in our own era) can be neither created nor destroyed. It may be variously combined and modified, but it remains the same in essence and unaltered in amount. Force, also, has recently been recognized as similarly conditioned; and in order that the bearings of food in relation to this principle may be understood, some preliminary considerations explanatory of the views now entertained regarding it are necessary.

To start, then, we may take it as accepted that, under present conditions, force, like matter, can neither be created nor destroyed. "Ex nihilo nihil fit" and "Nihil fit ad nihilum" form axioms that must be admitted to be incontrovertible. If we except the inconsiderable accession derived from the occasional descent of a meteoric body, the earth's matter remains fixed in amount. It is otherwise, however, with respect to force. Under the form of heat and light, force is constantly being transmitted to us from the sun; and it is from the force thus derived that, in a manner to be explained further on, life on earth originates and is sustained.

In enunciating his doctrine on the "Correlation of the Physical Forces," Grove demonstrated that one kind of force was capable of producing another. His views were first made known at a lecture delivered at the London Institution in 1842. The word "correlation" he employed as meaning "reciprocal production—in other words, that any force capable of producing another may in its turn be produced by it." The position sought to be established was that heat, light, electricity, magnetism, chemical affinity, and motion, are all correlative, or have a reciprocal dependence—that either might produce the others, and that neither could originate otherwise than by production from some antecedent force or forces.

Just at this time the same field of inquiry was being investigated by other workers. While Grove was asserting that the great problem awaiting solution in regard to the correlation of physical forces was the establishment of their equivalent of power, or their measurable relations to a given standard, Mayer, Joule, and Helmholtz were announcing the actual equivalents themselves.

Mayer, of Germany, had the priority in the publication of his re searches. As a member of the medical profession he approached the subject through its relation to physiology. In 1842 he propounded, in its full comprehensiveness, the doctrine of the " Conservation of Force."

Nearly at the same time Mr. Joule, of Manchester, discovered the equivalent of heat in mechanical motion. He had been led to prosecute researches in that direction, with the view of ascertaining the relative value of heat and motion for the advantage of engineering science. He found that what sufficed to raise the temperature of a pound of water one degree Fahrenheit would, under another mode of action, raise 772 pounds a foot high; or, putting it conversely, the fall of 772 pounds of water from a height of one foot would give rise to an amount of heat sufficient to elevate the temperature of one pound to the extent of one degree Fahrenheit. Thus the mechanical work corresponding to the elevation of 772 pounds a foot high, or, what comes to the same thing, one pound 772 feet high, forms the dynamic equivalent of one degree of heat of Fahrenheit's scale.

It is necessary to state here that the term " force," when used in a strict sense, is employed under a more limited acceptation now than formerly. Originally it represented what is now distinguished as both "force" and "energy." By "force," under a rigid signification, is understood the power of producing energy; by "energy" the power of performing work. To give an illustration : power has force, the cannon-ball energy; but to speak of the force of the cannon-ball is inexact. I may also remark that the words "actual" and "potential" are in frequent use to qualify the state in which energy is met with. By *actual* energy is meant energy in an active state—energy which is doing work. By *potential* energy, energy at rest—energy capable of doing work, but not doing it. In a bent cross-bow there is potential energy—energy in a state of rest, but ready to become actual, or to manifest itself when the trigger is pulled. Again, actual energy is evolved from the sun. By vegetable life this is made potential in the organic compounds formed. In these organic compounds the energy is stored up in a latent condition; potential energy is reconverted into actual energy when they undergo oxidation during combustion or in their utilization in the animal economy.

The doctrine of the "Conservation of Energy" implies that energy is as indestructible as matter, that a fixed amount exists in the universe, and that, however variously it may be modified, transferred, or transformed—in spite of all the changes of which it may be the subject throughout the realm of nature—it cannot be created or annihilated, increased or diminished. The doctrine further implies that the different forms of energy have their definite reciprocal equivalents; that so much chemical energy, for instance, will produce so much heat, which is the representative of so much motive power, and so on. The ascertained equivalents of heat and motive power have been already given.

Accepted as applicable to the physical forces, the doctrine of the "Conservation of Energy" next began to be applied to living nature. Grove, in his "Correlation of Physical Forces" (second edition, p. 89), suggested that the same principles and mode of reasoning adopted in his essay might answer equally for the organic as for the inorganic world, and that muscular force, animal and vegetable heat, etc., might, and one day would, be shown to possess similar definite correlations. He proceeded no further, however, remarking that he purposely avoided entering upon a subject not pertaining to his own field of science.

At this time the general belief prevailed that the processes going on in the living body were determined by "vitality" or the "vital principle." The physical forces, it was supposed, were overruled in the living by the vital principle. Without discussing whether we are to admit or deny the existence of this principle as a distinct operating force—a question which has been handled by some of the leading men of science of the day—we must, I think, concede, as a matter of experience, that in the living organism there are influences at play which have no existence in the dead matter around. Matter which has been impressed with life can produce effects which dead matter cannot. This does not conflict with the extension of the law of the "Conservation of Energy" to living nature. The effects produced may have their origin in the physical forces—the living matter forming the medium through which they operate. With artificial appliances force may be made to produce various effects, according to the nature of the instrument employed. With the same force in operation different kinds of work are performed, according to the character of the machine set in motion. Between the two—living matter and a machine—there exists an analogy which admits of being followed still further. It is only when in a certain state that matter is capable of forming the medium for the exercise of force in the production of living operations. Modify this state, and though there may be the same matter to deal with, yet it is no longer capable of fulfilling the same office it performed before. So in the case of an ordinary machine: it must possess a particular construction before it can form the medium for the operation of force. Disarrange this construction, and, although the matter remains unchanged, the application of force is without its proper effect. Thus a disarranged machine may be compared with living matter devitalized. In both, the capacity of being set in operation by force has existed, and in both that capacity has been lost. Further, it may be said that a machine in working order, but unoperated on by force—that is, in a state of rest—is like matter possessing vitality, but in a dormant state. Both are ready to move directly the proper force is applied.

Applying the law of the "Conservation of Energy" to living nature, the forms of force which we observe in operation are all primarily derived from the sun. When a weight is lifted by the hand it certainly seems a long way off to go to the sun for the muscular force employed in the act; yet the doctrine of the "Conservation of Energy" justifies, as I will proceed to show, the conclusion that its origin is there.

To begin with, the force evolved in muscular action has its source in the material which has been supplied to the body in the form of food. Now all food comes primarily from the vegetable kingdom, and vegetable products are built up through the agency of the sun's rays. It may be said that the energy contained in these rays, which has been employed in producing the compound, is fixed or rendered latent within it. When the cross-bow is bent, the force derived from the muscular action employed in bending it is stored up, ready to be again liberated when the trigger is pulled, no matter whether this be at once or a hundred years hence; and the force given to the arrow when it is launched is neither more nor less than that which has sprung from the muscular action employed in bending the bow. The same with vegetable products. Their formation is coincident with the disengagement of oxygen from oxidized principles and the development of combustible compounds. To effect this disengagement the operation of force is required. Now, the force so employed has its source in the heat and light evolved from the sun, and that which is used for the purpose may be said to become fixed and to exist in a latent condition—to exist stored up in the product, ready to be again liberated on exposure to conditions favorable to oxidation. Thus may these vegetable products be compared to a bent cross-bow, containing, as they do, a store of latent force, which may for an indefinite period remain as such, or may be liberated soon after it has been fixed. Whenever liberated, it is no more nor less than the equivalent of the force which has been used in the formation of the product. Our coal-fields represent a vast magazine of force drawn, ages ago, from the sun's rays, and capable at any moment of being set free by the occurrence of oxidation.

Vegetable products, then, may be regarded as containing a store of force accumulated from the vast supply continually emitted with the sun's rays; and, upon the principle of indestructibility enunciated, the force which has been employed in unlocking the elements in the combinations from which vegetable products are built up, and in forming the new compound, is contained in such compound in a latent state. Now, as above stated, animals either directly or indirectly subsist upon these vegetable products, and are thence supplied by them with accumulated force. By oxidation the force is set free in an active state under some form of manifestation or other. It matters not in what way—whether rapidly or slowly, or under what circumstances; whether inside or outside the living system—the oxidation occurs, the result is the same, so far as the amount of force liberated is concerned, it being implied in the doctrine of the "Conservation of Energy" that it should constitute the equivalent of the solar force originally made use of. This is presuming complete oxidation to occur; but in the processes of animal life, although fully oxidized compounds, like carbonic acid and water, are formed and discharged, yet others, like urea, are expelled in an imperfectly oxidized state, and carry with them a certain amount of latent or unutilized force.

Thus it is that the various forms of force manifested in the actions of animal life trace their origin to that emitted from the sun. Plants are media for fixing solar force—for converting actual into latent or potential energy. Animals reconvert latent into various forms of actual force. Thus, in the various forms of actual force liberated by the actions of animal life, we have the equivalent of that which has been fixed by plants from the sun. As there is a revolution of matter, so is there a revolution of force within and around us.

In the liberation of actual force, a complete analogy may be traced between the animal system and a steam-engine. Both are media for the conversion of latent into actual force. In the animal system, combustible material is supplied under the form of the various kinds of food, and oxygen is taken in by the process of respiration. From the chemical energy due to the combination of these, force is liberated in an active state; and, besides manifesting itself as heat, and in other ways peculiar to the animal system, is capable of performing mechanical work. The steam-engine is supplied with combustible material under the form of coal, which differs from our food in representing the result of the vegetative activity of a former instead of the present epoch. Air is also supplied, and from the combination which occurs between its oxygen and the elements of the combustible material, heat is produced, which in part is dissipated as such, but in part is applied to the performance of mechanical work.. According to Helmholtz, the animal economy, in respect of its capacity to turn force to account in the accomplishment of mechanical work, is a more perfect instrument than the steam-engine. His calculations lead him to conclude that whilst in the best steam-engine only one-tenth of the force liberated by the combustion of its fuel is realizable as mechanical work, the rest escaping as heat, the human body is capable of turning one-fifth of the power of its food into the equivalent of work. There is this, however, to be remarked, that the fuel of a steam-engine is a far less expensive article than the food of an animal being.

The animal body, then, may be regarded as holding an analogous position to a machine, in which a transmutation of chemical into other forms of force is taking place. Food on the one hand, and air on the other, are the factors concerned in the chemical action that occurs. It is through the interplay of changes between food and air that the manifestations of animal life, consisting of heat-production, muscular contraction, nervous (including mental) action, and nutritive or formative, secretory, and assimilative action arise. The egesta, or substances dismissed from the system, are metamorphosed products of the ingesta, or substances entering the system. The elements are the same, in nature and in quantity, in the two cases, but their forms of combination, and, with them, their force accompaniment, are different. The force employed in building up the organic compounds belonging to food is again evolved as they descend by oxidation into more simple combinations, and in the force evolved we have the representative of the active manifestations of animal life. If the products discharged from the system were fully oxidized principles, the force developed in the body would equal that contained in a latent condition in the food. Such, however, is not completely the case, a certain amount of latent force remaining, as has already been remarked, in some of the egesta. The position, therefore, may be formulated thus: The latent or potential force of ingesta equals the force developed in the body plus the force escaping with the egesta. In other words, the unexpended force in the egesta and the force disengaged by the operations of life, and manifested under the various forms of vital activity, equal the force contained in the ingesta.

What is required in food is matter that is susceptible of undergoing change in the system under the influence of the presence of oxygen. Life implies change, and the manifestations of life are due to the reaction of food, with the derivatives from it, and air upon each other. While in the inorganic kingdom a tendency to a state of rest prevails—while the closest affinities tend to become satisfied, and so establish equilibrium—in a manifestly living body rest is impossible. It is true, living organisms of certain kinds may exist in a state of rest, but then there is a suspension of vital manifestations. The state constitutes that which falls under the denomination of "dormant vitality." Animal organisms may exist in it, and the seed of a plant naturally remains for a while in it. Molecular rest, and, with it, an absence of any show of vital activity prevail. Concurrently, however, with the manifestation of vital activity, molecular change—change in a particular or prescribed direction—occurs. Organic compounds become resolved by the agency of oxygen into more simple combinations, as carbonic acid, water, and urea, and cease to be any longer of service. To maintain a continuance of vital activity fresh organic material is required: hence the demand for food. But food and the other material factor of life—oxygen—do not constitute all that is needed. It is further necessary that the two should be brought within the sphere of influence of living matter, in order that the changes may be made to pursue the particular line of direction resulting in the phenomena of life.

ON THE ORIGINATION OF FOOD.

Our food is in the first instance derived from the vegetable kingdom. Dumas at one time said, " L'animal s'assimile donc ou détruit des matières organiques toutes faites; il n'en crée donc pas." But, as he afterward admitted, this is not the case. The animal, it is true, is constantly consuming or destroying organic substances, and is incapable of forming them from the inorganic principles, but supplied with organic matter, organic compounds of various kinds are constructed.

Mulder's discoveries in 1838 led up to the doctrine that the albuminous compounds of plants and animals agree in composition and properties, whence it was inferred that the animal simply took the compound produced by the plant and made it a component part of its own body. Liebig was the first to maintain that animals possessed the power of forming one kind of organic compound out of another. A warm controversy was at one time carried on upon this point, turning particularly upon the formation of fat. While, on the one hand, it was held by Liebig that, in the animal system, fat could be formed from sugar, Dumas and Boussingault maintained, on the other, that whatever fat was found in an animal being was derived through its food from without. From the researches initiated by this dispute, it became incontestably established that Liebig was right, and the French chemists were ultimately compelled, even on the evidence of the results obtained by themselves, to abandon the doctrine they had advanced.

A moment's consideration will, further, suffice to show that one kind of albuminous compound is capable of being constructed from others. In the young mammal, subsisting solely on milk, it is to the caseine that we must look for the source of fibrine and albumen; and in the animal feeder, secreting milk, the caseine produced is derived from the fibrine and albumen. Gelatine, moreover, has no existence in vegetable food. At the present day we may waive the discussion of this matter, it being now established that none of these nitrogenous principles enter the system under the form in which they occur in food. They are all converted, during the performance of digestion, into a certain principle (albuminose), which is the principle that is absorbed, and that is subsequently transformed by the assimilative power of the animal into the various compounds met with.

The position, then, is this: That animals are not simply consumers of organic compounds, but are capable of exerting a constructive action as well. They must, however, be supplied with organic matter previously formed, and thus the capacity that really exists is that of transforming one organic compound into another. All organic matter has its primary source in the vegetable kingdom, from which kingdom, it follows, all our food must directly or indirectly be derived. The vegetable feeder goes directly for its food to the vegetable kingdom. The animal feeder is equally dependent upon the products of the vegetable kingdom for its pabulum. But it obtains it only at second-hand, so to speak, or in an indirect manner, its food consisting of the flesh of animals which have themselves been nourished upon vegetable products.

Now, it is only under exposure to the action of the sun's rays that plants will grow, and hence it is to the influence of these rays that we must refer the production of food in the first instance, and the primary source of all life upon our earth.

It has already been shown how the energy emitted from the sun, under the forms of heat and light, is capable, through the medium of the plant, of disengaging oxygen from its combination with carbon and hydrogen in carbonic acid and water, and leading to the formation of reoxidizable compounds; and how the energy evolved from the reoxidation of these compounds, whether by combustion or within the animal system, represents or forms the equivalent of that employed in effecting their construction.

What an immeasurable amount of force to be, and to have been, emitted from the solar centre! It is true that it must possess a store of heat altogether unrealizable by comparison with anything cognizable around us; for it has been shown, by recent investigations with the spectroscope, that iron and other metals, which cannot by any known method of heat-application be converted into the gaseous state upon our earth, exist in that state around the sun. It is true, also, that the sun is a body of almost inconceivable magnitude. To give the simile of Helmholtz, "its diameter is so great that if you suppose the earth to be put into the centre of the sun, the sun itself being like a hollow sphere, and the moon going about the earth, there would be a space of more than two hundred thousand miles around the orbit of the moon lying all interior to the surface of the sun." * But when we come to consider that, taking the view now held by philosophers, in that small pencil of rays which has impinged upon our earth at a distance of nearly ninety-five million miles from the sun has been contained all the energy or source of power which has been fixed by plants, and much besides which has escaped being so utilized, we cannot help being struck at the immensity of the store of power existing in the sun. Geology teaches us that at an early epoch in the history of our globe, this solar influence must have manifested itself to a much stronger degree then it does even at the present time. The vast coal-beds forming a portion of the earth's crust have originated in vegetable growth. During the carboniferous era, which comprised the period of this coal-formation, the atmosphere was probably laden with carbonic acid and humidity to a much greater extent than at the present day. But it is to the solar energy that we must look for the source of the luxuriant vegetation which evidently flourished at that time, and which must have existed in the Arctic Regions as well as in the lower latitudes, since coal-deposits are found there.

It has been already stated that it is only under the influence of the force contained in the sun's rays that organic compounds are built up by the agency of the plant; and it is found to be the green parts only of plants—those where chlorophyl exists—that effect the decomposition of carbonic acid and water—fixing the carbon and hydrogen and liberating the oxygen. This operation, it is the distinctive function of the plant to perform, and it fails to be carried on when either the influence of light is absent or chlorophyl is not present. Under these conditions—absence of light and chlorophyl—oxygen is absorbed and carbonic acid liberated instead, just as occurs in the animal. I have been informed that it is known to florists, as the result of practical observation, that in the case of the variegated-leaved geranium, a slip that may happen to be possessed of white leaves only will not grow alone like other slips. The absence of chlorophyl explains the non-capacity to effect the changes necessary for growth.

The solar beam is composed of rays possessing different properties and different degrees of refrangibility, and the question has been raised—What part of the solar spectrum exerts greatest power over vegetable growth? The colored rays produced by passing a pencil of light through a prism are arranged in the following order: violet, indigo, blue, green, yellow, orange, red.

The greatest illuminating power of the spectrum is in the bright yellow rays, and the greatest heating power in rays below the red, and therefore less refrangible than any of the colored rays; whilst the greatest chemical power—power of effecting chemical change—is in the rays at the other extremity of the spectrum, namely, the violet, and in the invisible rays just above, where the highest degree is encountered.

Draper, from experiments conducted in 1843, states that on causing plants to effect the decomposition of carbonic acid in the prismatic spectrum, he found the yellow rays by far the most effective. The relative power of the various colored rays he asserts to have been as follows: yellow, green, orange, red, blue, indigo, violet.

In opposition to the conclusion arrived at by Draper, it is affirmed by others that it is to the blue and violet rays that must be referred the maximum power of effecting the decomposition of carbonic acid through the medium of the plant. Helmholtz says: "The observations upon vegetable life have shown that plants can grow only under the influence of solar light, and as long as solar light, and principally the more refrangible parts of solar light, the blue and violet rays, fall upon the green parts of plants, the plants take in carbonic acid and exhale oxygen."* He further remarks, that in exerting this influence these rays are completely absorbed; for it can be shown that solar light which has passed through green leaves in full development is no longer capable of exerting any chemical influence.

I have spoken of light as a factor in the construction of organic compounds by the plant. The elements of which these organic compounds consist are drawn from the inorganic kingdom, and chiefly, as Liebig pointed out, from carbonic acid, water, and ammonia—principles which all exist to a greater or less extent in the atmosphere, and from the atmosphere are to a large extent, if not entirely, derived. In the case of the low vegetable organisms which become developed in moist situations as a green layer on the barren surface of rocks and stones, the elements required for their growth must have been derived solely from the atmosphere. In the case of the higher organisms, however, the elements of growth are drawn from the soil as well as the atmosphere. Humus, which forms the constituent of the soil which supplies these elements, consists

---

* Ibid., p. 473.

of the decaying remains of organic products. But it is not as organic matter that humus serves as food to the plants: that is, it is not the organic matter itself that is utilized. It is, on the other hand, as a source of carbonic acid and ammonia, principles resulting from its decomposition, that it owes its position in relation to the alimentation of plants.

The stages passed through in the history of vegetable life leading to the provision of a fitting supply of food for animal existence may be thus represented : Beginning, let us say, with a barren surface of rock, which may have been freshly exposed to the atmosphere from some subterranean, volcanic, or other agency, the germs of low vegetable organisms settling upon it, extract from the atmosphere their elements of growth. Passing through their term of life they die, and fresh ones spring up and similarly live and die. So the process goes on, higher and higher forms making their appearance. The decaying remains of this primitive growth encrust what was a barren surface with a layer of earth or mould, in which ultimately the highest plants find a suitable position for taking root and growing. Thus, clothed with vegetation, a fit locality is provided for the support of animal life, animal beings finding in the vegetable products now existing the necessary material for their subsistence.

It may be mentioned here that there is one class of vegetable organisms—the Fungi—which seems to occupy an exceptional position, and to resemble animals in being dependent upon organic products for their growth. It is possible, however, that the seeming appropriation of organic matter may be more apparent than real, and that the dependence upon organic matter may arise from a specially large and constant supply of carbonic acid and ammonia being required as a condition of growth. Still it must be said that these vegetable organisms are not dependent for growth upon light like others, that they have no green surfaces for decomposing carbonic acid, and, in fact, that, instead of absorbing carbonic acid and setting free oxygen, they agree with animals in doing precisely the reverse. Such circumstances, it is true, are strongly suggestive of the occurrence of growth from an appropriation of organic compounds; but there is this to be remarked, that the growth under consideration occurs only where decay is going on, and there is nothing, at all events, to show that any other than organic compounds in a state of decomposition can be made use of.

There are other vegetable organisms, such as Venus' fly-trap, the pitcher-plants, etc., which capture insects apparently with the view of deriving from their bodies organic matter for appropriation to the purposes of nutrition. In other respects, however, these plants agree in their mode of life with their fellow-organisms.

The chief elements of the various organic compounds built up by the agency of vegetable life, are carbon, hydrogen, oxygen, nitrogen, sulphur, and phosphorus; and the following may be regarded as the sources from which they are derived.

In the above enumeration, carbon is mentioned first, as being the element which occurs by far the most extensively in organic nature. Large as is the quantity of carbon entering into the composition of organic substances, the main, if not the entire, source from which it is derived is the carbonic acid in the atmosphere. According, however, to Saussure, the amount of carbonic acid contained in air is not, as a mean, more than one part, by volume, in two thousand; but then it must be remembered that it is constantly being generated, not only as a product of animal life, but from various processes carried on around us.

Now it appears that the leaves and other green parts of plants are continually absorbing the carbonic acid, and, with the aid of light, effecting its decomposition, the oxygen being exhaled and the carbon detained and applied to the production of organic substances. Whilst it is only by the leaves and green surfaces that carbonic acid is decomposed and oxygen liberated, it is probable that its absorption is not limited to those parts, but that some enters through the roots, this being derived from the process of decomposition going on in the organic matter of the soil, and from the carbonic acid carried down from the atmosphere with the rain.

Striking as it may seem, there yet are sufficient grounds for believing that the vast store of carbon contained in forests, of whatever extent we may encounter, has been derived in the manner above-mentioned. Geological investigations render it almost certain that at one time the atmosphere was far richer in carbonic acid than it is now, and that vegetation also was proportionately more luxuriant.

The absorption of carbonic acid and exhalation of oxygen which takes place in plants, under the influence of light, constitutes, then, a process of alimentation. The reverse process—the absorption of oxygen and exhalation of carbonic acid; a process which forms one of the principal phenomena of animal life—occurs also to some extent in plants, and stands out unconcealed during the night, when, from the absence of light, there is no decomposition of carbonic acid and liberation of oxygen going on. It also occurs as the result of certain operations of plant life, as, for instance, during germination, flowering, and fruiting.

Hydrogen and oxygen are supplied to an unlimited extent to plants under the form of water. In the production of the carbohydrate group of organic compounds; that is compounds such as starch, sugar, dextrine, gum, cellulose, etc., in which carbon is united with hydrogen and oxygen in the proportion to form water, it is possible that water is directly assimilated, although this is by no means an ascertained fact. In a large number of other compounds, however, it is evident from their composition that for water to serve for their production, its elements must undergo separation. The oleaginous compounds, for instance, chiefly consist of carbon and hydrogen. The amount of oxygen present is very much less than that required to form water with their hydrogen. For this element to be appropriated a deoxidation must occur, and it is believed that some of the oxygen exhaled by the plant under the influence of light has its source not only in carbonic acid, but likewise in water.

Although plants are freely surrounded with nitrogen—this element forming the large constituent it does of the atmosphere—yet it is not from the atmosphere that the nitrogen of organic matter is derived. The researches of Saussure and Boussingault have demonstrated that plants are incapable of appropriating the free nitrogen of the atmosphere and elaborating it into organic matter. Liebig's view, and it is one which is by common consent endorsed, is, that the nitrogen of organic matter is derived from ammonia. This able chemist was the first to show that ammonia is a constant constituent of the atmosphere. It is true that the quantity in which it is present is so small that it cannot be recognized except by extraction from a large volume of air. It may be removed and its quantity determined ("On the Estimation of Ammonia in Atmospheric Air," by Horace T. Brown: "Proceedings of the Royal Society," vol. xviii., p. 286) by passing a given volume of air through water slightly acidulated with sulphuric acid. It is also susceptible of recognition in rain-water, where it exists under the form of carbonate. Ammonia, like carbonic acid, forms a product of the decomposition of organic matter. The nitrogen of organic matter, indeed, is returned to the inorganic kingdom under the form of ammonia. Thus in humus we have a source of ammonia which, doubtless, combines with some of the carbonic acid also generated, and in this state is in great part dissipated into the atmosphere. The great volatility of the product would lead to this result. Diffused through the atmosphere, it would be abstracted by rain and snow, and in this way carried back to the earth, to be brought in contact with the roots of plants, through which its absorption is supposed to be effected. According to Liebig, ammonia enters the vegetable organism in combination with carbonic or sulphuric acid, while, according to Mulder, the combination is with the acids he describes as existing in humus.

Nitrogen is an element of the highest importance in regard to vegetable as well as to animal life. It is not only necessary that it should enter into the constitution of vegetable substances so that animals may obtain a supply of it with their food, but it forms an indispensable element in relation to the molecular changes of the plant as well as of the animal. Wherever living changes are carried on, nitrogenized matter is present. The proclivity of this to change forms one of its most characteristic qualities, and the changes it undergoes induce changes of a definite kind in other matter which *per se* has a tendency to remain at rest. Thus, in nitrogenized matter we have, as it were, the requisite starting-point for the various changes which result in the phenomena of life.

The four elements which have been referred to, viz., carbon, hydrogen, oxygen, and nitrogen, form by far the chief constituents of organic compounds, but sulphur and phosphorus are also present, to a small extent, bound up with the other elements in certain organic principles. Sulphur, for example, is met with in caseine, and both sulphur and phosphorus in fibrine and albumen. The probable sources of these elements are sulphates and phosphates, the acids of the salts undergoing deoxidation through the medium of the operations carried on in the plant, in the same manner as occurs in the case of carbonic acid.

As yet I have been referring merely to the *source* of the elements entering into the constitution of the organic compounds produced by plants, and upon this point it may be considered that our information is pretty definite. The precise mode, however, in which these elements are combined or elaborated into the infinite variety of organic compounds existing is quite another matter, and one which (it must be conceded) belongs as yet only to the domain of hypothesis. The point has been the subject of many laborious researches, conducted by some of the most distinguished observers, but, in spite of these attempts to elucidate it, we have at present little or nothing beyond conjecture to deal with. It may be fairly surmised, however, that the production of the higher compounds is effected step by step, or by a series of transition stages, and not by a direct or immediate union of the elements entering into their composition. Whatever the exact changes that ensue, there can be no doubt that they proceed in a definite and precise order. In organic nature we know that change induces change, and the change first set in motion in the act of growth may be regarded as starting the changes which produce the various organic compounds met with. Bodies in contact with changing matter are within the sphere of influence of a metabolic or metamorphosing force, and to the operation of this force is to be ascribed much that occurs as the result of living action.

It is the formation of organic compounds which constitutes the special province of the plant to effect in relation to the production of food. Food, however, to fulfil the requirements of animal life must contain certain mineral or inorganic as well as organic principles—a supply of the former being quite as indispensable as a supply of the latter. But we need not concern ourselves about a separate supply of mineral matter; for, wisely, the productions of nature contain in combination all that is wanted. It happens that, besides being furnished with carbonic acid, water, and ammonia for the formation of organic compounds, plants require for their growth a supply of saline principles. These they draw from the surrounding soil, and a portion of the advantage accruing to vegetable growth from the employment of manure is owing to the mineral matter it contains, and which is thereby given to the soil.

In appropriating mineral matter as an element of nutrition, the plant exercises a selective action. It is found, for instance, that some of the saline compounds belonging to the soil, and not others, are present, that they are present in different proportions as regards each other, and to a different extent in different parts of the plant. Mineral matter holds, in fact, a definite relation to the component parts of a plant, and probably enters into some sort of combination with the organic constituents.

Thus, in vegetable products we find not only the organic, but likewise the inorganic matter we require; and, in taking up and applying mineral matter as it does to its own purposes of growth as well as forming organic compounds, the vegetable organism contributes in a complete manner toward the supply of what is wanted for animal nutrition.

A reciprocal relation, however, it must be observed, in reality exists between what is supplied and what is wanted. We are as much adapted to the appropriation of the food supplied to us as our food is adapted to our wants. Were we not so adapted, existence would be impossible for us. In nature all things are mutually adapted to each other.

In what has been said about the production of food by the vegetable kingdom for animal subsistence, it is seen that animals and plants stand in direct antagonism to each other as regards the results of the main operations of life. Plants draw their food from the inorganic kingdom, and produce organic compounds. Animals find their food in these organic compounds, and, in applying them to the purposes of life, reconvert them into inorganic principles. In the appropriation of inorganic matter as food, plants absorb carbonic acid and set free oxygen. Animals, in their consumption of organic matter, absorb oxygen and give out carbonic acid. Thus animal life and vegetable life stand in complemental relation to each other, and it is in accordance with the requirements for the persistence of living nature upon the surface of our planet that it should be so. If the operations of animal and vegetable life proceeded in one and the same direction only, the effect would be a gradual alteration of the chemical arrangement of matter, until a state of things was arrived at unfit for the further continuance of life. Under the existing order of things, animals and plants in such a manner neutralize each other's effects upon surrounding matter that they balance each other's operations, and thereby maintain a state of uniformity.

THE CONSTITUENT ELEMENTS OF FOOD.

Of the various elements known to exist in nature, only a limited number enter into the constitution of living bodies. The following is a list of those found as constituents of the human body: Carbon, hydrogen, oxygen, nitrogen, sulphur, phosphorus, chlorine, sodium, potassium, calcium, magnesium, iron, fluorine, silicon, manganese, aluminium, copper. The first four, namely, carbon, hydrogen, oxygen, and nitrogen, exist in far larger quantity than any of the others. As for those which occur toward the end of the list, they are present only in exceedingly minute quantity, if, indeed, they are invariably present—it is more than doubtful if they are to be regarded as essential constituents.

The food being the source from which the elements forming the constituents of the body are derived, it follows that food must contain all the elements which are met therewith. No article can, as food, satisfy the requirements of life that fails to comply with this condition.

ALIMENTARY PRINCIPLES:

Their Classification, Chemical Relations, Digestion, Assimilation, and Physiological Uses.

Although it is necessary that our food should contain the elements that have been enumerated—and contain them in such proportion as to furnish the requisite amount of each to the system—yet it is not with these elements as such that, from an alimentary point of view, we have to deal. It is only in a state of combination that the elements are of any service to us as food; and, as has been already mentioned, the combination must have been formed by the agency of a living organism—the combination must, in other words, constitute an organic product.

Now, taking the different organic products which nature affords us as food, we find that they may, by analysis, be resolved into a variety of definite compounds. These constitute what are known as "alimentary principles," in contradistinction to "alimentary substances," or the articles of food as supplied to us by nature.

In a scientific consideration of food it is necessary to speak first of the alimentary principles. It is only, indeed, by looking at it through its constituent principles that we are in a position to discuss its physiological bearings, and I will begin by pointing out the most convenient division and classification to be adopted.

Popularly, the ingesta are looked upon as consisting of *food* and *drink*, the one supplying us with solid, the other with liquid, matter. Superficially, this appears a natural and convenient mode of primary grouping, but in a physiological point of view it is completely worthless. "Food" and "drink" constitute terms referring only to the particular state in which an article for consumption may happen to exist—viz., whether it is in a solid or liquid form. What is drunk, for instance, and this holds good particularly in the case of milk, may be rich in food or solid matter, and in the food we consume there is invariably a large proportion of liquid matter.

Physiologically, then, the separation of the ingesta into "food" and "drink" is unsuitable. The two material factors of life are food and air; and food may be considered as comprising that which contributes to the growth and nutrition of the body, and, by oxidation, to force-production. Regarded in this comprehensive light, food embraces both solid and liquid matter; and the primary natural division is into organic and inorganic portions; that is, combinations of elements producible only through the agency of life, and chemical combinations drawn simply from the mineral kingdom and incorporated with the others.

The inorganic portion of food consists of water and various saline principles. The organic portion may be subdivided into compounds of which nitrogen forms a constituent, and compounds from which it is absent; in other words, into nitrogenized and non-nitrogenized compounds. The non-nitrogenized alimentary principles are composed of the three elements — carbon, oxygen, and hydrogen, variously united together; whilst the nitrogenized likewise contain these three elements, but, in addition, nitrogen, and, for the most part, sulphur, or sulphur and phosphorus, as well.

Liebig, regarding the nitrogenized and non-nitrogenized principles as contributing to quite distinct purposes in the animal economy, referred to them as forming the basis of a physiological classification. The former he looked upon as destined for appropriation toward the growth and maintenance of the components of the body, and therefore he called them "plastic elements of nutrition." The latter he regarded as simply designed for undergoing oxidation, and, in this way, for serving as a source of heat. These he termed "elements of respiration," but the expression, it must be said, does not properly convey what is meant, and Dr. R. Dundas Thomson suggested that the term "calorifiant" should be employed instead. "Calorifacient," however, is a more appropriate word, and by general consent has been adopted.

It stands to reason, that for the growth and repair of the various textures of the body, as these have nitrogen forming an essential ingredient of their constitution, nitrogenized compounds must be supplied; but, from what is now known, it must also be said that these compounds are likewise susceptible of application to heat-production. They are truly, indeed, "histogenetic," or tissue-forming materials, but, by the separation of urea (which is known to occur in their metamorphosis in the animal system), a hydrocarbonaceous compound is left, which may be appropriated to heat-production. It may be asserted, in fact, that there is sufficient to show that the nitrogenized principles in reality subserve both purposes in the animal economy.

In fat, again, we have a non-nitrogenous principle, and one belonging, therefore, to the calorifacient group. There is every reason, however, to believe that fat is essential to tissue-development. It seems to be intrinsically mixed up with nitrogenized matter in the animal textures. Certainly it may be said to be directly applied toward the formation of adipose tissue. Fat, therefore, takes rank as a nutrient no less than as a calorifacient principle.

Hence Liebig's definition is not to be accepted in a rigid sense. Although nitrogenized principles constitute true "elements of nutrition," yet it neither follows nor appears likely that they are limited to this purpose. Fats are undoubtedly important calorifacient principles, and cannot *per se* supply what is required for tissue-development; they, nevertheless, take part in the process. According to our current views, which will be discussed more fully further on, fats are also concerned, in a manner not previously suspected, in muscular force-production. Taking all these considerations into account, Liebig's classification loses the scientific force it was originally supposed to possess. The subdivision of the organic portion of food, however, into nitrogenized and non-nitrogenized groups is still practically and physiologically convenient.

Prout proposed a classification which arranged food in four groups of principles, viz.: 1st, the aqueous; 2d, the saccharine; 3d, the oleaginous; and 4th, the albuminous.

It will be seen that this classification fails to include saline matter, which, as already stated, forms an element indispensable to nutrition. The saccharine and oleaginous groups comprise non-nitrogenized principles, while the albuminous comprehends the nitrogenized.

The classification that will be adopted in this treatise is one which involves no expression of physiological destination, but is based on the chemical nature of the principles. It is first assumed that food falls naturally into organic and inorganic divisions.

Next, that the organic is subdivisible into nitrogenous and non-nitrogenous; and further, that the non-nitrogenous is naturally and conveniently again subdivisible into fats and carbohydrates—the former consisting of carbon and hydrogen in combination with only a small amount of oxygen; the latter of carbon, with oxygen and hydrogen always in such relation to each other as to be in the exact proportion to form water. . To this latter group belong such principles as starch, sugar, gum, etc.

It must be observed that there are a few principles which do not strictly fall within either of the preceding groups. Such, for instance, as alcohol, the vegetable acids, and pectin or vegetable jelly. Alcohol occupies an intermediate place between the fats and carbohydrates, whilst the others are even more oxidized compounds than the carbohydrates—in other words, contain a larger amount of oxygen than is required for the conversion of their hydrogen into water. These principles are hardly of sufficient importance, in an alimentary point of view, to call for their consideration under a distinct head, and they will therefore be spoken of in connection with the carbohydrates.

Having said thus much upon the classification of the alimentary principles, I shall next speak of them in relation to their respective physiological bearings, taking the groups in the following order: 1st, nitrogenous principles; 2d, hydrocarbons or fats; 3d, carbohydrates; 4th, inorganic materials.

THE NITROGENOUS ALIMENTARY PRINCIPLES.

Nitrogen enters largely into the composition of the animal body. It therefore requires to be freely supplied from without. Although living in an atmosphere about four-fifths of which consists of nitrogen, yet it is not from this source (though the question was formerly entertained) that our supply of nitrogen is drawn. Nitrogen, to be available for us, must be supplied in a state of combination. It is not, indeed, with nitrogen in the form of an element that we have anything to do in the question of alimentation, but only with compounds containing it; and such compounds, it may be said (as regards animal alimentation), that have been produced under the influence of life—that is, compounds which answer to the name "organic."

Organic nitrogenous matter, then, and not nitrogen, is what we· require to have supplied to us, and what alone we have to deal with physiologically. Such nitrogenous matter must, therefore, constitute an essential ingredient of our food, and we find that it there exists under various chemical forms.

Chemists recognize several well-defined compounds amongst the nitrogenous matter found in different articles of food. Besides these, there may be some nitrogenous matter which is still susceptible of being used, but which has not yet been specialized, and which in an analysis would fall

2

amongst the extractives. This, however, cannot be sufficient in amount to be of much significance.

If we look at the nitrogenized alimentary principles which have been made known, some are characterized by yielding proteine when subjected to the action of an alkali and heat, whilst from others no proteine is similarly to be procured. The former comprise the albuminous group, and are often referred to as the proteine compounds; the latter constitute the gelatinous principles.

When the discovery of proteine was first of all made by Mulder, the substance was regarded as forming the base or radical of the albuminous principles. It contains the four elements—carbon, hydrogen, oxygen, and nitrogen; and each of the albuminous principles was regarded as simply resulting from the combination of the supposed base with different quantities of sulphur and phosphorus, or sulphur only. It must be stated, however, that there is nothing to show that proteine really exists in the compounds from which it is to be obtained. It can be regarded only as a product of the chemical process to which it is necessary to subject the compounds in order to obtain it. Looked at in this light, it constitutes a chemical and not a physiological principle. It therefore has no direct physiological bearing, but nevertheless it serves to link together certain important physiological compounds.

The albuminous or proteine compounds comprise albumen, fibrine, caseine, and certain other bodies which form modifications of these.

Albumen may be looked upon as the most important representative of the proteine group. It consists of the four elements—carbon, oxygen, hydrogen, and nitrogen, with the addition of some sulphur and phosphorus. As it is met with in animal productions, it is in such intimate union with fatty, alkaline, and earthy matter, that it is with some difficulty separable from them. It varies to some extent in its behavior, as it is obtained from different sources. The albumen of the blood, for instance, does not agree in all respects with the albumen of the white of egg. One of the most striking properties of albumen is its coagulability upon the application of heat. It therefore exists under two states, viz., soluble and coagulated albumen.

Albumen may be regarded as the pabulum in the blood from which the different animal tissues are evolved. That it can afford *per se* the nitrogenous matter required for nutrition is proved by its being the principle in the egg from which are developed the nitrogenous tissues of the chick.

Fibrine is characterized by its property of undergoing spontaneous coagulation. It is composed of the same elements as albumen, but contains a larger proportionate amount of sulphur, and also a rather larger quantity of oxygen.

Caseine forms the proteine compound of milk. It is distinguishable from fibrine by not undergoing spontaneous coagulation, and from albumen by not being coagulable by heat, and by being thrown down by organic acids which do not precipitate albumen. Besides the four elements —carbon, oxygen, hydrogen, and nitrogen—it contains sulphur, but no phosphorus. It is remarkable for the large quantity of phosphate of lime which it is capable of holding bound up with it, and the tenacity with which it retains it. There is, it should be stated, a little uncertainty regarding the chemical constitution of caseine. By some it is regarded, not as a simple, but as a compound body—a body composed (in reality) of a combination of two or more others.

Besides these well-known proteine compounds there are modifications of them which have been particularized by chemists, and the following may be referred to as connected with the subject of food.

Vitelline is the name given to the modified form of albumen which exists in the yolk of the egg. There are certain points in which this substance comports itself differently with reagents from ordinary albumen.

Globuline is the albuminoid matter existing in the fluid contents of the blood-corpuscle. It is there intimately associated with, but nevertheless quite distinct from, the coloring matter. The same principle is also found in the crystalline lens of the eye. Different opinions have been expressed regarding the true position it holds. Lecanu looked upon it as identical with albumen, and Simon with caseine, whilst Lehmann remarks that he would be disposed to place it by the side of vitelline, if the elementary analyses were not opposed to that view.

Myosine constitutes the insoluble principle of muscular substance, and is obtained by subjecting the tissue in a finely divided state to repeated washings with water. Another substance was described by Liebig as constituting muscle fibrine, and was named by him *syntonine*. It forms the principle dissolved from washed muscle by a weak solution of hydrochloric acid, and may be thrown down from this solution by neutralization with an alkali. It is present in and thereby increases the nutritive value of beef tea prepared according to Liebig's special directions. This principle has been lately regarded as nothing more than acid albumen; and it is said that if either albumen, myosine, vitelline, or fibrine be treated with dilute acids the formation of acid albumen occurs which is, or appears to be, identical with syntonine.

The proteine compounds have as yet been referred to only as they occur in animal productions. But vegetable productions also contain compounds which, in the language of Liebig, are not only similar to, but absolutely identical with, the albumen, fibrine, and caseine of the animal kingdom.

Vegetable albumen is contained in wheat and the other seeds of the *cerealia*. The juices of most vegetables, such as turnips, carrots, cauliflower, cabbage, etc., yield more or less precipitate with heat by virtue of its presence. It is also found in considerable abundance in association with vegetable caseine in the oily seeds, such as almonds, nuts, etc.

Vegetable fibrine, like albumen, is also found in the cereal seeds. It remains behind when flour is washed with a stream of water for the extraction of gluten. The albumen, starch, etc., are carried away with the water, and a tenacious mass is left, which is known as crude gluten. It is not this which constitutes vegetable fibrine, but vegetable fibrine forms a portion of it. By means of boiling alcohol the crude material obtained as above is resolved into two portions. The one which is dissolved consists of glutin and caseine, whilst that which remains is vegetable fibrine. Vegetable fibrine also exists in the juice of the grape and most vegetables.

Vegetable caseine can be obtained from peas, beans, and other leguminous seeds, and is sometimes specially denominated *legumine*. It also exists, with albumen, in the almond and such-like oily seeds.

The gelatinous principles constitute nitrogenous compounds, but do not yield proteine like the compounds that have just been referred to. They comprise *gelatine* and *chondrine*, and are obtainable only from animal products: gelatine from bone and other structures containing fibrous tissue, and chondrine from cartilage. The most striking property they possess is that of their aqueous solution gelatinizing upon cooling. It is gelatine which forms the basis of soups. Besides carbon, hydrogen, oxygen, and nitrogen, as constituent elements, a small amount of sulphur appears also to be present. They contain no phosphorus.

The question has been raised, and largely discussed, as to whether gelatine and chondrine exist in the tissues, or are formed in the process of obtaining them, viz., the prolonged boiling of the tissue in water. On looking at the chemical properties of gelatine, we notice that it forms an insoluble compound with tannic acid. Now, it is well known that a structure which yields gelatine, on being soaked in a solution of tannic acid, gives rise to the formation of the compound mentioned. It is this, indeed, which forms the basis of leather, a fact which is strongly in favor of gelatine really existing as a constituent of the animal body.

It has been stated that the gelatinous principles which have fallen under consideration are to be obtained only from animal products. No nitrogenous compound of the kind is met with in vegetable materials. The jelly yielded by fruits and some other vegetable substances is quite a different article. It consists only of the three elements—carbon, hydrogen, and oxygen, and is known chemically as pectine and pectic acid.

All the nitrogenous principles must undergo digestion before they can enter the system. Digestion, in fact, is simply a process which has for its object to fit substances for absorption into the system; and the nitrogenous principles are in a state to resist absorption, certainly to any material extent, until they have been liquefied and transformed by the agency of digestion.

Beyond being mechanically comminuted or reduced to a more or less finely divided state in the mouth, our nitrogenous food undergoes no change until it reaches the stomach. In this organ it is brought into contact with a secretion, the gastric juice, which has the effect of dissolving and transforming it into a principle which possesses the important property of being highly diffusible, and thereby readily transmissible from the alimentary canal into the blood-vessels. With all the nitrogenous alimentary principles the result is the same. They each, under the influence of the gastric juice, lose their characteristic properties and become converted into the highly soluble and diffusible product referred to.

Mialhe was the first to recognize this product of the digestion of the nitrogenous principles, and gave it the name of *albuminose*. *Peptone* is the name which has since been applied to it by Lehmann. Mialhe held that the substance obtained by the digestion of the proteine bodies was identical with that obtained by the gelatinous principles. This would bring the latter into precisely the same position with regard to nutrition as the former. Although our knowledge about the precise extent of the capacity of gelatine as an article of nutrition cannot be looked upon as complete, yet the information before us justifies the inference that it does not possess the same capabilities as an albuminoid substance. If such be true, the products of digestion of the two cannot be completely identical, however much they may resemble each other in their general properties.

It has been stated that, by the action of the stomach, the various principles composing our nitrogenous food lose their characteristic properties, and become converted into a substance which has received the designation of peptone from one, and albuminose from another. Fibrine is dissolved, and is not susceptible of again solidifying. Albumen in a fluid form is not precipitated, as has been asserted, and then redissolved, but simply transformed. Albumen in the solid or coagulated state is dissolved, and fails to be again coagulable. Caseine is first rendered solid, or curdled, and then redissolved. It is now no longer susceptible of being thrown down. Gelatine is liquefied, and cannot again be made to gelatinize.

No matter from what principle a digestive product or peptone has been obtained, the following are the characters which are found to belong to it. It is soluble to the highest degree in water, and it signifies nothing whether the liquid is in the acid, neutral, or alkaline state. It is not precipitable from its aqueous solution by heat. It is soluble in dilute alcohol, but absolute alcohol precipitates it. It is an uncrystallizable substance, devoid of odor and almost of taste. In a physiological point of view its most important property is the high degree of diffusibility it enjoys. It is designed for removal from the alimentary canal by absorption, and, by possessing the property referred to, a physically favorable disposition exists for the accomplishment of what is wanted.

The nitrogenous alimentary principles, then, on reaching the stomach, are fitted for absorption by undergoing transformation into a highly soluble and diffusible substance. The change, we know, is wrought by the secretion of the stomach, although the precise *modus operandi* cannot be explained. There are two indispensable ingredients of the gastric juice, viz., pepsine (a neutral nitrogenized principle) and an acid. Pepsine is a secretory product, peculiar to, and therefore obtainable only from, the stomach. About the acid there is nothing peculiar, and different views have been held regarding the kind of acid that is naturally present. With the combination of pepsine and acid, a liquid is obtained which dissolves nitrogenous matter in the same manner out of as within the stomach. According to Lehmann, it is only hydrochloric and lactic acids—and these, the same authority affirms, give the acidity to the natural secretion—which yield an energetic digestive fluid with pepsine; but, according to my own experiments on artificial digestion, other acids, such as the phosphoric, sulphuric, citric, and so on, will equally answer the purpose.

From the above statements it follows that the solution of nitrogenous food in the stomach is effected by the action of a liquid which owes its virtue to the presence of a couple of principles—pepsine and an acid. The action of this liquid is favored by the elevated temperature belonging to the body, and also by the movement to which the contents of the stomach are subjected by the action of the muscular fibres with which the walls of the organ are provided. As it is reduced to a fluid state the food is forced on into the upper bowel. Chyme is what this product of gastric digestion is called. Besides the nitrogenous matter in a dissolved state, it contains a portion suspended in a finely divided form which has not yet undergone solution, and likewise, in the same state, those constituents of the food which resist the solvent action of the stomach.

The nitrogenous matter which has escaped from the stomach in an undissolved state is submitted to a further digestion in the intestine. This may be shown by direct experimental observation. And it is not by a continued action of the gastric juice which passes on with the food in its course, but by an action exerted by the secretions poured into the intestine itself. It has been stated that the presence of an acid forms an indispensable factor in gastric digestion. The chyme as it passes on from the stomach is strongly acid. It contains nitrogenous matter which has not yet undergone solution, and also gastric juice whose power (it may be inferred) has not become exhausted. So far, we have conditions which suffice for a continuance of the process carried on in the stomach. It happens, however, that on reaching the small intestine the chyme encounters alkaline secretions. The pancreatic juice is, to a marked extent, alkaline, and so is also the intestinal juice. The bile likewise contains a quantity of alkali in feeble combination, and easily taken by the gastric juice acid. Thus it happens that the chyme becomes more or less neutralized as the small intestine is being traversed. As the result of observation, in fact, I have noticed that by the time the lower part of the ileum is reached, the intestinal contents may be found to present a neutral or even alkaline reaction. In this way, through contact with the secretions poured into the intestine, the energy of the unexhausted gastric juice contained in the chyme is destroyed, and whatever solution of nitrogenous food now occurs must be due to another agency.

Let us, therefore, inquire into the effect which the various secretions, as they become incorporated with the chyme, are capable of producing.

First, as regards the intestinal juice. This fluid, it is evident, possesses some solvent influence upon nitrogenous matter. Bidder and Schmidt ascertained by experiment that meat and coagulated albumen, contained in a muslin bag, undergo, on being placed in the empty small intestine, in which the bile and pancreatic juice are prevented by a ligature from descending, in from four to six hours' time a considerable amount of digestion. In an experiment performed by myself, in which the hind legs of a frog that had been separated from the body, were introduced into the empty small intestine, secured by a ligature from the descent of secretions from above, I found, after the lapse of six hours, the legs partially digested—a portion of the skin, for example, having been dissolved away, the muscles underneath it separated, and some of the bones, to a slight extent, exposed.

Next, as regards the pancreatic juice. Besides its other offices in the animal economy, this liquid acts upon and dissolves nitrogenous matters, as appears from the following considerations.

In 1836, Purkinje and Pappenheim asserted that the pancreas contained a principle capable of exerting a digestive action upon the nitrogenized elements of food. This statement attracted little attention, and soon dropped out of notice. More recently Lucien Corvisart, of Paris, having reopened the subject, proved, by a series of experiments, that the pancreas, as one of its functions, supplements the action of the stomach, and, after a copious meal, contributes to digest those nitrogenous matters which have escaped the stomachic digestion. As far as the result is concerned, the two kinds of digestion, he states, coincide, each leading to the production of albuminose. While acidity, however, is a necessary condition to digestion in the case of the gastric juice, the pancreatic secretion, it is affirmed, possesses the power of acting equally well, whatever the existing reaction—whether acid, neutral, or alkaline.

In support of his doctrine, Corvisart has adduced three sets of experimental results.

In the first place: if the pancreas of an animal be taken when its active principle is at its maximum of quantity and quality, that is, from the fourth to the seventh hour after digestion has begun, and it be then finely cut up and infused for an hour in twice its volume of water at a temperature of 20° Cent. (68° Fahr.), and the infusion be at once experimented with, it will be found, he asserts, to possess a power of dissolving the nitrogenized alimentary principles, and converting them into albuminose; and this with no evidence of putrefaction being perceptible, provided the experiment be stopped at the end of four or five hours, in which time, under a temperature of about 100° Fahr., the pancreatic principle will have effected all that it is capable of doing.

Secondly.—The pancreatic juice obtained during life from the duct of the gland is found, he affirms, to be capable of acting as a powerful solvent on the nitrogenized alimentary principles, when the requisite precautions are taken in conducting the experiment. The juice, that is to say, must be obtained from the fourth to the seventh hour after the ingestion of food, at which time it is charged to its maximum degree with the pancreatic principle; and must also be experimented with immediately after its collection. It dissolves, Corvisart says, fibrine more quickly and more largely than albumen. The heat being maintained between 42° and 45° Cent. (108° and 113° Fahr.), a specimen of pancreatic juice of ordinary energy dissolves, it is stated, if the mixture be agitated every quarter of an hour, all that it is capable of taking up of fibrine in two or three hours at the most, and of solid albumen in four or five hours, the experiment, up to this time, being attended with no evidence of ordinary decomposition, while at a subsequent period ordinary decomposition is found to set in.

Thirdly.—Nitrogenized substances introduced into the duodenum when pancreatic juice is flowing into it are found to be dissolved, notwithstanding the gastric juice and bile are precluded from entering by applying a ligature to the pylorus and bile-duct.

It is necessary to state that the evidence derivable from the last experiments must not be taken for more than it is really worth, viewed in relation to pancreatic juice *per se*. The bile and the gastric juice may, it is true, have been prevented entering the duodenum, and thereby precluded from contributing to the effect, but it is impossible to exclude from operation the secretions of Brunner's and the other glands of the duodenum.

My own experiments with the pancreatic juice at first inclined me to think that the effects producible on nitrogenous matter through the agency of the pancreas were rather like those which result from putrefaction than from true digestion.

On reperforming the experiments, however, I obtained results which certainly appeared to indicate that some digestive action had been at work. For example, upon operating with the pancreatic infusion, taken conformably with the instructions of Corvisart, I found that frogs' hind-legs (which, according to my experience, constitute one of the most, if not the most, sensitive and distinct tests of digestive action) were, upon some occasions, softened, so that the flesh broke down under very slight pressure, without any evidence of ordinary putrefaction being apparent. The effect, however, was not to be compared with what is observed after the use of artificial gastric juice, and ordinary decomposition tends quickly to occur, which is not the case in experiments conducted with gastric juice. Whatever the power actually enjoyed by the pancreatic juice in this direction, the chief point of interest to us, as regards the subject of food, is not whether this or that secretion poured into the intestine will dispose of nitrogenous matter, but whether nitrogenous matter really undergoes digestion in the intestine; and, thus framed, it will be presently seen that the question admits of being answered in a very positive manner.

The bile forms another secretion, which becomes incorporated with the alimentary matter after its exit from the stomach. There is nothing, however, to show that this fluid possesses any solvent power over the nitrogenized principles of food.

Remarks have been made upon the action of the secretions taken individually, but as regards the subject of food, the point of greatest interest to us, as has been already said, is what occurs within the intestine when all the secretions are allowed to enter. Experiment shows that there is a very powerful solvent action exerted, and, as I can state from personal investigation, a few hours suffice for nitrogenous matter, introduced directly into the upper part of the small intestine, to be completely digested. With reference, therefore, to the digestion of nitrogenous matter, the intestine may undoubtedly be regarded as performing a part supplementary to that of the stomach. Besides its other functions, it serves to complete the digestion of whatever nitrogenous alimentary matter may have escaped the digestive action of the stomach, and it may be remarked that the same result—namely, the production of albuminose or peptone—occurs as when the solution has been effected in the stomach.

Reviewing the stages that are passed through preliminary to the appropriation of nitrogenous matter within the system, we have seen that, through the agency of the stomach and of the intestine, it undergoes conversion into a principle which, from its diffusible nature, is readily susceptible of absorption, and it is in this form, viz., as albuminose, that the various nitrogenous alimentary principles reach the circulation.

The conversion of the nitrogenous alimentary matters into albuminose is necessary, it is further to be remarked, not only as a process preparatory to absorption, but also as fitting them for subsequent application to their proper destination. It cannot absolutely be affirmed that no absorption whatever occurs without previous conversion into albuminose; but this much is certain, that the amount so absorbed must be very trifling, and it can be shown that if they directly reach the circulation in any quantity, they visibly pass off without being applied to the purposes of the economy.

Bernard was the first to demonstrate that the albumen of egg, reaching the circulation without having previously undergone digestion, quickly passes from the system into the urine. If introduced directly into one of the blood-vessels, or even if injected into the subcutaneous tissue, it rapidly betrays its presence in the urine. This I can attest from my own experience. Both after injection into a vein and into the subcutaneous tissue, the albumen of egg, as I have often seen, is soon recognizable in the urine.

It has also been observed that a meal consisting largely of eggs, particularly if taken after prolonged fasting, has been followed by the appearance of albumen in the urine. Here, apparently, it has happened that some albumen has reached the circulation without having undergone the usual conversion, and, as when experimentally injected, has been thence discharged with the urine. Hence it may be concluded, not only that egg-albumen and blood-albumen differ strikingly from each other in a physiological point of view, but that egg-albumen, as such, is not fitted for entering the circulation.

The conversion of albumen into albuminose, therefore, not only bears on the facility of absorption, but on the adaptability for subsequent application in the system. The process of metamorphosis, in fact, is required not only with a view to adaptability for absorption, but to subsequent fitness for utilization in the system.

Caseine and gelatine I have found * comport themselves in the same

---

* Gulstonian Lectures (1862) on Assimilation and the Influence of its Defects on the Urine: Lancet, vol. i., p. 574, 1863.

manner as albumen, namely, pass off from the system with the urine when directly introduced into the circulation. The injection of three ounces of milk into a vein was observed in an experiment to be followed by the appearance of caseine in the urine. The injection of one hundred grains of isinglass, dissolved in two and a half ounces of water, also so charged the urine with gelatine as to give rise to the formation of a firm, solid jelly on côoling.

Thrown off as they thus are from the system, albumen, caseine, and gelatine are evidently not adapted for direct introduction into the circulation. Fibrine, on account of its solidity, cannot be similarly experimented with. Digestion, in its case also, is an indispensable condition to its introduction into the circulation. In respect, indeed, of all these principles, it may be said that their metamorphosis in the digestive system is needed as a preliminary step to their capability of appropriation in the body, and their application to the purposes of life.

We have followed the nitrogenous alimentary principles to the stage of albuminose. The precise nature of what next ensues is not yet known. There can be little or no doubt as to the progress from albuminose to the albumen of the blood, but as to what next occurs we have no data to show. With the ultimate products that are formed we are acquainted, but the steps of metamorphosis are as yet beyond our knowledge. The chain we have hitherto followed now wants one or more links, which we have as yet no means of discovering. As regards the seat of metamorphosis we have also no information of a precise nature to deal with, but we may, nevertheless, hazard the surmise that the liver is the viscus in which albuminose, like other nutritive matters absorbed from the alimentary canal, mainly, if not entirely, undergoes metamorphosis. The various nitrogenous principles of the body must be primarily derived from it ; but, whether by direct transformation into them, or by passing through the stage of albumen, we have not the means of deciding. That albumen is susceptible of metamorphosis, however, into the other principles, we know, from its forming in the egg the pabulum whence the various nitrogenous principles of the young bird take their origin.

Instead of wandering farther into the domain of conjecture as to the subject of metamorphosis, let us now turn our attention to the purposes fulfilled by the nitrogenous principles as alimentary matter.

Foremost in importance is the supply of material for the *development primarily, and for the renovation secondarily,* of the tissues. Wherever vital operations are going on, there nitrogenous matter is present, forming, so to speak, the spring of vital action. Although non-nitrogenous matter contributes in certain ways toward the maintenance of life, yet it is nitrogenous matter which starts and keeps in motion the molecular changes which result in the phenomena of life. Nitrogenous matter, it may be said, forms the basis, without which no life manifests itself. Life is coincident with molecular change. In non-nitrogenous matter the elements of the molecule are not, of themselves, prone to change; whereas in the molecule of nitrogenous matter there exists a greater complexity of grouping among the elements, and these cohere so loosely, or are so feebly combined, as to have a constant tendency to alter or to regroup themselves into simpler combinations. By this change in the nitrogenous, change is induced in the contiguous non-nitrogenous molecule, and, occurring as the whole does in a definite or prescribed order, the phenomena of life are produced. Nitrogenous matter, in this way forming the instrument of living action, is incessantly being disintegrated.

Becoming thereby effete and useless, a fresh supply is needed to replace that which has fulfilled its office. The primary object of nitrogenous alimentary matter may thereupon be said to be the development and renovation of the living tissues.

We have seen that nitrogenous matter forms an essential part of living structures. It holds the same position in the case of the *secretions*. These owe the active properties with which they are endowed, chiefly, if not entirely, to a nitrogenous constituent. This is drawn from the blood by the glands just as it is drawn by the tissues; and on passing from the blood it is modified or converted, by the agency of the gland, into the special principle encountered. Nitrogenous matter is thus as essential to the constitution of the active secretions as it is to the tissues; and, as the amount of the secretions required is in relation to the general vital activity, a corresponding demand for nitrogenous matter is created.

I now come to treat of *nitrogenous matter in relation to force production*.

The dependence of muscular and nervous action upon oxidation of the respective tissues is one of the many doctrines which have emanated from the inventive intellect of Liebig. According to the view propounded, nitrogenous matter alone constitutes the source of muscular and nervous power. The tissues being consumed in the exercise of their functional activity or the manifestation of their dynamic properties, fresh nitrogenous matter is alleged to be needed to replace that which has served for the production of power. Thus viewed, nitrogenous matter has been regarded as not only applied to nutrition and to the formation of the nitrogenous constituents of the active secretions, but also to the restitution of the loss incurred by the production of power. What wonder, then, if, with all these purposes to fulfil, the nutritive value of food should have been measured, as it latterly has been, by the amount of nitrogenous matter it contains?

Liebig's doctrine was at once accepted, and until recently has been looked upon as expressing a scientific truth. Like many other of its author's views, its plausibility was such that no one ventured to question its soundness. Gradually, however, experimental inquiry began to invalidate it, and the reactionary move has advanced till Traube has been led to express himself in directly opposite terms regarding the source of muscular and nervous power. According to this authority, for instance, the organized or nitrogenous part of a muscle is *not* destroyed or consumed in its action. The resulting force is affirmed to be due, instead, to the *oxidation of non-nitrogenous matter*—the muscle merely serving as a medium for the conversion of the generated force into motor power. The point has attracted much attention of late, and researches of an elaborate nature have been conducted with regard to it. Let us see the position in which these researches have placed it.

The argument representing the question to be solved may be thus expressed: Does the force evolved by muscular action proceed from destruction of muscular tissue? If so, nitrogenous matter would be needed to replace the loss incurred, and the result would be equivalent to nitrogenous matter through the medium of muscle being applied to the production of motor power. Now, if muscular action is coincident with the destruction of muscular tissue, there must, as a product of the destruction, be a nitrogen-containing principle eliminated. The elements of the compounds that have served their purpose in the economy do not accumulate, but are discharged from the system under certain known forms of combination. The nitrogen, therefore, belonging to a consumed nitrogenous structure should be recognizable in the effete matters thrown off from the body. Nay, more; as the force developed by muscular action cannot arise spontaneously—as it can be produced only by transmutation from another force—the destruction of muscular tissue (which through the chemical action involved supplies the force) should be in proportion to the amount of muscular work performed, and the nitrogen contained in the excreta in proportion also to the amount of muscular tissue destroyed.

Now, in proceeding to measure the extent of tissue metamorphosis by the nitrogen eliminated, it is necessary, in the first instance, to be sure of our data regarding the channels through which nitrogen finds its exit from the body—it is necessary, that is to say, to ascertain whether nitrogen escapes with the breath and perspiration, as was at one time asserted, as well as by the alimentary canal and the kidneys. We have no accessible means, it must be stated, of determining in a direct way whether nitrogen passes off by the lungs and skin. Our conclusions have to be based upon comparing the nitrogen ingested with that encountered in the urine and alvine evacuations. Formerly it was said that a deficiency in the latter existed, and it was put down to loss by pulmonary and cutaneous elimination. Barral, for instance, only detected half the nitrogen of the food in the urine and fæces, and thence inferred that the remainder was discharged with the breath and perspiration. In opposition to this, however, several trustworthy observers (amongst whom may be named Voit, Ranke, Haughton, and Parkes) aided by the improved methods of analysis introduced by modern experience, have recovered within a very close approach all the nitrogen of the food from the urinary and intestinal excreta. Dr. Parkes' observations are especially worthy of reliance, and he confidently asserts that it may be looked upon as established, that an amount of nitrogen is discharged by the kidney and intestine equivalent to that which enters with the food. Admitting this to be the case, we have only to look to the products that escape from these two channels for the information that is wanted about the discharged nitrogen in relation to the question before us.

Next comes the determination of the relation respectively held by the urinary and intestinal nitrogen to the point under consideration. It has long been known that the chief portion of the escaping nitrogen is to be met with in the urine. Lehmann, for instance, found, while subsisting on a purely animal diet (eggs), that a daily average of 30.3 grammes (467 grains) of nitrogen entered his system, and that a daily average of 24.4 grammes (376 grains) was discharged by the urine. Here, therefore, it was ascertained that an amount equal to five-sixths of the ingested nitrogen escaped by the kidneys.

But more recent and precise evidence has been afforded by a series of very carefully conducted observations made upon two soldiers by Dr. Parkes.[*] The observations extended over sixteen consecutive days, and the results not only bear on the ingestion and egestion of nitrogen generally, but likewise show that the great bulk of outgoing nitrogen is to be met with in the urine. The men were both of almost precisely the same weight at the end of the time as at the beginning, so that the ingoing and outgoing matter must have been closely balanced. They were subjected to varying conditions of rest and exercise, but consumed ex-

---

actly the same allowance of food every day. The nitrogen in the food taken during the sixteen days amounted to 313.76 grammes; and, from the urine of one of the men (distinguished as S.) there were recovered 303.660 grammes, and from that of the other (distinguished as B.) 307.257 grammes. Thus, the amount of nitrogen discharged from the kidneys was, in the case of S., only about ten grammes, and in that of B., six grammes less than that admitted with the food. The alvine evacuations were collected and analyzed only upon three occasions. Taking the mean of the results then obtained as representing the daily average, and calculating from this for the sixteen days, the quantity of nitrogen discharged from the bowels amounted in S. to 25.8 grammes, and in B. to 17.2 grammes, thus somewhat exceeding the difference between the ingested nitrogen and that excreted in the urine, or giving, in other words, rather more nitrogen discharged than nitrogen ingested.

The nitrogen discharged from the bowels may be said to have been found to form, upon an average, from about one-eighth to one-twelfth or one-thirteenth of the total nitrogen voided. Owing its origin, as it does, to the nitrogen belonging to the undigested food on the one hand, and that contained in the unabsorbed intestinal secretions on the other, it is constantly liable to incidental variation. There is this, also, to be remarked, that the nature of its source excludes it from possessing any relation to the question under consideration. We have, therefore, only the urinary excretion to look to as forming the channel through which the exit of nitrogen, resulting from the metamorphosis of nitrogenous matter in the system, takes place; and observation has shown that in the human subject it is mainly under the shape of urea that the escape occurs.

What, now, is the state of the urine in relation to rest and exercise? If muscular disintegration forms the source of muscular work, the quantity of urinary nitrogen ought to increase in proportion to the amount of muscular work performed.

Lehmann, imbued with Liebig's views, as his writings show, speaks of there being an actual increase in the elimination of urea in proportion to muscular exercise, and yet he gives it as the result or observation upon himself that, while under ordinary circumstances he passed about 32 grammes (493 grains) of urea in the twenty-four hours, the quantity passed after severe bodily exercise was upon one occasion 36 grammes (555 grains), and upon another 37.4 grammes (577 grains)—only this insignificant disparity to correspond with the difference in the amount of muscular work performed.

Voit experimented upon a dog, and determined the amount of urea voided during rest and the performance of mechanical work, in association with abstinence and a regulated diet of meat. The work imposed upon the dog was running in a tread-mill. The results, both during abstinence and feeding, exhibited no material excess in the urea voided during work over that voided during rest.

Dr. E. Smith, also, in his observations on the elimination of carbonic acid and urea during rest and exercise, found, in the case of the prisoners at Coldbath Fields, that, in the absence of food, the labor of the tread-wheel did not, to any material extent, increase the nitrogen discharged under the form of urea. Like others have done, he noticed a distinct relation between the urea discharged and the food ingested. At the same time he regarded—and this was several years ago, when our knowledge stood in a very different position from what it does now—the relation between the urea and muscular work as far less established then than it had been held to be for some time before.

The theory that muscular work is dependent on and proportioned to the destruction of muscular tissue by oxidation, received its decisive blow from the now celebrated observations of Drs. Fick and Wislicenus, professors of physiology and chemistry respectively at Zurich.* These experimentalists subjected themselves to a measurable amount of work by ascending a mountain of an ascertained height. They argued that if the work performed be due to destruction of muscular tissue—seeing that the nitrogenous product of destruction is discharged in great part,, if not entirely, with the urine—the collection of the urine, and the determination of its nitrogenous contents, ought to show the amount of nitrogenous matter destroyed. Again, as the mechanical work to be performed must be represented by an equivalent of chemical action to produce it, the destruction of nitrogenous matter, as measured by the nitrogen appearing in the urine, ought to accord with the amount of work performed. To simplify the experiment, the food consumed by the experimentalists consisted solely of non-nitrogenous matter, so that the nitrogen appearing in the urine might be derived exclusively from that belonging to the system.

Drs. Fick and Wislicenus chose for ascent the Faulhorn, near the Lake of Brienz, in the Bernese Oberland, a steep mountain of about 2,000 metres (6,561 feet) above the level of the lake, and furnished with hotel accommodation on the summit, enabling them to rest over-night and make the descent next day.

On the 30th of August, between ten minutes past five in the morning and twenty minutes past one in the afternoon, the ascent was made. From the noon of the 29th no nitrogenous food had been eaten by the experimenters, their diet consisting solely of starch and fat (taken in the form of small cakes), and sugar as solid matter, and tea, beer, and wine as drink. After ascending the mountain, Drs. Fick and Wislicenus rested, and took no other kind of food till seven in the evening, when they partook of a plentiful repast of meat and its usual accompaniments.

They began to collect their urine for examination from six P.M. of the 29th; that is, six hours after the commencement of their non-nitrogenous diet. The urine secreted from this time till ten minutes past five A.M. of the 30th, when the ascent began, was called the " before-work " urine. The urine secreted during the ascent was called the " work " urine; and that from twenty minutes past one P.M. to seven P.M. (from the completion of the ascent to the cessation of the non-nitrogenous diet) the " after-work " urine. Finally, the urine secreted during the night spent on the Faulhorn up to half-past five A.M. was also collected, and denominated " night " urine.

Each specimen was measured, and both the quantity of urea and the absolute amount of nitrogen contained in it determined. For the object before us it will suffice to confine our attention to the nitrogen; and the quantity of this element secreted per hour (calculated from the amount contained in the respective specimens and the time passed in secretion), stood thus for the several periods:

---

* On the Origin of Muscular Power, by Drs. Fick and Wislicenus : Philosophical Magazine (Supplement), vol. xxxi., 1866.

Quantity of Nitrogen Excreted per Hour.

	Fick. Grammes.	Wislicenus. Grammes.
Before work,	0.63	0.61
During work,	0.41	0.39
After work,	0.40	0.40
Night,	0.45	0.51

A glance at these figures shows the agreement that existed in the two cases. The result proved that, whilst the nitrogenous excretion was related to the food ingested, it was not so to muscular action. Less nitrogen, it is noticeable, was voided during the " work " and " after-work " than during the " before-work " period, and this was plainly attributable to the absence of nitrogenous food from the diet. During the night, after the meal of mixed food, there was an increase, greater in Wislicenus's than in Fick's case; but the one meal did not bring the amount of nitrogen up to the point at which it stood shortly after the commencement of their abstinence from nitrogenous food.

The conclusion, then, that in the first place may be drawn from this experiment is, that muscular work is not accompanied by the increased elimination of nitrogen that might be looked for if it resulted from the oxidation of muscle. But let us inquire whether the disintegration of nitrogenous matter which actually occurred during the " work " and " after-work " periods, as measured by the nitrogen excreted, would account for the generation of an amount of force equivalent to that expended in the work performed.

Knowing that the nitrogenous matter of muscle contains—say, in round numbers, fifteen per cent. of nitrogen—it is easy to calculate to how much muscular tissue the excreted nitrogen was equivalent; and taking the muscular tissue thus represented, an approximate, if not an absolute, estimate can be given of the amount of mechanical work which its oxidation would be capable of performing.

The height of the ascended mountain, likewise, being known, the amount of muscular force actually employed in raising the weight of the body to the summit can also be definitely expressed.

We have, therefore, these data supplied:

First.—From the nitrogen excreted the amount of nitrogenous matter oxidized;

Second.—The amount of force that this oxidation would generate; and

Third.—The expenditure of force required to raise the bodies of the experimenters to the height they reached.

Now if the work performed were due to the oxidation of muscle, the second factor ought to equal the third; that is, the force producible from the muscle oxidized ought to be equivalent to the force that was expended. The results of the calculation, however, show, as will be presently seen, that the force expended considerably exceeded the amount derivable from the nitrogenous matter consumed.

Nor is this all. Besides the force expended in simply raising the body-weights of the two men to the elevation reached, there would also be occurring, during the performance of the work, an expenditure of muscular power in keeping up the circulation, in respiratory action, and the other life-processes. The calculations on these points have been carefully worked out by Fick and Wislicenus; and though the data for the process are scarcely precise enough to warrant our regarding the results as scientifically exact, still they may be admitted as affording a basis for a safe general conclusion to be drawn. We are also told that wherever a doubt existed about the data, figures were taken as favorable as was allowable to the old hypothesis, which referred the source of power to muscular oxidation.

In giving the conclusion furnished, it is not necessary to introduce the details of the calculation. It will suffice to say, that summarily stated, the result of the calculation showed that the measured work performed during the ascent exceeded by about one-half in Fick's case, and more than three-fourths in that of Wislicenus, the amount which it would be theoretically possible to realize from the amount of nitrogenous matter consumed.

It has been shown by Professor Frankland * that the results of Fick and Wislicenus in reality afford stronger evidence than they have contended for. Fick and Wislicenus were obliged to estimate the force-value of the nitrogenous matter, shown by the nitrogen in the urine to have been destroyed in the system, from the amount of force known to be producible by the oxidation of its elements, because the actual determination for the compound itself had not been made. Professor Frankland, however, has since experimentally ascertained, with the calorimeter, the amount of energy or force evolved under the form of heat during the oxidation of a given quantity of nitrogenous matter, as the oxidation occurs within the living system, in which position a portion, it must be borne in mind, of the carbon and hydrogen escapes being consumed, on account of being carried off by the nitrogen in the shape of urea. Frankland's results give as the actual amount of energy producible from the nitrogenous matter consumed in the bodies of the experimentalists, about half the quantity they had reckoned in their calculations. Thus, the results tell so much the more in Fick and Wislicenus' favor. Frankland considers, taking all points into consideration, that scarcely one-fifth of the actual energy required for the accomplishment of the work performed in the ascent of the mountain could have been obtained from the amount of muscle (nitrogenous matter) that was consumed. Assuming, therefore, the foregoing conclusions to be entitled to credence, the doctrine which ascribes muscular action to oxidation of muscular tissue becomes utterly untenable.

Dr. Parkes has conducted, in a most careful manner, a series of investigations on the influence of rest and exercise, under different diets, upon the effete products of the system, and, more particularly, to test the accuracy of the results arrived at by Fick and Wislicenus. He says, "Although these results (Fick and Wislicenus') are supported by the previous experiments of Dr. Speck, who has shown that if the ingress of nitrogen be restricted, bodily exercise causes no or a very slight increase in the elimination of nitrogen by the urine, it appeared desirable to carefully repeat the experiments, not only because the question is one of great importance, but because objections might be, and, indeed, have been, reasonably made to the experiments of Professors Fick and Wislicenus, on the ground that no sufficient basis of comparison between periods of rest and exercise was given, that the periods were altogether too short, and that no attention was paid to the possible exit of nitrogen by the intestines."

---

* On the Origin of Muscular Power: Philos. Magazine, vol. xxxii., 1866.

Dr. Parkes' experiments were conducted upon perfectly healthy soldiers, men who, when steady and trustworthy, as were the soldiers made use of, form, as Dr. Parkes observes, highly suitable subjects for experiments of the kind, their regularity in diet and occupation, and their habits of obedience, affording a special guarantee for the precision with which they will carry out the instructions given. There can, indeed, be little or no doubt, from the harmony observable all through, that the results furnish as exact and reliable information as can be hoped to be obtained.

The total nitrogen contained in the urine was determined, as well as the urea; and by this step more conclusive evidence is supplied than by the simple determination of urea, as had only been done in the experiments of Fick and Wislicenus and others; obviously so, because it might be said that nitrogen escaped (as is really to some extent the case) in other forms than that of urea.

The experiments consisted of two series, and extended, in each case, over several successive days. In the first series * a comparison is instituted of the products of excretion during rest and exercise under a non-nitrogenous diet. In the second † the same comparison is made under a fixed diet, containing an ordinary admixture of nitrogenous and non-nitrogenous food.

In drawing conclusions regarding the destruction of muscle from the nitrogen eliminated, it is, of course, of the first importance that the whole of the voided nitrogen should be presented to our notice. Dr. Parkes is convinced, from his experiments, that no nitrogen escapes either by the breath or perspiration, but that it is all to be found in the excreta from the kidneys and bowels. The nitrogen discharged by the bowels forms a comparatively small and varying proportion, and being derived from the undigested food and the unabsorbed digestive secretions, has no bearing in reference to the point before us. There remains, therefore, only the urinary nitrogen to consider as a measure of the tissue-metamorphosis occurring in the system. Thus prefaced, let us now see what light is thrown upon the matter under consideration by Dr. Parkes' experiments. For the sake of simplicity, notice will only be taken of the total urinary nitrogen voided, as this gives in a more reliable manner than the urea the information that is wanted.

The men forming the subjects of the first series of experiments are distinguished as S. and T. T. was a much smaller man than S. (S. weighing one hundred and fifty and T. one hundred and twelve pounds), and it will be observed that he, throughout, passed a less amount of urinary nitrogen. He did not consume *quite* so much food; and as it was found that he discharged rather more nitrogen from the intestine, it may be assumed that he did not so fully digest and absorb what he ingested.

For six days the men were kept upon an ordinary mixed diet, and pursued their customary occupation. The urine was collected and examined during four out of the six days, and the following is the mean amount of the total nitrogen passed *per diem:*

	Mean urinary nitrogen per diem.—Grammes.
Mixed diet, with customary occupation, ...	S. 17.973
	T. 13.409

---

* Proceedings of the Royal Society, No. 80, vol. xv., January, 1867.
† Ibid., No. 94, vol. xvi., June, 1867.

During the following two days the diet was restricted to non-nitro-genous food consisting of arrow-root, sugar, and butter. The only nitro-gen ingested—and this may be regarded as too insignificant to require being taken into account—was in the tea the men were allowed to drink, it being thought desirable not to deprive them of this beverage. Through-out the two days they remained as much at rest as was practicable; they were allowed to get up, but not to leave the room.

Non-nitrogenous diet, with rest, ... $\left\{ \begin{array}{l} \text{Mean urinary nitrogen} \\ \text{per diem.—Grammes.} \\ \text{S. 9.176} \\ \text{T. 7.} \end{array} \right.$

The men were now put back, for four days, upon a mixed diet, with customary occupation, just as at the beginning of the experiment.

Mixed diet, with customary occupation, . . $\left\{ \begin{array}{l} \text{Mean urinary nitrogen} \\ \text{per diem.—Grammes.} \\ \text{S. 12.988} \\ \text{T. 11.095} \end{array} \right.$

Next they were restricted again for two days to the same non-nitro-genous food as before, but this time it was accompanied with active walking exercise. During the first day the distance walked was 23¾ miles, and during the second 32¾ miles. The diet, it is stated, satisfied hunger, and there was no sinking or craving for other kinds of food.

Non-nitrogenous diet, with active exercise, . . $\left\{ \begin{array}{l} \text{Mean urinary nitrogen} \\ \text{per diem.—Grammes.} \\ \text{S. 8.971} \\ \text{T. 8.034} \end{array} \right.$

To complete the experiment, four more days were passed under obser-vation with the ordinary mixed diet, accompanied by ordinary exercise. Rather more nitrogenous food was taken during these four days succeeding the two days' active exercise than during the four days succeeding the two days' rest, the men feeling more hungry after the " work" period than after the period of " rest." The mean for T., it is mentioned, is for three days instead of four, one analysis having failed.

Mixed diet, with customary occupation, . . $\left\{ \begin{array}{l} \text{Mean urinary nitrogen} \\ \text{per diem.—Grammes.} \\ \text{S. 13.361} \\ \text{T. 11.658} \end{array} \right.$

From this series of results we find that there was no material variation in the amount of urinary nitrogen discharged during the two days when a distance of 56¼ miles was walked, as compared with the two days spent in as complete a state of rest as possible, on both occasions restriction to non-nitrogenous food being enjoined. Comparing both these periods, however, with those in which nitrogenous food was taken, we recognize a marked exemplification of the well-established fact that diet, on the other hand, exerts a striking influence over the amount of nitrogen eliminated with the urine. During each of the non-nitrogenous diet periods the quantity of nitrogen eliminated was considerably less than during the others; it is also noticeable that the influence of the non-nitrogenous food was extended into the subsequent ordinary diet periods, less nitrogen being voided during these than at the commencement of the experiment, ·

3

before any restriction from nitrogenous food had been imposed. This point, however, will be further alluded to hereafter.

In the second series of experiments, the amount of nitrogen eliminated was determined under the conditions of rest and exercise, combined with a *mixed* diet. One of the two men, S., was the same who had been made use of in the former experiment; the other, B., was a fresh man, weighing one hundred and forty pounds, and therefore nearer in size to S., who weighed one hundred and fifty pounds, than T., of the former experiment, who weighed one hundred and twelve pounds. During the sixteen days over which the observations extended, each man took *precisely* the same allowance of food in the twenty-four hours: the food consisting of weighed quantities of meat, bread, potatoes, and the other constituents of an ordinary mixed diet. For the first four days the men pursued their customary employment. The next two days were passed in rest. Then followed four days of ordinary employment; after this, two days of active exercise; and finally, four days again of ordinary employment. The amount of nitrogen eliminated by the kidneys during the several periods is shown in the following table:

	Urinary nitrogen per diem.—Grammes.
Ordinary employment (mean of four days),	S. 17.857 B. 18.502
Rest (mean of two days),	S. 19.137 B. 19.471
Ordinary employment (mean of four days),	S. 17.612 B. 18.485
Active exercise—walking on level ground, 24 miles the first day, and 35 the second—(mean of two days),	S. 19.046 B. 19.959
Ordinary employment (mean of four days),	S. 21.054 B. 20.092

In these results it will be seen that there is nothing to sanction the doctrine that the source of muscular power resides in the destruction of muscular tissue. In two persons subsisting on an identical and unvarying daily diet, and subjected to varying conditions of muscular exertion, we find nearly the same quantity of nitrogen eliminated during two days' hard walking as during two days of rest. It is curious, and also, it must be owned, does not appear explicable, that during the periods of both rest and active exercise the daily amount of nitrogen eliminated was in excess of that eliminated during the first two periods of ordinary employment, the figures at the same time for the associated periods respectively agreeing very closely with each other. In the third period of ordinary employment—that is, after the two days of walking exercise—the nitrogen voided was greater in quantity than at any other time. Such excess, however, did not amount to anything particularly marked.

Comparing in detail the nitrogen eliminated during the corresponding portions of the two day-periods—those of rest and active exercise—Dr. Parkes observes, with respect to the results furnished : "On the first day of exercise, the nitrogen in each man fell below the corresponding day of rest by 1.626 and 1.131 grammes. In the next twelve hours, which were almost entirely occupied in exercise (this period extending from 8 A.M. to 8 P.M.), the diminution was still greater, being 2.498 and 1.225 grammes, which would be equivalent to 5 and 2½ grammes for twenty-four hours. In the last twelve hours (8 P.M. to 8 A.M.) of rest after work, the elimination increased greatly, so that 5.142 and 3.331 grammes more were excreted than in the corresponding rest period." Seeking to reconcile his results in relation to muscular action, Dr. Parkes observes: " It appears to me that we can only express the facts by saying that a muscle during action appropriates more nitrogen than it gives off, and during rest gives off more than it appropriates."

But must we, I would suggest, look only to the muscles for the source of the variation in the amount of nitrogen discharged in these experiments? The results, in the first place, conclusively show that the nitrogen eliminated forms no measure of muscular work performed, and hence it may be inferred as a corollary that muscular work is not a result of muscular destruction. But taking the variation in the voided nitrogen that was observable, independently of that occasioned by diet, why should we seek its source exclusively in the muscles ?

On looking at the several daily amounts discharged, I remark the existence of instances in which considerable variation occurs within the periods themselves. Thus, during the first day of the first period, when the men were engaged in ordinary employment, B. discharged 20.417 grammes of nitrogen, and during the third day only 17.090, a difference approaching to 3½ grammes. Again, during the last period, which was also spent in ordinary employment (it will be remembered that the daily diet was the same throughout the experiment), the urinary nitrogen voided by both men stood as follows:

	S. Grammes.	B. Grammes.
First day,	21.25	20.25
Second day,	19.942	19.273
Third day,	23.488	19.248
Fourth day,	19.536	21.597

On the third day, it thus appears, S. discharged nearly 4 grammes of nitrogen in excess of that on the fourth, and about 3½ in excess of that on the second. No corresponding fluctuation, it will be remarked, was observable in the case of B. Here, then, are marked variations in the elimination of nitrogen without a variation of muscular action

In a more recently performed experiment,* Dr. Parkes' results show, with a fixed daily ingress of nitrogen, a variation in the daily exit amounting in the extreme to seven and a half grammes.

Now we know that the nitrogen of the urine is derivable from the metamorphosis of the nitrogenous ingesta within the system. It is true the food taken was every day the same throughout the experiment that has been forming the subject of consideration, but it does not follow that the rate of metamorphosis was every day similarly identical. Doubtless, like other processes of life, it is influenced by various internal conditions. We know also, as the result of observation in the case of starvation, that, notwithstanding an absence of ingoing nitrogen, an elimination of this element still continues, and that the nitrogen eliminated is drawn from the nitrogenous principles of the body, belonging alike to the solids and fluids. There is a general waste or loss occurring, and the only difference noticeable is that the loss goes on with different degrees of rapidity in the different parts of the system. In the muscles it certainly occurs somewhat more rapidly than elsewhere, but this is all. With these con-

* Proceedings of the Royal Society, March, 1871.

siderations before us, it appears to me that we are taking an unjustifiably narrow view in looking only to the muscles to account for the variation in question in the voided nitrogen. Exercise cannot fail to influence the processes going on in the system generally, as well as in the muscles, and, in accounting for the results observed, instead of limiting ourselves, with Dr. Parkes, to the assertion that "we can only express the fact by saying that a muscle during action appropriates more nitrogen than it gives off, and during rest gives off more than it appropriates," I think what we ought rather to say is, that during exercise the *system* appropriates more nitrogen than it gives off, and during rest gives off more than it appropriates.

Voit, however, disputes the reality of exercise producing *any* influence over the elimination of nitrogen, and has taken exception to some of Dr. Parkes' experiments, on the ground, more particularly, that the daily ingress of nitrogen could not be kept sufficiently stable. This elicited from Dr. Parkes his further series, the results of which are recorded in the "Proceedings of the Royal Society" for March, 1871. In these it appeared that there was no change induced, either at the time or afterward, by a moderate amount of additional exercise under a mixed regulated diet; but, under a non-nitrogenous diet, the increase in the nitrogen on the following day to the performance of a hard day's march was exceedingly striking. The non-nitrogenous diet was continued through five successive days. During the first three it was associated with the ordinary work of a soldier; on the fourth, with a march of thirty-two miles, performed with a load of 43¼ lbs.; and on the fifth with rest. As the ordinary result of abstinence from nitrogenous food, the eliminated urinary nitrogen underwent a steady decrease during the first four days; on the fifth, however, it showed a marked ascent, the amount being then in considerable excess of that discharged on the first.

In the *New York Medical Journal* for October, 1870, Dr. Austin Flint, Jun., records the result of the examination of the urine secreted during the performance of, perhaps, an unprecedented amount of muscular work within the space of time occupied. A Mr. Weston, aged thirty-two, of medium height, and weighing ordinarily 122 lbs. without his clothes, celebrated as a pedestrian of the United States, undertook to perform the astonishing feat of walking one hundred miles in twenty-two consecutive hours. The feat, it appears, was accomplished within the time — namely, in twenty-one hours and thirty-nine minutes. The food consumed during the period was taken in small quantities at short intervals, and consisted of between one and two bottles of beef-essence, two bottles of oatmeal-gruel, and sixteen to twenty raw eggs, with water. Mr. Weston drank, it is said, a little lemonade and took water very frequently, but only in quantity sufficient to rinse his mouth. While walking the last ten miles he took, it is further stated, two or three mouthfuls of champagne, amounting to about three fluid ounces, and about two and a half fluid ounces of brandy in ten-drop doses. The head and face were sponged freely at short intervals, and the food and drink were taken mainly on the walk, which was conducted within a covered enclosure.

The urine passed during and at the completion of the walk measured 73½ fluid ounces, and presented the specific gravity of 1011. According to Dr. Flint's analysis it contained 424¾ grains of urea. Now 500 grains form about the average daily quantity of urea discharged under an ordinary mixed diet; and as the diet during the performance of the pedestrian feat was rich, as the account shows it to have been, in nitrogenous matter, the quantity of urea, apart from any other consideration, was even less than might have been expected. And yet, on the strength of a comparison with another examination of the urine conducted three months later, when only 191 grains of urea are stated to have been discharged in the absence of exposure to muscular exertion, Dr. Flint argues that muscular exercise notably increases the elimination of urea. To take a solitary result of so exceptional a kind as the discharge of only 191 grains of urea in the twenty-four hours, and use it as a ground of comparison for reasoning upon, as Dr. Flint has done, is surely to violate all rules of sound induction, and it is to be hoped that we shall not find the observation quoted by writers as bearing out what Dr. Flint has contended for.

During November, 1870, Mr. Weston undertook another pedestrian feat, and this time a very elaborate examination was made of the ingesta and egesta, and of various conditions of the body, by Dr. Flint and a staff of associates. The results are recorded in detail in the *New York Medical Journal* for June, 1871. The feat proposed was to walk 400 miles in five consecutive days, and upon one of the days 112 miles were to be walked in twenty-four consecutive hours. Mr. Weston commenced the undertaking on the 21st of November. The examination of the ingesta, egesta, etc., had been conducted for five days before; it was also carried on during the five days of the walk, and continued for five days afterward. Thus, the result for three periods—before, during, and after the walk—were obtained. The subjoined tabular representation will give a summary view of the leading points noted. The walk was undertaken over a measured track, marked out in the form of a parallelogram, within a large covered space—namely, the Empire Skating Rink in New York. It appears that Mr. Weston failed this time to accomplish the feat he had attempted, the distance walked during the five days amounting to 317½ miles, and the greatest distance on any one day to 92 miles.

Notwithstanding the figures to be presented, Dr. Flint still holds to his former opinion, and looks upon the results as showing, to use his own words, that " excessive and prolonged muscular exertion increases enormously the excretion of nitrogen, and that the excess of nitrogen discharged is due to an increased disassimilation of the muscular substance."

DR. FLINT'S *Observations on the Effects of the Five-day Pedestrian Feat Performed by* MR. WESTON.

BEFORE THE WALK.

	Weight of body (nude).	Temperature.	Pulse.	Miles walked.	Nitrogen in ingesta.	Nitrogen in egesta.	Excess or deficiency in nitrogen egested.
	Lbs.	Deg. Fahr.			Grains.	Grains.	Grains.
First day, . .	120.5	99.7	75	15	361.22	323.26	— 37.96
Second day, . .	121.25	98.4	73	5	288.35	301.18	+ 12.83
Third day, . .	120	98.0	71	5	272.27	330.36	+ 58.09
Fourth day, . .	118.5	99.1	78	15	335.01	300.57	— 34.44
Fifth day, . .	119.2	99.5	93	1	440.43	320.06	— 120.37

DURING THE WALK.

	Weight of body (nude).	Temperature.	Pulse.	Miles walked.	Nitrogen in ingesta.	Nitrogen in egesta.	Excess or deficiency in nitrogen egested.
	Lbs.	Deg. Fahr.			Grains.	Grains.	Grains.
First day, . .	116.5	95.3	98	80	151.55	357.10	+ 205.55
Second day, . .	116.25	94.8	93	48	265.92	370.64	+' 104.72
Third day, . .	115	96.6	109	92	228.61	397.58	+ 168.97
Fourth day, . .	114	96.6	68	57	144.70	348.53	+ 203.83
Fifth day, . .	115.75	97.9	80	40.5	383.04	332.77	− 50.27

AFTER THE WALK.

First day, . .	118	98.6	76	2	385.65	295.70	− 89.95
Second day, . .	120.25	98.4	73	2	499.10	358.81	− 140.29
Third day, . .	120.25	99.3	70	2	394.83	409.87	+ 15.04
Fourth day, . .	123.5	98.8	78	2	641.71	382.89	− 258.82
Fifth day, . .	120.75	97.5	76	3	283.35	418.49	+ 135.14

Let us accept Dr. Flint's estimates of the ingoing and outgoing nitrogen. It is true, during the first four days of the walking period the exit of nitrogen was in considerable excess of the entrance; but why should this be referred specially and exclusively to muscular disintegration? There was during these few days a progressive decline in the weight of the body, the loss reaching a little over five pounds. From the account given, considerably less solid food was taken then than before and after. There existed a state of marked disturbance of the bodily functions, as shown by the depression of temperature and elevation of pulse; but little sleep was obtained; and on the third day, when an attempt was made to walk the one hundred and twelve miles in twenty-four consecutive hours, drowsiness, it is stated, prevailed to such'an extent that it was found impossible to make the necessary time to accomplish what had been intended. On the fourth day Mr. Weston actually broke down for a time altogether, becoming dizzy, staggering, and at last failing to be able to see sufficiently to turn the corners of the track.

Now, apart from the fact that a marked deviation from the physiological state existed when the results upon which the conclusions are based were yielded, is there anything in the results to show that in reality we have more to deal with than simply a consumption of nitrogenous material within the system beyond the supply for the time from without? Taking the figures throughout, there is not much more to be seen than a difference occasioned by a falling off in the amount of nitrogen ingested during the first four days of the walk; and it is well known that when the ingesta do not furnish what is wanted for meeting the expenditure going on (as during inanition), the resources of the body are drawn upon, and the nitrogenous matter existing in the various parts—both solids and fluids—wastes or yields itself up as well as the rest. On the fifth day, after a prolonged sleep, which appears to have restored the flagging powers, the previous relation was reversed. The food ingested afforded more than enough to meet the requirements. There was a gain of 1¾ pound in body-weight, and, according to the figures, the nitrogen discharged fell short by 50.27 grains of that which entered, notwithstanding a walk of forty and a half miles was performed.

The distance walked during the five days amounted to 317½ miles, and the excess of nitrogen eliminated during the time, over that ingested, appears to have been 633 grains. Presuming, for sake of argument, this to have represented the nitrogen of muscle disintegrated in the accomplishment of the work performed, we have before us the data for ascertaining how far the force producible in this way would correspond with the expenditure that must have occurred.

According to Mulder's analysis, albuminous matter contains 15.5 per cent. of nitrogen. Reckoning from this proportion, 633 grains of nitrogen will correspond with 4,083 grains of dry albumen, and the composition of the nitrogenous matter of muscle is closely analogous. Now the force producible from the oxidation of albuminous matter has been experimentally ascertained by Frankland, and as it occurs within the body, the oxidation of 4,083 grains of dry albumen would give rise to the evolution of an amount of power equal to lifting 1,540 tons one foot high.

Here we have one side of the question—the amount of work obtainable from the nitrogenous matter presumed to have undergone disintegration as muscular tissue; and so far the information in our possession may be regarded as sufficiently authentic to enable us to frame a reliable conclusion. As regards the work accomplished, we may assume, with Professor Haughton, that the force expended in walking or progressing on level ground is equal to that required to lift one-twentieth of the weight of the body through the distance traversed. The distance walked amounted to 317½ miles, and if we take the weight of the body and clothing at, say, 120 pounds, this will give the performance of an amount of work equal to lifting 4,490 tons one foot high, or about two-thirds more work than the oxidation of the nitrogenous matter representing the 633 grains of nitrogen could accomplish. And, in this calculation, only the external work has been taken into consideration. There is, in reality, also a considerable amount of internal work constantly being performed— viz., that employed in keeping up the circulation, in respiration, and in various other essential actions of life.

I have entered thus minutely into the question of the elimination of nitrogen in relation to muscular work because it bears in so forcible and direct a manner upon the question immediately before us, viz., the uses to which the nitrogenous alimentary principles are applied in the system. Briefly represented, the position of the matter may be said to be this:

Many years ago it was asserted by Liebig that muscular action involved the destruction of muscular tissue. The plausibility of the doctrine, and the readiness with which the views of its author were then received, must be considered as having led to its being at once generally accepted as though it formed a scientific truth, although, in reality, only constituting a speculative proposition, unsupported by anything of the nature of proof. It was further argued that, if muscular action involved the destruction of muscular tissue, the excretion of the nitrogenous product of destruction—urea—ought to be in proportion to the amount of muscular work performed. This seemed to follow as a necessary sequence, and the one being accepted, the other was taken for granted also. Thus, notwithstanding the absence of anything in the shape of proof, we find physiologists reasoning and writing as though the doctrine had been actually proved.

If the theory of Liebig were true, we should have to look upon nitro-

genous alimentary matter as forming, through the medium of muscular
tissue, the source, the only source, of muscular power. The renewal of
muscular tissue for subsequent oxidation in its turn, and evolution of muscular force, would thus constitute one of the functions of nitrogenous
alimentary matter; and on its supply would, accordingly, depend our
capacity for the performance of muscular work.

It is only lately that the doctrine has been submitted to the test of experiment, and with what result the foregoing account of the researches
of various observers has shown. Even Liebig * was brought to assert
that muscular action is not attended by the production of urea. He admitted that the question as to the source of muscular power had been
complicated by an inference which had proved erroneous, and for which
he acknowledged himself as responsible—the inference, namely, that
muscular work is represented by the metamorphosis of muscular tissue,
and the formation of urea as a final product. While admitting this much,
however, Liebig still looked to changes in the nitrogenous constituents
of muscle as the source of muscular power. He assumed the presence in
muscle of nitrogenous substances in a much higher state of tension than
syntonine and albumen, and to these he referred the performance of
muscular work, taking shelter under the proposition that it is due to the
liberation of the tension thus presumed to have been accumulated in
them during their formation.

The application of food to the genesis of muscular power will form
the subject of further consideration hereafter, when we reach the head of
non-nitrogenous matter. Suffice it here to reiterate that muscular action
is not to be considered as the result of muscle-destruction, as was formerly supposed, and hence that nitrogenous matter is not applied through
muscle—in the manner hitherto maintained—to the development of
muscular force. Thus much, from the evidence before us, may be said,
but, at the same time, common experience seems to show that a plentiful supply of nitrogenous matter in the food tends to increase the capacity for the performance of muscular work. If, however, it does so in any
other way than by supplying material for nutrition and the secretions,
and so contributing to the production of a fully nourished and vigorous
state of the system, we have no data before us to indicate how.

Let me next draw attention to the application of nitrogenous matter
to force-production by the direct utilization of the carbon and hydrogen
it contains. Liebig's doctrine, which, until recently, has formed the accepted one on this point, was that nitrogenous food, to be turned to
account for force-production, *must* pass through the condition of living
tissue. This brings us back to the discussion that has preceded, with the
addition that our nitrogenous food must perform work as tissue to enable
it to be susceptible of application to force, or—say—heat-production.
Thus, in his work on "Animal Chemistry," at page 60, Liebig says, "the
flesh and blood consumed as food yield their carbon for the support of the
respiratory process, whilst the nitrogen appears as uric acid, ammonia, or
urea. But, previously to these final changes, the dead flesh and blood
become converted into living flesh and blood, and it is, strictly speaking,
the carbon of the compounds formed in the metamorphosis of living tissues that serves for the production of animal heat." Again, at page 77,
we find: "Man when confined to animal food respires like the carnivora

---

* Proceedings of the Royal Bavarian Academy of Science, 1869 ; Pharmaceutical
Journal, 1870.

at the expense of the matter produced by the metamorphosis of organized tissues; and just as the lion, tiger, and hyena, in the cages of a menagerie, are compelled to accelerate the waste of their organized tissues by incessant motion, in order to furnish the matter necessary for respiration, so the savage, for the very same object, is forced to make the most laborious exertions and go through a vast amount of muscular exercise. He is compelled to consume force merely in order to supply matter for respiration." Once more, in speaking of the derivation of urea from the metamorphosis of nitrogenous matter, he says, at page 144: "There can be no greater contradiction with regard to the nutritive process than to suppose that the nitrogen of the food can pass into the urine as urea, without having previously become part of an organized tissue."

Liebig's idea, then, upon this point is very precise. He considers that nitrogenous matter may contribute toward heat-production, but that it must first pass into the condition of tissue before it can do so, and that it is in the wear and tear of tissue that occurs the splitting up of the compound, so as to lead to the production of urea for secretion on the one hand, and the liberation of carbon and hydrogen for oxidation on the other.

The facts which have been already adduced, suffice to refute this doctrine. Indeed, it may be considered as now abundantly proved that food does not require to become organized tissue before it can be rendered available for force-production. But Liebig himself, in language not less precise than that which he at first employed, has recently * given utterance to words which directly contradict his original view, inasmuch as he now asserts that muscular work and the production of urea bear no immediate relation to each other, and that among the products formed as the result of muscular action, urea certainly does not even constitute one.

If the elimination of urea, as has been shown, is not related, as was formerly supposed, to muscular action, it is, on the other hand, in a very direct manner influenced by the food ingested. As far back as 1854, Messrs. Lawes and Gilbert, in opposition to the views then prevailing, showed by the results obtained in their observations on the feeding of cattle, that the nitrogen in the urine is related to that in the food, and not to the muscular work; and, since then, the concurrent testimony of numerous observers, as has been already pointed out, may be held as completely establishing this position. Lehmann's well-known experiments upon himself strikingly illustrate the extent to which this influence is manifested. The results he obtained were as follows:

While living on a purely animal diet, namely, almost exclusively on eggs, Lehmann passed 53.2 grammes (820 grains) of urea in the twenty-four hours as the mean of twelve observations.

Upon a mixed diet, the urea amounted to 32.5 grammes (501 grains) as the mean of fifteen observations.

Upon a vegetable diet, the urea given as the mean of twelve observations was 22.5 grammes (347 grains).

And, lastly, upon a purely non-nitrogenous diet (fat, sugar of milk, and starch) he voided, as the mean of three observations, only 15.4 grammes (237 grains) of urea.

It is thus seen that upon an animal diet, which is the richest in nitrogenous matter, the voided urea more than doubled that eliminated upon a vegetable diet, while the amount of urea voided upon a mixture of the

---

* Proceedings of the Royal Bavarian Academy of Sciences, 1869.

two kinds of food held an intermediate position. When no nitrogenous matter was ingested, the area was at its minimum. What was then passed would be derived from the metamorphosis of the nitrogenous matter belonging to the blood and the other constituents of the system.

Some experiments of Schmidt show, also, in accordance with the results obtained by Lehmann, that the amount of urea passed is related to the *quantity* of food ingested, the *nature* of it remaining the same. Schmidt found that a cat excreted the following relative amounts of urea to body-weight under the consumption of different amounts of meat:

Daily amount of meat eaten. Grammes.	Daily amount of urea excreted per kilogramme body-weight. Grammes.
44.188	2.958
46.154	3.050
75.938	5.152
108.755	7.663

From these results it may be computed that a cat, living on a flesh diet, discharges by the kidneys on an average 6.8 parts of urea for every hundred parts of meat consumed.

The great bulk of the nitrogen belonging to the food ingested, thus passes out of the system in the form of urea. If all escaped in this way the quantity of urea discharged would amount to (say) 7.88 per cent. of the weight of the meat: the nitrogen contained in 100 parts of flesh corresponding with that contained in 7.88 parts of urea. There were, then, 6.8 parts of urea produced instead of the 7.88 parts, which may be spoken of as representing the actual equivalent, as far as contained nitrogen is concerned, of 100 parts of flesh.

Lehmann, from his observations on himself, asserts that as much as five-sixths of the nitrogen of the ingested food were found in his urine under the form of urea. For example, while living upon a purely animal diet, consisting of thirty-two eggs daily, he ingested about 30.16 grammes of nitrogen, and, in the urea voided, discharged about 25 grammes of nitrogen.

The discharge of urea being thus proportioned to the amount of the nitrogenous matter ingested, it follows that nitrogenous matter must undergo metamorphosis of such a nature within the system as to lead to the production of urea. Further, it may be said that this metamorphosis must take place rapidly, as it is found that the effect upon the excretion of urea quickly follows an alteration in the food ingested. Lehmann, for example, again drawing from his observations on himself, noticed in the morning, after he had lived exclusively on animal food, that his urine was so rich in urea as to throw down a copious precipitate of the nitrate on the addition of nitric acid. In Dr. Parkes' observations, also, upon the two soldiers S. and T., before referred to, the alterations in the food ingested speedily influenced the amount of urea escaping. These men were, first of all, kept for four days upon a regulated mixed diet; next, for two days upon a non-nitrogenous diet; then again for four days upon a mixed diet; afterward for two days on a non-nitrogenous diet; and, lastly, for four days on a mixed diet. S. during the first four days on the mixed diet passed 35 grammes of urea as the daily mean. During the first day of the non-nitrogenous diet he passed 20, and during the second, 13.52 grammes. Resuming the mixed diet, he passed on the first day, 20.67; on the second,

25.68; on the third, 26.29; and on the fourth, 29.67 grammes of urea. Changing again to the non-nitrogenous diet, he passed on the first day 19.12, and on the second, 15 grammes of urea. On the next four days, the diet being a mixed one, he passed, during the first day, 20.8; the second, 26.36; the third, 28.32; and the fourth, 30.10 grammes of urea. With T. (a much smaller man. than S.) the mean for the first four days of mixed food was 25.92 grammes of voided urea. During the next two days, upon non-nitrogenous food, he passed on the first day, 17.3; and on the second, 12.65 grammes. On the following four days, upon a diet of mixed food, he voided 14.40 the first day; 23 the second; 25.20 the third; and 22.99 grammes the fourth. During the next two days, resuming the non-nitrogenous diet, he voided 16 the first day, and 13.20 grammes the second. With a return to a mixed diet, during the following four days the urea stood at 23 on the first; 24.36 on the second; 24.57 on the third; and 21.36 grammes on the fourth.

Although conducted for settling another point, it will be seen that these observations very clearly and consistently throughout show that the production and elimination of urea are speedily affected by the ingestion of nitrogenous matter.

With the view of obtaining more precise information regarding the time required for the metamorphosis of nitrogenous matter to occur and lead to an increased elimination of urea, Mr. Mahomed, whilst formerly assisting me in my laboratory, carried out, with laudable zeal and self-denial, two series of experiments upon himself, the particulars of which I will introduce here. It may be mentioned that he was twenty-two years of age, 6 feet in height, and 11st. 11lb. in weight.

The method of procedure had recourse to was to diminish the elimination of urea by limiting in one experiment, and withholding in the other, the introduction of nitrogenous matter, and then note within what space of time the ingestion of nitrogenous matter showed its effects upon the urine.

The first experiment was commenced on April 16, 1871. Mr. Mahomed had been previously living upon an ordinary mixed diet, and took his dinner of mixed food, as usual, at 1.30 P.M. From this time he restricted himself to rice, arrow-root, butter, sugar, and tea. Rice was allowed that he might not suffer too much privation, and as being one of the least nitrogenous of the natural food products. The diet was continued throughout the 17th, and at 8 A.M. on the 18th, four eggs—purposely to supply nitrogenous matter—were eaten. This was the only deviation from the diet of the preceding day, so that an opportunity was given for the urea to be again at a low point on the following morning, when a meal, consisting mainly of meat, was taken. On page 44 is a representation of the results obtained, arranged in a tabular form.

On looking at the results obtained, it appears that under the restricted diet the urea pretty steadily decreased in amount from 21 to 9.05 grains per hour. The ingestion of four eggs caused an ascent, within the four succeeding hours, to 13.82 grains, and having thus immediately risen, the rate of elimination only underwent a little further increase through the remainder of the day. The urea having again descended to 10.62 grains per hour by the following morning, the ingestion of a meal in which steak was eaten plentifully, led to a rise for the next four hours to 21.16 grains per hour, and, with the repetition of the nitrogenous food, the elimination of urea continued to increase throughout the day.

First Experiment on the Determination of the Time Required for Urea to be Produced and Pass off After the Ingestion of Nitrogenous Matter.

Date, and period of day.	Amount of urine secreted.	Amount of urea present per fluid ounce.	Mean amount of urea secreted per hour.	Food consumed.
	Fluid ounces.	Grains.	Grains.	
April 16th 1.30 p.m. to 5.30 p.m.	6	14	21	1.30 p.m., ordinary mixed food
5.30 " 11.30 "	9	13.78	20.67	5.30 " Arrow-root, rice, butter, sugar, and tea. 9 " "
April 17th 11.30 p.m. to 8.30 a.m.	11	11.59	14.16	8.30 a.m.,
8.30 a.m. " 2 p.m.	16.5	5.68	17.06	Ditto.
2 p.m. " 8 "	14	6.16	14.37	8 p.m.,
8 " " 11.30 "	21.5	1.66	10.19	
April 18th 11.30 p.m. to 8 a.m.	11	7	9.05	8 a.m., four eggs, rice, butter, sugar, and tea.
8 a.m. " 12 noon	8	6.91	13.82	
12 noon " 4 p.m.	7	8.96	15.68	6 p.m., rice, arrow-root, butter, sugar, and tea.
4 p.m. " 8 "	21.875	2.66	14.54	
8 " " 12 midnight	20.50	2.53	12.96	9 " rice, butter, sugar, and water.
April 19th 12 midnight to 8 a.m.	20.25	4.20	10.62	8 a.m., mixed food, comprising a large proportion of meat
8 a.m. " 12 noon	4.50	18.81	21.16	
12 noon " 4 p.m.	7.25	12.68	22.98	1 p.m.
4 p.m. " 8 "	7	14.43	25.25	6.30 " Ditto.
8 " " 12 midnight	7	16.40	28.70	10.30 "

Second Experiment on the Determination of the Time Required for Urea to be Produced and Pass off After the Ingestion of Nitrogenous Matter.

Date, and period of day.	Amount of urine secreted.	Amount of urea present per fluid ounce.	Mean amount of urea secreted per hour.		Food consumed.
	Fluid ounces.	Grains.	Grains.		
May 5th					
8 a.m. to 1 p.m.	13	8.13	21.14	8 a.m.	Ordinary mixed food.
1 p.m. " 4 "	10.375	6.78	23.45	1 p.m.	
4 " " 8 "	10	9.75	24.37	7 "	
8 " " 1 a.m.	10.625	11.81	25.09	9 "	
May 6th					
1 a.m. to 8 a.m.	12.375	12.03	21.26	8 a.m.	Non-nitrogenous food, consisting of arrow-root, sugar, and butter, with tea and water.
8 " " 12 noon	7.25	12.38	22.44	2 p.m.	
12 noon " 4 p.m.	4.875	12.64	15.40	6 "	
4 p.m. " 8 "	4.50	13.12	14.76	9 "	
8 " " 12 midnight	11	3.85	10.59		
May 7th					
12 midnight to 8 a.m.	14.75	5.90	10.88	8 a.m.	Same non-nitrogenous food as on preceding day.
8 a.m. " 12 noon	5.50	8.09	11.12	11.30 "	
12 noon " 4 p.m.	15.50	4.15	16.08	1.30 p.m.	
4 p.m. " 8 "	9.375	4.37	10.24	7.30 "	
8 " " 12 midnight	14	3.93	13.75	9.30 "	
May 8th					
12 midnight to 8 a.m.	13	5.46	8.87	8 a.m.	egg and milk beaten together.
8 a.m. " 11 "	4.375	8.53	12.43	8.30 "	meat, bread, butter, and coffee.
11 " " 2 p.m.	3	14.13	14.13	2.30 p.m.	
2 p.m. " 5 "	3.375	13.78	15.50	6 "	Ordinary mixed food.
5 " " 8 "	3.625	14	16.91	9	
8 " " 11 "	4.125	14.87	20.44		

During the performance of the experiment the accustomed mental and bodily work was undertaken. Mr. Mahomed did not notice that the 2½ days' dietetic restriction produced any other sensation than an increase of the appetite and a slight feeling of faintness experienced the last morning before breakfast. The urine, before the experiment, had been frequently noticed to be loaded with lithates. During the period of restricted diet it was perfectly clear, and the table shows that the quantity was considerably larger than whilst animal food was being consumed. It is a noteworthy fact, indeed, and one which gives increased weight to the results, that the augmented elimination of urea was associated with a fall in the amount of urine, for, had the quantity of urine been increased instead, it might have been questioned whether the alterations in the urea might not have been simply due to more being carried off as a consequence of the greater urinary flow.

In the second experiment a complete restriction (excepting the insignificant amount of nitrogenous matter contained in the tea) from nitrogenous food was practised for two days, and then the diet suddenly changed to one rich in nitrogenous matter. To begin the experiment, an observation was made for one day upon ordinary food. The table on page 45 shows the results obtained.

It will be seen that the results harmonize with those obtained in the first experiment, and show that the ingestion of nitrogenous matter is followed by a speedy metamorphosis and production of urea. Under the two days' restriction to non-nitrogenous food the urea fell from a range of 21 to 25 grains per hour to 8.87 grains per hour. Nitrogenous food was now taken, and the form of egg and milk beaten together was selected, that, on account of its fluidity, absorption might be rapid. Half an hour later an ordinary breakfast with cold meat was eaten. During the *three* hours succeeding the first ingestion of nitrogenous matter, the urea secreted amounted to 12.43 grains per hour against 8.87 grains per hour, the mean amount given for the eight hours previously. During the next three hours it stood at 14.13 grains per hour, and afterward showed a steady increase throughout the day. It is true between 8.87 and 12.43 grains per hour there is not the difference that was noticeable on the morning of April 19th in the first experiment; but I think it may be fairly assumed that evidence is afforded of the production and elimination of urea within the three hours from the nitrogenous matter ingested at the commencement of the time. Throughout the day the urea was less in quantity than during the corresponding period in the first experiment, which may be due to the more complete restriction having led to a greater exhaustion of nitrogenous matter, and thereby, owing to the greater demand for the requirements of the system, a less surplus having existed for metamorphosis into urea and the complemental hydrocarbonaceous portion.

For supplying solid food during the restriction, the arrow-root was made into biscuits with butter, sugar, and water. Mr. Mahomed remarked, on rising on the morning of the 7th, that he felt depressed, and experienced a general want of tone. Before the meal in the middle of the day he felt very hungry and thirsty, but these sensations disappeared after partaking of a basin of arrow-root, two of his arrow-root biscuits, and a cup of tea. He walked afterward between five and six miles without any distress. Between the 5th and the 8th he lost one pound in weight. The urine, it may be observed, as in the first experiment, underwent a marked diminution in quantity with the return to nitrogenous food. It is a noteworthy point that between noon and midnight of the second day's restriction the urine presented an alkaline reaction. The same feeling of weakness was experienced upon rising on the morning of the 8th as on that of the preceding day.

Although it has been clearly ascertained that a more or less large proportion of the nitrogenous matter ingested undergoes metamorphosis attended with the production of urea, yet, as to the precise seat of metamorphosis, our information at present warrants, it must be said, little more than a surmise being formed. According to the old doctrine of muscular action, the chief portion was thought to be produced in the muscles; but even Liebig now argues (abstractedly from the doctrine in question) that the absence of urea as a constituent of muscular tissue may be taken as affording presumptive evidence of its production occurring elsewhere. While absent from flesh, or if present only so to a barely appreciable extent, it is, according to Meissner and others, to be detected in mammals in considerable quantity in the substance of the liver; and in birds, where uric acid holds the position of urea, this has been similarly found in the liver. Other considerations have been also advanced in support of the liver forming the seat of metamorphosis of nitrogenous matter attended with the production of urea, but the point is one which requires to be further investigated.

Having brought the subject before us to this point, the next question for consideration is, What purpose is subserved by the metamorphosis of nitrogenous matter that has been shown to occur?

It has been hitherto the custom to look upon the nitrogenous matter which undergoes this transformation as holding the position of superfluous alimentary material—"luxus consumption," as it has been styled. Thus, Lehmann writes : "In the present state of our knowledge we may say that urea is formed in the blood, and that it is produced from materials which have become effete—the detritus of the tissues—as well as from unserviceable and superfluous nitrogenous substances in the blood." As albumen fails under natural circumstances to pass off as such from the system, it was thought that, when introduced in excess of the requirements of nutrition, it underwent a retrograde metamorphosis of such a nature as would admit of the escape of its elements. It is perfectly true that the process which occurs does constitute a retrograde metamorphosis; but the question presents itself whether it is simply designed as a means of exit of surplus matter, or whether it is not preparatory to some useful purpose being fulfilled by a part of the nitrogenous compound.

The fundamental fact to be dealt with is, that nitrogenous matter undergoes a metamorphosis in the system attended with the production of urea. Now let us look at the chemical constitution of these bodies, and see what this transformation implies. The percentage composition and chemical formulæ are at our disposal to appeal to, but the former is the most suitable for our purpose; for although the atomic constitution of urea has been agreed upon, yet, as regards the albuminous molecule, it cannot be considered that we know with any degree of certainty the exact number of atoms of the different elements belonging to it, much less the precise mode in which these atoms are grouped. The formula, therefore, that can be given for it is only hypothetical. The percentage composition, however, has been ascertained with sufficient precision to serve as a trustworthy basis for the calculation about to be made, and the deduction to be drawn from it.

Let us take, for our calculation, Mulder's analysis of albumen, which is as follows:

Carbon, ...	53.5
Hydrogen, ...	7.0
Nitrogen, ...	15.5
Oxygen, ...	22.0
Sulphur, ...	1.6
Phosphorus, ...	0.4
	100.0

On looking at these figures, it will be seen that the nitrogen belonging to albumen amounts to 15.5 parts in 100. Now, let us suppose, as it is not very far from being actually the case, that the whole of the nitrogen of the ingoing albumen escapes from the system under the form of urea. In thus escaping as urea, the nitrogen carries with it a certain portion of the other constituent elements of albumen, and by ascertaining of what this portion consists, we shall see what remains behind to be disposed of in another way.

To obtain the information required, we must first be in possession of a knowledge of the relative proportion in which the elements exist in urea. This is supplied by its percentage composition, which stands as follows:

Carbon, ...	20.000
Hydrogen, ...	6.666
Nitrogen, ...	46.667
Oxygen, ...	26.667
	100.000

Now, to give to 15.5 parts of nitrogen (the quantity of nitrogen existing in one hundred parts of albumen) the due proportion of the other elements required to form urea, we shall have to supply 6.64 parts of carbon, 2.21 of hydrogen, and 8.85 of oxygen. In other words, the 15.5 parts of nitrogen contained in 100 of albumen, in escaping as urea, will carry with it 6.64 parts of carbon, 2.21 of hydrogen, and 8.85 of oxygen; leaving a residuary portion, consisting, of 46.86 parts of carbon, 4.79 of hydrogen, and 13.15 of oxygen, besides the sulphur and phosphorus, for utilization and exit in another way. Thus 33.20 per cent. (or, as nearly as possible, one-third) of the albumen will be turned into urea, and 66.80 per cent. (or, as nearly as possible, two-thirds) of complemental matter will be left.

Urea must be regarded as constituting the unutilizable portion of the albuminous principle. Whether it is formed as a primary product of the splitting up of albumen—that is, whether the elements at once group themselves from the albuminous compound into the combination representing it—or whether it forms the final product of a series of changes, cannot be stated. From comparing the egesta with the ingesta we know that it is produced. But what constitute the actual steps of metamorphosis within the system remains for physiological chemistry to disclose.

It may be remarked incidentally that, taking urea as an effete product of the metamorphosis of albuminous matter within the system, and looking at its composition under a certain point of view, we discern a relation to other products of the decomposition of nitrogenous matter that does not suggest itself on looking at its composition as ordinarily represented. Carbonic acid, ammonia, and water are the final products into which all nitrogenous matter of an organic nature is constantly tending to resolve itself. Now the formula for urea is $C_2H_4N_2O_2$ $[CH_4N_2O]$, which is equivalent to two atoms of carbonate of ammonia minus two atoms of water $(2NH_4CO_2-2HO = C_2N_2N_4O_2)$ $[(H_4N_2)$ $CO_2-2H_2O=CH_4N_2O]$. Its composition is, therefore, not exactly that of carbonate of ammonia, but we have only to add the elements of water to get the formula for carbonic acid and ammonia—two of the products into which, as we have seen, the nitrogenous matter tends by ordinary decomposition to resolve itself. It may further be remarked that not only does the above-indicated relation exist as to composition, but urea and carbonate of ammonia are mutually convertible, with the greatest facility, the one into the other. Urea, indeed, is very prone, under the influence of the action of heat, acids, alkalies, and decomposing organic matter, to pass into carbonate of ammonia, and, conversely, it has been somewhat recently discovered that carbonate of ammonia, when subject to a high temperature in a closed receptacle, is transformed into urea. It is, to say the least, a notable and significant fact that the above-mentioned relation should exist between carbonic acid and ammonia—final products of the ordinary decomposition of nitrogenous matter—and urea, a product designed for excretion arising from the metamorphosis of nitrogenous matter within the living system. It is not difficult to see why the unutilizable portion of nitrogenous alimentary matter should pass off under the form of urea, and not of carbonate of ammonia. It would scarcely be compatible with life that a powerful irritant like carbonate of ammonia should be produced to any extent within the animal system, while urea presents itself as a neutral body, quite destitute of irritating properties, and, therefore, an eligible compound as a product of metamorphosis for excretion.

The residual portion of an albuminous compound, after the separation of the nitrogen with the necessary quantities of the other elements to form urea, amounts, as has already been shown, to 66.80 per cent. of the whole. This consists of 46.86 parts of carbon, 4.79 of hydrogen, and 13.15 of oxygen, with small quantities of sulphur and phosphorus, which, in reference to the point now about to be discussed, viz., the application of this portion to force-production, may be left out of the question. It will be seen that we have here to deal with a considerable surplus of carbon and hydrogen, which represents latent force.

The 13.15 parts of oxygen will appropriate 1.64 parts of the hydrogen to exhaust its oxidizing capacity in combination as water. Reckoning this amount of hydrogen, then, as appropriated by the oxygen present, we shall have 3.15 parts of hydrogen and 46.86 parts of carbon in a free state for undergoing oxidation.

It thus appears, if we take away the nitrogen and the elements it carries off as urea, and also abstract from the hydrogen the amount which the residual oxygen would oxidize, that from 100 parts of albumen there remain 46.86 parts of carbon and 3.15 parts of hydrogen free to undergo chemical combination with oxygen supplied from without. These quantities of carbon and hydrogen will require, for their conversion into carbonic acid and water, 150 parts of oxygen, and this is tantamount to saying, according to the calculation given, that one hundred parts of albumen

4

will be capable of consuming this quantity of oxygen in undergoing oxidation. As the force produced is in proportion to the amount of chemical action, we may measure the value of different articles for force-production by the amount of oxygen they will relatively consume in undergoing complete oxidation. Regarded in this light, albumen stands in the following position in relation to grape-sugar (anhydrous $C_{12}H_{12}O_{12}$ [$C_6H_{12}O_6$]), starch, and fat:

	Amount of oxygen appropriated in oxidizing 100 parts as consumed within the body.
Grape-sugar (anhydrous),	106
Starch,	120
Albumen,	150
Fat,	293

Thus, as a force-producing agent, if we are right in taking capacity for oxidation as a measure, albumen has about half the value of fat, and a greater value than both sugar and starch.

It is true Liebig contends * for the existence of some hidden source of power in nitrogenous compounds. Arguing from the fact that alcohol in combustion gives off more heat than its corresponding amount of sugar, although a certain amount of heat has been evolved in the act of fermentation or conversion of the sugar into alcohol, he urges that force may be held stored up in the nitrogenous molecule, and liberated when the elements of the molecule are split asunder, and that thus more force may manifest itself than that derivable from chemical action.

Professor Frankland,† however, has experimentally determined the actual amount of force evolved during the breaking up by oxidation of various organic products (see table below); and unless nitrogenous matter is capable of liberating force under oxidation within the system in a manner different from that occurring outside it, there is no alternative but to look to chemical action as the source of the force produced.

Frankland's process consisted in deflagrating the substance with a mixture of chlorate of potash and manganic peroxide in an apparatus specially devised for such experiments, and called a calorimeter. The heat evolved was measured by ascertaining the elevation of temperature occurring in a known quantity of surrounding water. The results were brought to uniformity by being reduced into units of heat, the unit constituting the amount of heat required to raise the temperature of one gramme (15.432 grains) of water one degree Centigrade (1.8° Fahrenheit).

Subjoined are Professor Frankland's results for grape-sugar, starch, albumen, and fat. The ratio of the figures does not differ much from the ratio of those representing the amount of oxygen consumed in oxidation.

	Units of heat evolved by oxidation of one gramme (15.432 grains) as consumed within the body.
Grape-sugar (commercial),	3277
Starch (arrow-root),	3912
Albumen (purified),	4263
Fat (beef-fat),	9069

---

* Pharmaceutical Journal, September 3. 1870.
† Philosophical Magazine, vol. xxxii., 1866.

In the case of sugar, starch, and fat, it has been taken that the heat evolved under oxidation in the calorimeter represents the heat given off when consumed within the body, there being every reason to conclude that the ultimate products are, in both instances, the same. With regard to albumen, however, it is known that complete oxidation is not undergone within the system. The nitrogen, in escaping as urea, carries off some of the combustible portion of the compound unconsumed. "The actual energy," remarks Professor Frankland, "developed by the combustion of muscle in oxygen represents more than the amount of actual energy produced by its oxidation within the body, because, when muscle burns in oxygen, its carbon is converted into carbonic acid, and its hydrogen into water, the nitrogen being to a great extent evolved in the elementary state; whereas when muscle is most completely consumed in the body the products are carbonic acid, water, and urea—a substance which still retains a considerable amount of potential energy." The data for determining the force-value of albumen, as consumed within the body, were furnished by experimentally ascertaining the amount of heat evolved in the oxidation of urea, and knowing that almost exactly one-third of the weight of dry albumen is yielded as urea. Thence is supplied the deduction that has to be made from the full combustion-value of albumen to give the result required.

It appears that about one-seventh of the potential (latent) energy—capacity for force-production—belonging to nitrogenous matter is carried off by urea, and thereby escapes in an unexpended state when nitrogenous matter is consumed within the body.

Albumen has been selected for illustration, but what has been said for albumen applies also to the other nitrogenous alimentary principles, with the requisite variations for the slight difference in elementary composition that exists.

I have looked at the matter which has just formed the subject of consideration by the light of percentage composition, because, as I have already remarked, it supplies us with authentic data for our calculation, and because it cannot be said that we know with certainty the formulæ for the nitrogenous alimentary principles. But still we are not precluded from surveying the change under the light of the formulæ; and, if we do not know the precise number of atoms of each element entering into the composition of the proteine molecule, or the exact manner in which they are grouped, we do know that in the formula given a correct relative proportion is expressed. Now, taking the generally received formula for proteine, and showing what is left on the removal of the nitrogen under the form of urea, the surplus carbon and hydrogen available for force-production is brought very conspicuously into view. Thus Mulder's formula for proteine is $C_{48}H_{39}N_6O_{14}+2HO$. Abstract from this 2 atoms of urea, viz., $C_4H_8N_4O_4$, and 8 atoms of water, H_8O_8, and we get an available residue of 32 atoms of carbon and 11 of hydrogen, according to the old notation, or 16 of carbon and 11 of hydrogen according to the new, thus: $C_{48}H_{39}N_6O_{14} + H_8O (2CH_4N_2O + 4H_2O) = C_{16}H_{11}$.

From the relation already shown to exist between urea discharged and nitrogenous food ingested, it is not to be inferred that the nitrogenous matter which constitutes an integral part of the blood and other parts of the system is not also susceptible of metamorphosis—of being similarly split up into urea for excretion, and into carbon and hydrogen for force-production. After prolonged abstinence urea is still discoverable to some extent in the urine, and Lehmann found the same at the end of three days' subsistence upon a strictly non-nitrogenous diet. It may, therefore, be concluded that the nitrogenous matter belonging to the system may be utilized for force-production after the same manner as has been set forth for the nitrogenous matter of food.

Seeing that nitrogenous matter is broken up, 1st, into a nitrogenous portion—urea—which is eliminated as useless, and, 2d, a hydrocarbonaceous residue which represents capacity for force-production, the question next confronts us, whether this hydrocarbonaceous residue, instead of being oxidized and applied at the moment of its production, presents itself under a form (that of fat, for example) for retention in the system, and for application as necessity may demand.

Without any actual proof being available, there has long been a prevailing disposition to infer that fat may be formed as a product of the metamorphosis of proteine compounds within the animal economy. All attempts, it is true, have heretofore failed to produce fat by chemical means from proteine compounds; but there is nothing in a chemical point of view to render the possibility of such production unlikely. Indeed Liebig has argued on chemical grounds in favor of its occurrence. There are these considerations, also, bearing on the question:

It is well known that, under certain conditions, the organs and tissues of the animal body are prone to undergo deviation from the natural state, and to become the seat of a deposit of fat in place of the natural histological element, such deviation constituting what is termed "fatty degeneration." Now this change is susceptible of two explanations: it may be due to a deposition of fat during the performance of the nutritive process, in lieu of the material that has been removed; or, on the other hand, may proceed from a chemical transformation—a downward metamorphosis of the nitrogenous substance—the nitrogen disappearing under the form of an ammoniacal salt, urea, or some other simple combination, and a fatty compound being left to occupy the site.

Virchow, who has closely studied the process of fatty degeneration, and whose opinion is entitled to weight on the subject, is strongly in favor of the latter hypothesis, viz., that the fat accumulated is a product of the metamorphosis of the nitrogenous portion of the affected tissue.

Attempts have been made to find whether the transformation of nitrogenous matter into fat could be demonstrated by experiment. Excised animal structures were introduced into the peritoneal cavity of birds, and allowed to remain for some time, and were then examined in relation to the amount of fat discoverable. At first it was thought that evidence was afforded of a fatty metamorphosis of nitrogenous matter occurring, but on further investigation the evidence was found to be inconclusive.

Thus much it can be considered may be said: that what is observed in the mode of the occurrence of fatty degeneration is strongly suggestive of the doctrine that fat is producible by the metamorphosis of nitrogenous matter in the living economy, although nothing absolutely demonstrative can be adduced in support of it.

In the production of adipocere it has also been contended that evidence is afforded in favor of the origin of fat from nitrogenous matter. Adipocere is a peculiar substance, somewhat spermaceti-like, into which the animal solids are sometimes found to be converted when exposed in a humid situation to putrefaction. Fourcroy first described it in 1789, in a communication to the Academy of Sciences of Paris, having noticed its existence in certain bodies which had been interred in one of the Parisian cemeteries. The bodies appeared shrunk and flattened, and the soft solids, instead of having undergone the ordinary putrefactive change, were found to be converted into a brittle, cheesy matter, which softened and felt greasy when rubbed between the fingers. This material has since been recognized by other observers in dead bodies, and likewise in refuse-heaps of animal matter. It is also said to be obtainable by immersing flesh in a stream of water. It has been regarded as a product of the metamorphosis of nitrogenous matter; but, on the other hand, some chemists of authority, as Gay-Lussac, Chevreul, and Berzelius, have contended that it simply represents the fat which has originally existed in the animal substance, the nitrogenous matter having undergone putrefaction and been removed. Here, again, therefore, it forms a debatable point whether or no the fat encountered is a product of the metamorphosis of nitrogenous matter.

It must, in fact, be said, with regard to the evidence as to the production of fat as a result of the splitting up of nitrogenous matter, that we have nothing of the nature of proof to deal with, but that it is highly probable that such production takes place, not, perhaps, as an immediate result, but as the last link in a chain of metamorphoses passed through by the hydrocarbonaceous portion which stands in complemental relation to the urea.

Before bringing this subject to a close, it may be stated that Messrs. Lawes and Gilbert,* in a series of experiments on the feeding of animals, and the subsequent determination of the respective increase occurring in the component matters of the body, have adduced, if not actual proof, at least strong evidence in favor of fat being formed from the nitrogenous portion of food. They first of all show that, for various reasons, the pig is the most appropriate animal for yielding information upon the point in question, and hence its selection as the subject of their experiments. Their results, they say, demonstrate that when pigs are fed on good ordinary food for periods of not less than eight or ten weeks, the amounts of total increase and of fat stored up are so great in proportion both to the original weight of the animal and the food ingested, that the data given may be safely relied on for furnishing a means of estimating from what constituent or constituents of the food the fat of the animal has been derived. In their experiments, the increase in body-weight ranged between 51.3 and 68.9 per cent. when the feeding was conducted eight weeks, and between 85.4 and 106.8 per cent. when conducted ten weeks. From 59.9 to 79 per cent. of this total increase was reckoned to consist of fat. From the nature of the food, the proportion of the stored-up fat that could possibly have been derived from the ready-formed fat ingested, even supposing the whole of what was supplied had been assimilated, was so small as to leave no doubt that a very large proportion must have originated from some other source. According to the figures given, the proportion of fat which must have so originated ranged from about two-thirds to eight-ninths of the total amount stored up.

Thus, then, it was shown that fat must have been formed from the food ingested. The next question for solution was whether the fat produced originated from the nitrogenous or non-nitrogenous elements of the food, or from both.

That fat must have been produced from the non-nitrogenous matters —the carbohydrates—was easily susceptible of proof, for in some of the experiments the nature of the food was such that the carbon contained

* On the Sources of Fat of the Animal Body: Philosoph. Mag , vol. xxxii. 1866.

in the fat that was formed amounted to more than could have been derived from the nitrogenous matter ingested.

As regards the origin of fat from nitrogenous matter, the question is
not to be disposed of in so simple a manner, but Messrs. Lawes and Gilbert conclude that its production from this source may be looked upon,
as shown by the following train of reasoning, to occur. In their experiments they purposely varied the relative proportion of the nitrogenous
and non-nitrogenous parts of the food given to the several pigs. In some
they were in the proportion existing in what may be considered the staple
fattening food of the animal. In others the proportion of nitrogenous
matter was raised considerably in excess of this standard. Now, from
the results obtained, it appeared that there was no material difference in
the amount of fat produced; although if fat were capable of originating
only from the carbohydrates it would be reasonable to expect that, on
diminishing their supply, as in replacing a portion of them by nitrogenous matters—in other words, by increasing the proportionate amount of
nitrogenous matter in the food—the amount of fat developed would have
been less. Looking at the evidence furnished, it seems only rational to
infer that, under the diminution in the proportion of the carbohydrates,
the nitrogenous matter, through the hydrocarbonaceous portion which
remains after the separation of urea, took their place in supplying material for fat production, and thus led to there being no falling off observable in the quantity of fat produced.

The precise position held by the gelatinous principles as alimentary
matter must be considered, in spite of the numerous investigations that
have been specially conducted on the subject, as involved in some degree
of uncertainty. These principles, while forming highly nitrogenized
compounds, stand apart from the albuminous group in not yielding proteine. Hence they are classed as the non-proteine compounds. Whilst
the albuminous or proteine compounds exist in both animal and vegetable kinds of food, these, the non-proteine, are encountered only in substances derived from the animal kingdom. They consist of gelatine and
chondrine—the former obtainable from bones, ligaments, tendons, skin,
mucous and serous membranes, in fact wherever fibrous tissue exists;
and the latter from cartilage.

By subjecting these tissues to the action of boiling water the respective principles are obtained; but whether they have been formed during
the process or existed preformed in the tissues has been a disputed
point, although the weight of evidence is in favor of the latter view.
The chief characteristic, which they possess in common, is the property
belonging to the hot aqueous solution of solidifying into a jelly on cooling. To some extent, in elementary composition and also in some minor
chemical points, these principles differ from each other.

With reference to the alimentary power of gelatinous matter, the
great point of uncertainty is as to whether it is applicable to histogenetic or tissue-forming purposes. It may be concluded that gelatinous
matter is producible from albuminous substances, because the food of the
herbivorous animal is entirely devoid of anything of the nature of gelatine, and because, while gelatinous matter is obtainable in abundance
from the body of the chick, none can be produced from the original constituents of the egg. The proteine compounds, therefore, appear to be
evidently capable of becoming the source of gelatinous matter, but the
point to be determined is, how far gelatinous matter is capable of contributing to the production of the nitrogenous compounds met with in

the body. It has been contended that it certainly is unsusceptible of application toward the formation of muscle and the other tissues having as their basis an albuminous compound; and it is doubtful if it is even capable of contributing to the formation of the tissues, such as skin, bone, tendon, etc., whose basis consists of gelatinous matter, and which are hence styled the gelatinous tissues.

The fact of its not being recognizable in the blood, while the blood constitutes the source from which all the tissues draw their nutrient supply, has been adduced as an argument against its having any histogenetic capacity. But this, in reality, tells for nothing, because under any circumstances it is not to be expected that the gelatine should be recognizable in the blood, as it is converted by digestion into albuminose before its absorption occurs.

The nutritive value of gelatine was made the subject of special inquiry several years back, by a committee appointed by the French Academy of Sciences, to ascertain if bones could be turned to account for yielding an article of food for human consumption. The results arrived at by this committee, which passes under the designation of the Gelatine Commission, have attained a widely spread notoriety. Among the conclusions drawn up by Magendie in the name of the commission, it is stated that by no known method of procedure could there be extracted from bones an aliment which either alone or mixed with other substances could be substituted for meat. It was found that dogs fed solely on raw bones and water for three months continued in perfect health, and maintained their original weight. Fed on the same kind of bones which had been previously subjected to the change induced by boiling with water, the dogs died at the end of two months with all the signs of inanition. The general issue of the inquiry was to throw doubt upon the nutritive capacity of gelatine as an individual organic principle. Before accepting such a conclusion, however, it is necessary that we should take a more comprehensive survey of the matter, and look to the weight to be attached to investigations conducted upon the nutritive value of an isolated organic principle, and in doing so it is found that in no case will it supply what is requisite for supporting life. Neither this nor that chemical principle will suffice. There must be a combination of principles furnished; such, indeed, as exists in the objects of nature around us, which we instinctively consume as food.

In opposition to the inference to which the conclusions arrived at by the Gelatine Commission pointed, Bischoff and Voit, from their researches on nutrition, are of opinion that gelatine possesses real nutritive value; that to some extent it forms a substitute for other plastic matter, and that, therefore, by its admixture with the food, the quantity of the other nitrogenous matter may, without disadvantage, be diminished.

If uncertainty prevails as to the precise capacity of gelatine as an agent of nutrition, there can be no doubt that it behaves like a proteine compound in relation to force-production. It has been ascertained that the elimination of urea is augmented by the copious ingestion of gelatine, just as happens in the case of the proteine compounds. It is evident, therefore, that the same kind of splitting up occurs in the two cases; and, with the separation of urea from the gelatine molecule, a residue of available carbon and hydrogen will be left, in accordance with what has been before explained, for application toward force-production. There is this further analogy between these compounds, as regards the phenomena of metamorphosis, that leucine is yielded by both under the influence of boiling with a solution of potash.

THE NON-NITROGENOUS ALIMENTARY PRINCIPLES.

While nitrogenous matter may be regarded as forming the essential basis of structures possessing active or living properties, the non-nitrogenous principles may be looked upon as supplying the source of power. The one may be spoken of as holding the position of the instrument of action, while the other supplies the motive power. Nitrogenous alimentary matter may, it is true, by oxidation contribute to the generation of the moving force, but, as has been explained, in fulfilling this office there is evidence before us to show that it is split up into two distinct portions, one containing the nitrogen, which is eliminated as useless, and a residuary non-nitrogenous portion which is retained and utilized in force-production. It is true also, as will be shown hereafter, that non-nitrogenous matter may be applied to tissue formation, but it is probable that, in doing so, it is simply for the purpose of being stored up for subsequent appropriation to force-production, according as circumstances may require.

The non-nitrogenous alimentary principles comprise—
First.—The hydrocarbons or fats,
Second.—The carbohydrates, starch, sugar, etc.; and
Third.—Principles such as alcohol and the vegetable acids, which do not strictly fall within either of the preceding groups.

Hydrocarbons or Fats.—These principles constitute compounds consisting of carbon and hydrogen, combined with only a small proportion of oxygen. Represented in round numbers, the following may be given as the percentage composition of the chief fatty principles:—

Carbon, ...	79
Hydrogen, ...	11
Oxygen, ...	10
	—
	100

The formula answering to the above composition that has been framed consists of $C_{10}H_9O$ [$C_{16}H_{16}O$].

This, it will be seen, might be considered as representing a pure hydrocarbon, in which every tenth atom of hydrogen is replaced by an atom of oxygen.

Fats are supplied to us in both animal and vegetable articles of food. Chemically, they consist of a principle possessing acid properties—a fatty acid—in combination with a radical. When acted upon by alkalies, and also by contact with bodies of the nature of ferments, and by decomposing animal substances, the fatty acid is separated, and a sweet principle known as glycerine makes its appearance. Glycerine, however, it would seem, has not pre-existed in the fat. It is found that the united weight of the glycerine and fatty acid produced exceeds that of the fat originally employed. The elements of water are appropriated, and glycerine is thereupon formed by an addition to the hypothetical radical in combination with the fatty acid in the neutral fat.

There are three compounds—stearine, palmitine, and oleine—which make up the great bulk of the fatty matter met with.

Stearine is the most solid fat of the three. It exists largely in mutton suet, and gives rise to the firmness by which this kind of fat is characterized. Requiring a temperature of about 145° Fahrenheit to melt it, at ordinary temperatures it is always solid. It occurs to a larger or smaller extent in most animal fats; but still there are some in which it has not been recognized. It is never found in vegetable fat.

Palmitine holds an intermediate place between stearine and oleine as regards consistence. It is the chief component of most animal fats, and occurs largely in vegetable fats. What was formerly described as margarine proves to be a mixture of palmitine and stearine.

Oleine is always met with in a fluid state, unless the temperature is very low. It occurs in both vegetable and animal fats, but vegetable fats are richer in it than animal.

The digestion of fat takes place in the small intestine. It traverses the mouth without undergoing any change beyond that induced by the mechanical action of mastication.

In the stomach the nitrogenous matter which may be incorporated with and invest the fatty, as occurs in the natural alimentary product, is dissolved, and the latter set free. Passing from the stomach, it is prepared for absorption in the small intestine by emulsification or reduction to a minute state of subdivision. As regards animal and vegetable fats, it appears that the former are easier of digestion and absorption than the latter.

The emulsification of fat is effected by the pancreatic juice, and probably also by the secretion of Brunner's glands. The bile has no influence over neutral fats, *i.e.*, fats in the state in which we consume them; but according to Dr. Marcet it possesses the power of emulsifying the fatty acids, and he says there is some liberation of fatty acid effected while the fat is contained in the stomach. The process of emulsification is one of a purely physical nature. The fat is separated into very minute globules, just as it exists in milk, and in this state it is taken up by the special absorbing organs of the small intestine, viz., the villi.

It was noticed by Bernard that when fat is delayed for some hours in contact with pancreatic juice, an acidification of it, or chemical conversion into fatty acid and glycerine, is found to have taken place. The delay, however, in the intestine is not long enough for this chemical change to occur as a physiological phenomenon. Bernard thought originally that it did—that the digestion of fat was attended with acidification; but fat contained in the lacteals—the absorbed fat, that is to say—has been found to be in precisely the same chemical condition as that contained in the intestine. It is thus evident that digestion and absorption of fat do not involve its chemical change.

The villi—little projecting bodies limited in situation to the small intestine—are the organs through the agency of which the fat is absorbed. While absorption is going on they are to be seen in a densely white state, from the quantity of fatty particles with which they are charged. It is not precisely understood how the fatty matter passes from the intestine and reaches their centre. From what is to be seen on microscopic examination, conducted immediately after death, it would seem that it is by cell-agency that the fatty matter is picked out from the intestinal contents. During fasting the epithelial cells investing the villi are club-shaped and devoid of fat-globules. During absorption, on the other hand, they are charged with fat-globules, and many are found of a spheroidal, instead of a columnar form. The process of absorption may be thus far likened to that of secretion. As the secreting cells of the glands separate from the blood the particular materials required for each individual secretion, so these cells of the villi pick out or separate from the chyme or intestinal contents the fatty matter which is subsequently found in the lacteals. A branch of the lacteal system existing in the centre of the villus receives the product of absorption. Thus much is certain—what remains to be made clear is the manner in which the transmission to the lacteal is effected. By the lacteal system the absorbed fat is conducted to and poured into the circulation. Mixing with the alkaline blood, the fat becomes saponified and dissolved, and in this state it is mostly met with in the circulation. Should a rapid entrance, however, have been effected, as happens for a while after the ingestion of food rich in fatty matter, free fat exists in the blood; and a specimen withdrawn under these circumstances, and afterward allowed to remain at rest, presents, after a short time, a distinct cream-like layer upon the surface.

Having pointed out how the fat belonging to the food reaches the circulation, we have next to consider the purposes to which it is applied in the system.

I will first speak of it as contributing to the construction of one of the anatomical elements of the body. The adipose tissue consists of nucleated vesicles filled with fatty matter. These vesicles are closely packed together and surrounded by capillary blood-vessels. The fat contained in them is evidently drawn, as in nutrition generally, from the blood circulating around, and, when so separated, a tissue is formed which is turned to account for mechanical, physical, and chemico-physiological purposes.

For instance, it fills up interstices between muscles, bones, vessels, and the other anatomical structures, and by its accumulation under the skin, it gives a regular and rounded form to the outer surface of the body.

As a bad conductor of heat, the layer of adipose tissue beneath the skin contributes toward retaining the animal warmth. This function it most conspicuously fulfils in the aquatic warm-blooded animals, such as the seal, porpoise, whale, etc., in which a coat of hair would prove of no service from the nature of the circumstances that exist. The very great thickness of the subcutaneous layer of adipose tissue met with in these animals is evidently designed to meet the demand occasioned by the unsuitableness, in this particular instance, of the ordinary provision.

Accumulated within the vesicles and susceptible of reabsorption into the blood, the fat forms a store of force-producing material to be drawn upon as circumstances may require. Hence it is that life is sustained longer in a fat animal under abstinence from food and with a supply of water than in a thin one.

In vol. xi. of the " Transactions of the Linnæan Society," an account is given by Mr. Mantell (afterward Dr. Mantell, the celebrated geologist); a Fellow of the Society, under the form of a letter to the secretary, of an instance of extraordinary prolongation of life in a fat animal under absence of food. So extraordinary, indeed, is the account, that I should scarcely feel disposed to allude to it here did not the source from which it is derived entitle it to credit. It appears that on December 14, 1810, a pig was buried in its sty by the fall of part of the chalk cliff under Dover Castle. On May 23d—160 days afterward—Mr. Mantell was told

.

by some workmen employed in removing the fallen chalk that they had heard the whining of the pig, and although he had great doubt of the fact, he urged them to proceed in clearing away the chalk from the sty, and was soon afterward surprised to see the pig extricated from its confinement alive. At the time of the accident the pig was in a fat condition, and supposed to have weighed about 160 lbs. When extricated it presented an extremely emaciated appearance, and weighed no more than 40 lbs. The sty consisted of a cave about six feet square, dug in the rock, and boarded in front. There was neither food nor water in it, it was asserted, when the fall of the cliff took place. The door and other wood in front of the sty was much nibbled, and the sides of the cave looked very smooth, as though the animal had been constantly licking them to obtain the moisture exuding through the rock.

In the hibernating animal, a great accumulation of fat takes place during the autumn, which is favored by the oily nature of the nuts, seeds, etc., then obtainable as food. At the end of the winter sleep, the animal is reduced to a comparatively emaciated condition. The fat accumulated may be looked upon as designed to form an internal store for consumption when the supply from without is suspended.

In an emaciated animal, the fat vesicles, under the microscope, betray the process of absorption that has been going on. They are shrunken in appearance, and the fatty contents of the vesicle, receding from the envelope, leave a space which is filled with watery fluid.

Besides forming the basis of a tissue fulfilling the functions referred to, fatty matter occurs in intimate incorporation with the nitrogenous elements of most, if not all, of the various anatomical structures. Lehmann remarks that no animal cell or fibre can be formed without the co-operation of fat, and insists strongly on the fat constituting an active agent in exciting the metamorphosis of nitrogenous matter. Lehmann, however, wrote under the influence of the formerly prevailing notion that the manifestation of vital energy, as under muscular and nervous action, was due to a destructive metamorphosis of the nitrogenous constituents of the tissues. This, as has already been pointed out, stands opposed to the results of modern research; and instead of (as suggested by Lehmann) the fatty matter operating by inducing a metamorphosis of the nitrogenous, it may now be considered that, in undergoing oxidation, it constitutes, itself, the source of the power manifested. But this is a point that will be more particularly adverted to hereafter.

Lehmann has also asserted that fat assists the action of the digestive fluid. He goes so far as to say that he has ascertained that a certain, though small, amount of fat is indispensable to the metamorphosis and solution of nitrogenous articles of food during the process of gastric digestion. I do not think that experiment is found to bear out this statement of Lehmann; at all events I have seen nothing from my own experiments on artificial digestion to warrant the belief that the action of the gastric juice is even influenced, much less determined by, the presence of fat.

We now come to the consideration of fat with reference to the functions fulfilled by its oxidation within the system, and here we have to deal with functions associated with its final destination. It is the fatty matter existing in the blood that may be looked upon as being thus applied, and when this fails to be adequately replenished by a supply from the food, then absorption occurs from the store which the adipose tissue of the body represents.

Under Liebig's classification, fat is held to be a so-called "element of respiration," or, to speak more correctly, a calorifacient or heat-producing agent. An exalted temperature is required for a high manifestation of vitality, and amongst the higher members of the animal kingdom, in which the processes of life are carried on with much greater activity than amongst the lower, provision is made for the generation of heat within the body. Notwithstanding exposure to great external cold, so long as a healthy condition prevails, a certain uniform temperature is maintained; and for this end the oxidation of combustible material is constantly going on. Hence arises a demand for food capable of undergoing the process of oxidation. Liebig holds the non-nitrogenous alimentary principles to be specially devoted to this purpose. That they *do* contribute to it there can be no doubt; but it will be for us presently to consider whether they do not also contribute to the production of other manifestations of energy besides heat.

The capacity of a material for heat-production depends upon the amount of unoxidized carbon and hydrogen it contains; and of all elementary materials the fats hold the highest place in this respect. While in starchy, saccharine, and such-like matters, a sufficient amount of oxygen exists in the compound to oxidize all the hydrogen present, leaving only the carbon in an oxidizable condition; in the fats not only is the carbon, but also the chief portion of the hydrogen in an unoxidized state.

To illustrate the difference existing, it may be stated that starch contains, in round numbers, 45 per cent. of carbon and 6 per cent. of hydrogen, making 51 per cent. of carbon and hydrogen together. The remainder consists of oxygen, amounting to as much as 49 per cent. of the whole. Sugar, and gum likewise, in round numbers, contain 43 per cent. of carbon and 6 per cent. of hydrogen, making 49 per cent. of carbon and hydrogen together, and leaving 51 per cent. to be made up by oxygen. Fat, on the other hand, contains about 90 per cent. of carbon and hydrogen—79 per cent. of carbon and 11 per cent. of hydrogen. Only 10 per cent., therefore, remains to consist of oxygen.

The respective values of these compounds, as regards capacity for oxidation, may also be displayed by reference to their chemical formulæ. The formula for starch, for instance, consists of $C_{12}H_{10}O_{10}$ [$C_6H_5O_5$], and in all the other allied compounds the hydrogen and oxygen exist similarly in the proportion to form water. Fat may be represented by the formula C_9H_9O [C_8H_8O]. Here only one atom of hydrogen has its combining equivalent of oxygen contained in the compound. The remaining eight atoms, as well as the carbon, are in a free state for oxidation.

The amount of oxygen consumed in oxidizing a given quantity of an alimentary principle will necessarily vary with the amount of surplus or uncombined carbon and hydrogen it contains. Hence the relative value of these principles as heat-producing agents (it being upon the amount of chemical action that the quantity of heat produced depends) may be further represented through the medium of the oxygen for which there is the capacity for appropriating; and, looked at in this light, fat, starch, and sugar hold the following positions with regard to each other. The figures show the amount of oxygen required to oxidize fully 100 parts:

Fat, ... 293
Starch, ... 120
Sugar ($C_{12}H_{12}O_{12}$) [$C_6H_6O_6$], ... 106

According to what is here shown, a given quantity of fat will have the power of appropriating about 2.4 times as much oxygen as the same quantity of starch; or, stated in other words, will develop about 2.4 times as much heat in the process of oxidation, and hence has about 2.4 times as much value as a heat-producing agent.

The conclusions which have up to this point been set forth are based on calculation. But the actual value in respect of capacity for heat-production has been determined experimentally by means of the calorimeter, and the following are the figures obtained by Professor Frankland. It will be seen that they accord with the conclusions otherwise arrived at:

Actual Heat, Expressed in Units [the unit representing the heat required to raise 1 gramme (15.432 grains) of water 1° Cent. or 1.8° Fahr.], Developed by 1 Gramme when Burnt in Oxgyen.

	Heat units.
Beef-fat, ...	9069
Starch (arrow-root), ...	3912
Cane- (lump) sugar, ...	3348
Commercial grape-sugar, ...	3277

Such is equivalent to saying that 1 lb. of beef-fat by oxidation will generate heat sufficient to raise the temperature of 9,069 lbs. (about 4 tons weight) of water by 1.8° Fahr. (1° Cent.); that the oxidation of the same quantity of arrow-root will similarly raise the temperature of only 3,912 lbs. of water; cane-sugar, 3,348 lbs.; and commercial grape-sugar, 3,277 lbs.

Looking at this difference in the relative value of fatty, starchy, and saccharine matters as heat-producers, we see the wisdom of the instinctive consumption of food abounding in fatty matter by the inhabitants of the arctic regions. The Esquimaux and other dwellers in the frigid zone devour with avidity the fat of whales, seals, etc., and find in this the most efficient kind of combustible material. In the tropics, on the other hand, the food consumed by the native inhabitants consists mainly of farinaceous and succulent vegetable matter. On account of the elevated temperature of the surrounding air, less heat is required to be produced within the body, and a less efficient combustible material is able to supply what is needed for the maintenance of the ordinary temperature.

I now arrive at the appropriate place for discussing the question of the application of fat to the production of muscular and nervous force, and what I have to say upon the point will apply, not to fat merely, but to other forms of non-nitrogenous alimentary matter.

Until of late years, Liebig's doctrines have been very generally received. These, as is well known, assign to non-nitrogenous matters, in respect of their *chemico*-physiological office, the part simply of heat-producers. Believing that muscular and nervous action involved a destruction of the respective tissues, and that in this destruction was to be sought the development of the power manifested, Liebig maintained that the nitrogenous alimentary matters constitute the primary source of the power, these being the principles out of which the tissues are in the first instance formed and subsequently renewed.

Under such a view, the nitrogenous matters eliminated as products of disintegration should vary according to the amount of work performed, and this was at one time believed to be the case. Even as recently as 1865, Dr. Lyon Playfair (on "The Food of Man in Relation to his Useful Work") writes in support of Liebig's doctrine, and reasons on the assumption that the work is expressed by the elimination of urea. "The normal function," he says, "of nutrition is to build up plastic food into tissues, to be transformed by internal and external dynamical work into carbonic acid, water, and urea." He elsewhere asserts that he considers Liebig as amply justified in viewing the non-nitrogenous portions of food as mere heat-givers; and, with reference to the oxidation of fat forming the source of muscular action, the conception, he says, "can only have arisen from the false analogy of the animal body to a steam-engine. But incessant transformation of the acting parts of the animal machine forms the condition for its action, while in the case of the steam-engine it is the transformation of fuel external to the machine which causes it to move." Dr. Playfair even furthermore reproduces and endorses Liebig's representation of the wild beast in confinement being obliged to consume its tissues by incessantly pacing backward and forward in its den, in order that the opportunity may be afforded for its food, which abounds in nitrogenous matter, to be turned to account.

These assertions, it must be said, are not in accord with the results of recent investigations. It has been amply shown (*vide* p. 26 *et seq.*) that the elimination of urea, or to speak more generally—nitrogen, does not bear the relation which it was formerly supposed to do to muscular work; and, as a corollary, it may be taken that muscular action is not the result of and is not to be measured by muscular destruction. If not, then, to an oxidation or consumption of muscular tissue, to what is the energy manifested to be ascribed? The known laws about force, lead us to look to chemical action of some kind as the source of the manifestation in question.

An examination of the outgoings from the system may, therefore, be rationally appealed to for information regarding the nature of the materials that are consumed in the production of the energy that is manifested. Now, if urea is not a measure of muscular work, it is noticeable that carbonic acid is; and it is upon this fact that is founded the doctrine of the present day, which refers the source of muscular power to the oxidation of non-nitrogenous matter. So thorough has been the modification of views upon this point, that Traube, as mentioned on a former page, has gone as far as directly to invert the doctrine of Liebig. While Liebig considered that mechanical work could only be produced from the oxidation of nitrogenous matter, Traube has asserted that, in such work, non-nitrogenous substances exclusively are consumed, and that the metamorphosis of the organized nitrogenous part of a muscle is neither involved in nor increased by its action.

It has, for some time past, been generally believed that the elimination of carbonic acid is increased by muscular work. Thus Lehmann says that bodily exercise increases the exhalation of carbonic acid in the same manner as a state of rest diminishes it. Vierordt, he states, convinced himself that the absolute as well as the relative quantity of carbonic acid was increased after moderate exercise, and this result, he says, is in perfect conformity with the experiments of Scharling. H. Hoffmann, he continues, found that the sum of the products of exhalation of the skin and lungs was much more considerable after prolonged motion than after prolonged rest; and every one, he further says, who has instituted experiments on the respiration of animals, must be aware that they exhale far more carbonic acid when they are lively and active than during a state of repose. ✱

The older observations upon this point, however, were attended with some lack of uniformity in the results, and it has been reserved for more recent inquiry, with improved means and modes of investigation, to put the matter in a thoroughly satisfactory position, and to show that the exhalation of carbonic acid holds a direct relation to the amount of work performed.

Dr. Edward Smith, in the "Philosophical Transactions" for 1859, has given the results of an extensive series of experiments upon the elimination of carbonic acid under various conditions. They were mostly practised upon himself, and carried out with zealous self-denial. A mask was closely fitted to the face, and a tube passing off from it conducted the expired air to an apparatus in which the carbonic acid was abstracted and absorbed by means of potash, and afterward estimated by weighing. The amounts of carbonic acid exhaled by Dr. Smith, under varying conditions of exertion, stood as follows:

	Carbonic acid exhaled per minute, in grains.
During sleep,	4.99
Lying down and almost asleep (average of three observations),	5.91
Walking at the rate of two miles per hour,	18.10
Walking at the rate of three miles per hour,	25.83
Working at the treadmill, ascending at the rate of 28.65 feet per minute (average of three observations),	44.97

Dr. Smith's results are drawn from the carbonic acid exhaled during limited periods of time. Pettenkofer, assisted by Voit, has instituted experiments whereby the observation extended through a period consisting of many hours. An air-tight chamber, sufficiently large to enable a man to live, move about, and sleep in, was provided. To this was adapted an arrangement for maintaining an ingress and egress of air, and for diverting a definite proportion of the latter for the purpose of analysis, in order that the amount of carbonic acid escaping might be determined. In this chamber, upon one occasion, July 31, 1866,* a watchmaker remained for twenty-four hours, passing a day of rest; that is, he occupied himself only so far as not to feel dull, reading newspapers and a novel, and repairing and cleaning a watch which he had taken with him into the chamber. He went to bed at eight P.M., and slept well till five A.M., when he was aroused by some one on the outside. Three days later the same man entered the chamber, and passed a day of work; the work consisting of turning a wheel with a weight attached to it. Rest and meals were taken at the periods usual with workmen, and work was stopped at half-past five P.M. The food taken was exactly the same as on the day of rest; but 600 grammes more water, which had been allowed *ad libitum* on both days, were consumed. The quantities of carbonic acid and urea eliminated are shown by the subjoined figures:

Day of Rest.

	Carbonic acid. Grammes.	Urea, Grammes.
6 A.M. to 6 P.M.,	532.9	21.7
6 P.M. to 6 A.M.,	378.6	15.5
Total,	911.5	37.2

* Medical Times and Gazette, vol. ii., p. 680. 1866.

Day of Work.

	Carbonic acid. Grammes.	Urea. Grammes.
6 A.M. to 6 P.M.,	884.6	20.1
6 P.M. to 6 A.M.,	399.6	16.9
Total,	1,184.2	37.0

It will be noticed from the above results that no effect was produced upon the elimination of urea. The food consumed was, as mentioned, similar on the two days, and, in accordance with this fact, there was a close agreement in the respective amounts of urea voided. The carbonic acid discharged during the actual period of work greatly exceeded that discharged during the corresponding period of rest. During the two night-periods when similar conditions prevailed, no material difference in the amount of carbonic acid was perceptible. The quantities, of course, represented the exhalation from both the lungs and the cutaneous surface.

It is impossible by experiment to ascertain anything about the oxidation of hydrogen and production of water in relation to muscular work. It having been shown, however, that work is associated with an oxidation of carbon, it may be assumed that it is similarly associated with, and producible from, an oxidation of hydrogen.

To this point, then, are we brought by the progress of experimental research. The facts connected with the elimination of nitrogen show that muscular work is not to be referred—as taught by Liebig, and till lately generally believed—to an oxidation of the nitrogenous basis of muscular tissue; and if this holds good for muscular, it may be assumed also to do so for nervous tissue. The relation, on the other hand, which has been shown to exist between the elimination of carbonic acid and the performance of work entitles us to consider that to the oxidation of hydrocarbonaceous matter may be referred the production of power.

Just as matter is indestructible and cannot be created, so, it is now understood, is force. Force may be transmuted from one form into another—from chemical energy into heat, mechanical power, and so on; but this, it is considered, is all that occurs; and what holds good for the world around us is considered also to apply within the living organism. Physiologists refer the chief source of heat to the oxidation of carbon and hydrogen, and to the same source is now ascribed the production of mechanical power. The energy set free by chemical action manifests itself under the form of mechanical work. The following simile has been suggested by Fick and Wislicenus: *

"A bundle of muscle-fibres is a kind of machine, consisting of albuminous material, just as a steam-engine is made of steel, iron, brass, etc. Now, as in the steam-engine coal is burnt in order to produce force, so in the muscular machine fats, or hydrates of carbon, are burnt for the same purpose. And, in the same manner as the constructive material of the steam-engine (iron, etc.) is worn away and oxidized, the constructive material of the muscle is worn away, and this wearing away is the source of the nitrogenous constituents of the urine. This theory explains why, during muscular exertion, the excretion of the nitrogenous constituents of the urine is little or not at all increased, while that of carbonic acid is enormously augmented; for, in a steam-engine moderately fired, and ready

---

* On the Origin of Muscular Power, Philosophical Mag., vol. xxxi., p. 501.

for use, the oxidation of iron, etc., would go on tolerably equably, and would not be much increased by the more rapid firing necessary for working, but much more coal would be burnt when it was at work than when it was standing idle."

Looking, then, at the evidence adduced, the result of modern research goes to show that the non-nitrogenous alimentary principles are applied not only to the production of heat, but likewise to other forms of force. It may be considered that nitrogenous matter, which constitutes the basis of the various organs and textures, forms the instrument of action, whilst the oxidation of non-nitrogenous matter supplies the motive power.

Fick and Wislicenus, in their celebrated mountain ascent, ascertained that severe labor might be performed for a while without the use of nitrogenous food. As a result of their experience they remark: "We can assert from our own experience in the ascent of the Faulhorn, that, in spite of the amount of work, and the abstinence for thirty-one hours from albuminous food, we neither of us felt in the least exhausted. This could hardly have been the case," they proceed to say, "if our muscular force had not been sustained by the non-nitrogenous food of which we partook."

The two soldiers, in one of Dr. Parkes' experiments,* who were subjected to a couple of days' pretty severe walking exercise on a non-nitrogenous diet, were questioned as to how they felt in performing it. The distance traversed amounted to 23¾ miles on the first day, and 32¾ miles on the second, on level ground. The diet satisfied hunger. There was no sinking nor craving for other kinds of food, but it was monotonous, and neither man wished to continue it. The first day's walking was borne pretty well. On the second day, both men accomplished the first twenty miles well, but felt very much fatigued during the last thirteen. They could have both marched on the following day, had it been necessary. One man would give no opinion as to the amount of fatigue experienced in comparison with walking on other occasions, as he had no fair basis, he said, to go by. The other, however, was decidedly of opinion that he sustained much more fatigue than when walking upon other food.

In a previous part of this work (vide p. 40 et seq.), it has been fully pointed out how, without coinciding with the doctrine formerly entertained, the nitrogenous alimentary principles are, like the non-nitrogenous, rendered applicable to force-production. Instead of passing into the state of tissue, and thence by oxidation giving rise to the evolution of force, they undergo (probably by the action of the liver) a splitting up into urea for the one part, which carries off the nitrogen as an unavailable element, and into a slightly oxygenated hydrocarbonaceous residue for the other, which may be looked upon as applicable in the same way as primarily ingested non-nitrogenous matter to force-production.

That energy capable of resulting in the performance of mechanical work is produced in the animal system by the oxidation of carbonaceous matter may be considered as an established fact. Whether, however, this energy arises from the occurrence of oxidation in the blood as it is circulating through the capillary vessels of the muscle, or whether from the oxidation of hydrocarbonaceous matter existing in the muscular tissue, is a point which it is not easy to see the way to settle; but the latter proposition, it may be said, appears the more probable of the two.

As is the case with reference to heat, the amount of mechanical energy producible is in proportion to the amount of chemical action occurring.

* Proceedings of the Royal Society, vol. xv., p. 346. 1867.

5

A given amount of an organic compound, for example, will, as is well known, by oxidation give rise to the generation of a definite and ascertainable amount of heat. In the same manner, when the energy set free is manifested under the form of mechanical power instead of heat, a fixed amount of work is capable of being performed. The energy produced may present itself under the form of a certain amount of heat, or, on the other hand, may lead to the accomplishment of a certain amount of work; not only so, but heat and mechanical power are known to be mutually convertible, and a definite expression can be given of their relative value in representative equivalents.

According to the English system, work is measured by pounds or tons lifted a foot, and the measurement is expressed as foot-pounds or foot-tons.

Now, Mr. Joule, of Manchester, has ascertained, and his conclusions are very generally acquiesced in, that the amount of energy which under the form of heat will raise the temperature of a pound of water 1° Fahr. will, if manifested as mechanical force, raise 772 pounds a foot high, or what, of course, amounts to the same, 1 pound 772 feet high. Thus the dynamic equivalent of 1° Fahr. of heat is said to be 772 foot-pounds. Adopting the Centigrade scale of thermal measurement, the mechanical equivalent of 1° (1.8° Fahr.) will be 1,389 foot-pounds; that is, the energy which, as calorific power, will raise the temperature of a pound of water 1° Cent. (1.8° Fahr.) will be capable, as motive power, of raising a pound weight 1,389 feet high.

Under the Continental system the mechanical equivalent of heat is expressed in kilogrammetres—a kilogrammetre constituting one kilogramme (2.2046 pounds avoirdupois) raised to the height of a metre (3.2808 feet). Thus represented, and following Mr. Joule's formula, 1° Cent. of heat may be said to be equivalent to 423½ kilogrammetres, which means that the heat which will raise the temperature of a kilogramme of water 1° Cent. will be equivalent to the mechanical power required to raise a kilogramme weight 423½ metres high.

Applying this to the utilization of food, the value of the various principles as mechanical-power-producers will correspond with their value as heat-producers. As heat-production is related to the amount of chemical action ensuing, so likewise is mechanical power-production. Such alimentary principle as will by oxidation give rise to the greatest amount of heat will have the greatest capacity for the production of working power.

At p. 61 the calorific value of fat, starch, cane-sugar, and grape-sugar is to be found according to the actual determinations of Professor Frankland. Looked at in relation to the performance of work, and taking Mr. Joule's estimate of the mechanical equivalent of heat as the basis of calculation, the capacity of these articles will stand thus:

Amount of Mechanical Work obtainable from the Oxidation of One Gramme (15.432) grains.

	(*Frankland.*)	
	In kilogrammetres (kilogrammes lifted a metre).	In foot-pounds * (pounds lifted a foot).
Beef fat, . . .	3,841	27,778
Starch (arrow-root), .	1,657	11,983
Lump sugar, . .	1,418	10,254
Grape sugar, . .	1,388	10,038

* Kilogrammetres are convertible into foot-pounds by multiplying by 7.232 : one kilogrammetre being equal to 7.232 foot-pounds.

Nitrogenous matters, as has been previously explained, do not undergo complete oxidation within the body, a portion of the compound being separated and eliminated under the form of urea in an unoxidized condition. Taking lean beef, and viewing it as oxidized to the extent which occurs in the animal system, one gramme (15.432 grains) in a dried state will develop energy capable of raising 2,047 kilogrammes a metre high, or 14,803 pounds a foot high.

Such is the modern way of regarding food in reference to its application to force-production.

THE CARBO-HYDRATES,

Forming a second systematic group of non-nitrogenous alimentary principles, are compounds in which the hydrogen and oxygen exist in the proportion to form water. Hence, these compounds have been designated hydrates of carbon or carbo-hydrates. It must not, however, be inferred that the elements are in reality grouped as the name would imply. There is no ground for such a conclusion. All that can be said is that the respective quantities of the elements are such as would form water. But from this it does not follow that they exist in combination as water, to be then linked as such to the carbon. Comprised in the group of compounds we have starch, cane-sugar, grape-sugar, lactine (sugar of milk), inosite (muscle-sugar), amyloid substance, gum, dextrine, cellulose, woody fibre, lactic acid, acetic acid.

Starch ($C_{12}H_{10}O_{10}$) [$C_6H_{10}O_5$].—Starch may be regarded as the most important alimentary principle of the group, on account of its entering so largely as it does into some of our staple articles of food. It is met with only in vegetable products, and is found stored up in the form of little granules, or solid particles, in many seeds, roots, stems, and some fruits. Each granule is made up of a series of concentric layers, the external being of a firmer or more indurated nature than the rest. In cold water the granules remain unaltered, but when subjected to the influence of boiling water they swell up, burst, and form a mucilage which assumes a gelatinous nature on being allowed to cool.

Starch constitutes a principle which, as long as it remains as such, resists absorption from the alimentary canal. At least, all that can be said is that a few particles, like finely divided particles of other kinds, as of charcoal and sulphur, have been known to find their way, in some manner or other, through the walls of the alimentary canal into the blood-vessels. To serve, therefore, as an alimentary article, it must undergo a preliminary metamorphosis to fit it for absorption, and this is effected by the process of digestion.

The influence exerted upon starch in the digestive system leads to its conversion, in the first instance, into dextrine, which has only a very transitory existence, and then into sugar—an agent which possesses the property of being easily susceptible of absorption. Thus it is that starch is prepared by the digestive apparatus for undergoing absorption.

There are various secretions that are endowed with the power of transforming starch into sugar. I will speak, in the first place, of the action of the saliva in this respect.

When starch has been brought into the most favorable condition for metamorphosis, as by subjection to the influence of boiling water, it is very speedily converted into sugar upon being brought into contact with human saliva. In the solid form, however, or whilst the granules remain in an unruptured state, the transformation is much less speedily effected. Now, it happens that our food is not long delayed in the mouth, and that the starch, as we usually consume it, is not in the most favorable condition for metamorphosis. It may, therefore, be considered that during the accomplishment of the first step of the digestive process, viz., the action which is exerted while the food is in the mouth, little, if any, conversion of starch into sugar takes place. Moreover, although the human saliva enjoys the property above mentioned, yet the saliva of many of the lower animals fails, it has been found, to possess a similar capacity.

The transformative power of saliva is also checked by the presence of an acid. Hence, when the stomach is reached, and the food arrives in contact with its acid secretion, any change that might occur from the prolonged admixture of starch and saliva is prevented. In the ruminant animal, however, the food, after being a first time swallowed, is retained for a while in a simple receptacle, a favorable condition being here presented for the exercise of the transformative action of the saliva. The same likewise holds good in the case of the crop of the bird.

It has been suggested by Dr. Bence Jones that the secretion of the stomach, by virtue of the acid belonging to it, is capable of effecting some conversion of starch into sugar. The amount of change, however, that can be thus exerted is probably not sufficient to warrant our looking upon it as possessing any material extent of physiological significance.

Passing from the stomach, the food reaches the small intestine—the part of the alimentary canal which may be regarded as forming the main seat of the digestion of starch. The secretion both of the pancreas and of the glands of the intestinal walls possesses the power of acting energetically upon starch, and within the intestinal canal there exist the most favorable conditions for the exercise of the transformative power enjoyed by these fluids. The food, for instance, has been reduced to a semifluid state before reaching the intestine, where its admixture with the secretions in question takes place. The two are then urged slowly along by the peristaltic movement of the intestinal canal, and thus cannot fail to become thoroughly incorporated together. Subjected in this way to prolonged contact with each other, and at the same time exposed to the equable and elevated temperature which belongs to the locality, nothing could be more favorable for the occurrence of the metamorphosis. As the transformation of the starch is accomplished, the resulting sugar is removed by absorption, passing, simply by virtue of its diffusibility, into the circulating current within the blood-vessels.

Microscopic examination shows that in this conversion of starch into dextrine, in the first place, and afterward into sugar, the granules become softened and gradually broken up. Individual lamellæ have been seen to become detached and subsequently to undergo disintegration—isolated shreds having been brought into view with the aid of the iodine test. The farther the starch is traced onward in the intestinal canal the smaller do the granules become, in consequence of the gradually advancing disintegration and solution which they undergo from the surface inward.

The power of digesting starch is not by any means such as to secure the digestion of all that enters the alimentary canal as food. Starch-granules, especially when the starch has been ingested in the raw state, have been frequently shown to pass off from the alimentary canal in considerable numbers with the evacuations, both in man and in the lower animals.

Cane-sugar $(C_{12}H_{11}O_{11})$ $[C_{12}H_{22}O_{11}]$.—There are various kinds of sugar, and this is the crystallizable variety, which is so extensively employed as an article of food. It is produced only by the vegetable kingdom, and is contained in the juice of the stems, roots, and other parts of various plants. It is present in a dissolved state in these juices instead of existing in a solid form, as is the case with starch.

The properties of solubility and diffusibility which cane-sugar possesses dispense with the necessity of any aid to absorption being afforded by the digestive process. All that is required is that it should be either dissolved or that there should be liquid to dissolve it, and its diffusibility will enable it, without any preparatory process, to pass by absorption from the alimentary canal into the current of fluid contained in the blood-vessels.

Although cane-sugar, however, requires no digestion to fit it for absorption, it may be considered probable that it undergoes conversion into grape-sugar, certainly in part, if not wholly, before leaving the alimentary canal. If cane-sugar be introduced into one of the vessels of the general circulation, it passes off from the system without being utilized, and escapes, still in the form of cane-sugar, with the urine. If, however, cane-sugar be introduced into the alimentary canal beyond the capacity, say, for subsequent assimilation, sugar similarly passes off with the urine, but now in the form of grape-sugar instead of cane-sugar; and if this conversion is not effected in the alimentary canal, the liver must be the organ in which it occurs. Lehmann asserts that he has ascertained, as the result of repeated experiments, that when rabbits are fed with beet-root, which contains cane- and not grape-sugar, grape-sugar is to be found in the stomach and intestine, and no cane-sugar. Even when large quantities of cane-sugar were dissolved in water and injected into the stomach of rabbits, grape-sugar was the only kind of sugar which he could detect in the stomach and intestine. Similar results, Lehmann adds, were obtained in numerous experiments of a like nature, conducted by Von Becker, and it was only rarely that cane-sugar could be traced as far as the middle of the small intestine, even in those cases in which large quantities had been introduced into the stomachs of cats and rabbits. Since neither the saliva nor the gastric juice, he continues, is able to effect an immediate conversion of cane-sugar into grape-sugar, it only remains to be assumed, as suggested by Von Becker, that the transformation is produced by the action of the substances in a state of change which are always present in the alimentary canal.

There is nothing surprising in the convertibility, under these circumstances, of cane-sugar into grape-sugar, seeing with what facility the change is effected by chemical and other agencies. Boiling, for instance, with a little sulphuric acid, causes an immediate metamorphosis. Cane-sugar in the form of syrup, maintained long near the boiling-point, and without the aid of any chemical agent, undergoes partial conversion into grape-sugar. In the case of beet-root, also, I have noticed that grape-sugar has made its appearance simply as a result of keeping, and more strikingly so when it has been reduced to a pulp and mixed with a decomposable liquid like saliva, or even with water.

Grape-sugar $(C_{12}H_{12}O_{12}+2HO)$ $[C_6H_{12}O_6,H_2O]$.—Grape-sugar is met with extensively as a vegetable product in the juices of many fruits and other parts of plants, and is also readily obtainable from other carbohydrates by chemical means, and likewise by the metamorphosic influence of organic bodies in a state of change. It may, perhaps, be set down as representing the lowest, in a chemico-physiological point of view, of the *neutral* compounds of the carbohydrate group, as it constitutes that form into which they are all easily convertible, and into which they appear to have a tendency to descend. It may also be considered as having its elements in looser combination, as it yields to oxidizing influences which the others resist. Upon this depends the reaction which specially occurs in this form of sugar when in contact with the oxide of copper and some other metallic oxides, at a temperature of ebullition—a reaction which is turned to account for analytical purposes.

Grape-sugar may constitute a product arising in the animal system from the transformation of another form of carbohydrate—amyloid substance—to be presently referred to, which exists as a deposit in the liver and some other structures of the body.

It is a substance which requires no preliminary process of digestion to fit it for absorption, and it may be considered that the main part of that which is received into the alimentary canal passes without modification into the blood-vessels, by virtue of the physical property of diffusibility which it enjoys.

Grape-sugar, however, is readily convertible, by organic bodies in a state of change, into lactic acid, a principle in which the elements are combined in precisely the same relative proportion as in anhydrous grape-sugar, one atom of sugar corresponding with two atoms of the acid. Now, such bodies freely exist within the alimentary canal, and probably occasion a transformation of some of the ingested sugar into lactic acid— through what is styled, in fact, the lactic-acid fermentation. Lehmann comments upon the exceptionally acid condition of the contents of the stomach, and likewise of the intestine, after the introduction of sugar or starch in quantity into the alimentary canal. In the case of some experiments of my own on rabbits which had been fed exclusively on starch and sugar for a few days previous to being killed, I was struck with the remarkably acid state of the contents of the stomach. In some experiments, also, upon rats which had been for some days kept upon sugar only, I noticed a strongly sour smell on laying open the abdominal cavity directly after death.

It is known that in some cases of dyspepsia there is an undue presence of acid in the stomach. The secretion of the organ being of an acid nature, the condition in question might be ascribable to an inordinate discharge by the secreting structures, and such, it may be considered, is not unfrequently the case. There are grounds, however, for believing that the undue acidity is sometimes attributable to a development of acid from the contents of the stomach. When digestion is carried out in a natural way the tendency to ordinary decomposition and fermentation is held in check; but when the process is defectively performed, changes of an ordinary nature are allowed, to a greater or less extent, to proceed. Now, saccharine material in this way undergoing the lactic-acid fermentation, would suffice to account for the unnatural condition in question ; and, in accordance with the view expressed, it is noticeable that articles of food impregnated with sugar are particularly apt to give rise to acidity where a disposition to the derangement exists.

When saccharine matter is metamorphosed into lactic acid in the manner above referred to, the latter (it may be assumed) becomes absorbed, and subsequently undergoes, in the system, more or less complete oxidation, in the manner that will be pointed out as occurring with organic acids in general.

The sugar which is absorbed from the alimentary canal will be subsequently traced on in the system when I have gone through the list of carbohydrates. The fitting time will then have arrived for speaking of the assimilation and destination of the group taken altogether.

Lactine, *or sugar of milk* ($C_{12}H_{12}O_{12}$) [$C_{12}H_{24}O_{12}$, or $C_{12}H_{22}O_{11}$, H_2O].—This variety of sugar constitutes an animal product, and its only source is the milk of mammals. Very closely allied in its properties to grape-sugar, it appears to comport itself in precisely the same manner as this principle in the alimentary canal. Nothing, therefore, requires to be further said about it.

Inosite, *or muscle-sugar* ($C_{12}H_{12}O_{12}+4HO$) [$C_6H_{12}O_6$, $2H_2O$].—This is another animal carbo-hydrate. It was not long since discovered by Scherer amongst the constituents of the juice of flesh. According to Lehmann, it has hitherto been obtained from the flesh of the heart. With so limited a source it can have little or no significance in an alimentary point of view. Unlike grape-sugar, it does not reduce the cupro-potassic solution, nor does it undergo the vinous fermentation with yeast, but in the presence of caseine it becomes tranformed into lactic and butyric acids.

Amyloid substance ($C_{12}H_{12}O_{12}$, or $C_{12}H_{10}O_{10}+2HO$) [$C_6H_{12}O_6$, or C_6H_{10} O_5, H_2O].—This is also an animal product. It was discovered by Bernard as the material yielding the sugar obtainable from the liver, and was designated by him *glycogen*. Besides the liver, where it may occur largely, some other structures yield it. It has a much more extensive existence and distribution among the tissues in the fetal state than afterwards. It is also discoverable in the placenta.

One of its most noteworthy characters is the striking facility and rapidity with which it undergoes conversion into sugar under the influence of a ferment operating under appropriate conditions. This principle possesses an important bearing in relation to the assimilation of sugar, as will appear from what is shortly to be mentioned.

Gum ($C_{12}H_{11}O_{11}$) [$C_{12}H_{22}O_{11}$].—Gum, like starch, extensively pervades the vegetable kingdom. It is met with in the juices of nearly all plants, and occurs in its purest form as an exudation upon the bark of certain trees. With water it produces a tasteless, ropy, mucilaginous liquid, possessing strongly adhesive properties, which render it a useful article for various purposes. It is convertible into sugar by boiling with dilute sulphuric acid.

Gum is, doubtless, susceptible of being utilized as an alimentary principle, although nothing definite is known about what becomes of it when introduced into the alimentary canal. Although soluble, it is of very low diffusibility, and, belonging to the class of colloids, is, according to Graham, only two and a half times more dialyzable than albumen.

- Its properties, therefore, are such as to preclude its passage to any great extent, by absorption into the blood-vessels. We have no tangible evidence that, like starch, it undergoes conversion in the alimentary canal into sugar. In the first place, none of the secretions are found to possess the power of effecting the conversion, and, in the next, no sugar is discoverable in the alimentary canal after gum has been administered. I have experimented both upon rabbits and dogs with reference to this point. In rabbits, to which nothing else but gum in solution had been administered for a few days before death, no sugar was subsequently discoverable in either the stomach or intestine. After the administration of gum, also, in conjunction with animal food, to a dog, no trace of sugar was to be detected in the alimentary canal.

Lehmann, in one part of his "Physiological Chemistry," goes as far as to say that gum remains unabsorbed. Farther on he speaks of its absorption as being extremely limited, if, indeed, it occurs at all. There are considerations, however, which, I think, must be held as indirectly showing that, under some form or other, its elements, to some, if not to a large extent, reach the circulation.

The first consideration is this. Amyloid substance, which has been before referred to as forming a constituent of the liver, is evidently derivable from the absorbed products of the food, and under the absence of food it is noticeable that it entirely disappears from the organ. Now, when substances like starch and sugar have been exclusively administered, the liver is found to be charged with amyloid substance, and in a series of experiments which I some time ago conducted I observed, after the exclusive administration of gum, a similar existence of amyloid substance in the liver. It is true the amount present was not very large, but, nevertheless, there was a notable quantity to deal with.

The next consideration is that the carbohydrates, which are absorbable and convertible within the system into sugar, increase the sugar eliminated with the urine in cases of diabetes. To a patient suffering from this disease, and under very strict regimen and observation, gum was administered, and a distinct, although not a large, augmentation in the eliminated sugar was noticed.

Dextrine ($C_{12}H_{10}O_{10}$) [$C_6H_5O_5$].—Dextrine does not occur as a natural product, but constitutes an artificial gum, derivable from the transformation of starch, with which, in composition, it is identical. It is producible from starch by the action of heat, the mineral acids, and the ferment—diastase, which is developed during the process of fermentation. It has been suggested that it behaves in the alimentary canal like gum; but, being readily convertible, in the same manner as starch, by some of the digestive secretions into sugar, it is probable that, when it happens to be consumed, it is transformed into sugar, and in that state absorbs.

Cellulose ($C_{12}H_{10}O_{10}$) [$C_{12}H_{10}O_{10}$].—This constitutes the basis of the structure forming the walls of the cells, fibres, and vessels of plants. It is presented in a nearly pure form in cotton, linen, and elder pith. It offers strong resistance to solution, but yields, however, to the more powerful chemical agents. It is convertible first into dextrine, and then into sugar, by boiling with dilute sulphuric acid.

Closely allied to cellulose of the vegetable kingdom is a principle which was discovered by C. Schmidt in the outer tunic of some of the lower mollusca. It is known as *animal cellulose*, or *tunicine* ($C_{12}H_{10}O_{10}$) [$C_6H_5O_5$], and possesses significance from furnishing an instance in which a carbohydrate enters into the composition, if even it does not form the basis, of an animal texture.

From the resistance offered by cellulose to solvents, it can scarcely constitute an article of any decided alimentary value for the generality of animals. It seems, however, that in the case of the beaver a special aptitude exists for digesting this principle.

Lignine or woody fibre ($C_{12}H_{10}O_{10}$) [$C_6H_5O_5$].—Lignine forms the pervading solid matter which is deposited within the vegetable fibre, and gives to wood the property of hardness. It is of an exceedingly insoluble nature, and it is only in exceptional instances that it can do otherwise than escape the action of the digestive juices.

Lactic acid $(C_6H_6O_6)$ $[HC_6H_5O_6]$ and *acetic acid* $(C_4H_4O_4+HO)$ $[HC_4H_3O_4]$ also belong chemically to the group of carbohydrates according to the old formulæ, but in a physiological point of view they probably stand in quite a distinct position. They will be subsequently considered in connection with the next group of substances, which will be found to include other organic acids.

I now come to speak of the *assimilation and utilization of the carbohydrates.*

It has been stated that some conversion of saccharine matter into lactic acid may occur within the alimentary canal. It can scarcely be considered, however, that this transformation takes place to a sufficient extent to be deserving of much consideration as regards the question of utilization. It may be assumed that the lactic acid so produced becomes absorbed, and is subsequently mainly disposed of by undergoing oxidation within the system, as happens with the organic acids in general.

It is as saccharine matter that the carbohydrates, in the ordinary course, reach the circulation, and the saccharine matter thus derived is conveyed by the portal system of vessels to the liver, where it can be shown to be detained and subjected to metamorphosis—a process which may be regarded as forming its first step of assimilation.

That the saccharine matter is detained, as has been asserted, in the liver, is attested by the fact that if it should reach the general circulation it will immediately become recognizable in the urine.

Under natural circumstances, for instance, the urine, on being examined in the ordinary way, gives no reaction with the tests for sugar, although, it is true, when large quantities are operated upon, and evaporation and separation of the other ingredients effected, sugar, to a *minute* extent, is found to exist. On introducing sugar, however, into the general circulatory system, it is found to pass off with the urine, and to be more or less strongly recognizable by the ordinary mode of testing.

It used to be thought that sugar was capable of being oxidized on being conveyed by the blood through the lungs. Liebig suggested this view on theoretical grounds, and Bernard's experiments supported it. With regard to the theoretical proposition, it does not appear to me to demand consideration, and Bernard's experiments I have shown, in another place,* to have received a fallacious interpretation. There is no appreciably recognizable destruction of sugar, in fact, anywhere effected within the circulatory system; hence, sugar in any way reaching the general circulation will be carried in due course to the kidney, and by virtue of its property of diffusibility will escape with the urine.

Lehmann's experiments and my own are in accord upon this point. Lehmann, for instance, states that, without including previous experiments, he had recently injected grape-sugar into the jugular vein of thirty-seven rabbits and dogs, and in no single instance was grape-sugar absent from the urine. He further remarks that sugar passes so quickly into the urine that it may frequently be detected five minutes after its injection, and this even when only one-tenth of a gramme (1½ grain) has been injected.

If, then, sugar passes off in this way with the urine when introduced into the general circulation, and sugar is not similarly to be detected in the urine by ordinary examination under natural circumstances, it becomes

---

* Researches on Sugar Formation in the Liver, Philosophical Transactions, 1860.

evident that the sugar absorbed from the alimentary canal must be stopped on its transit before reaching so far.

Such is what occurs when ordinary circumstances exist; but if sugar be ingested in excessive quantity, and particularly after fasting, when absorption is at the height of its activity, sugar in notable amount is to be recognized in the urine. It may be here inferred that its rapidity of entrance exceeds, for the time, the capacity of the liver for detaining and assimilating it, and that thereby some passes through the organ and reaches the general circulation. In illustration of what has been mentioned, it may be stated that the urine has been observed to have been rendered temporarily saccharine in man by the ingestion of a considerable quantity of syrup the first thing in the morning, before any food had been taken. Also, in my experiments, where rabbits have been fed for a few days solely on starch and sugar, and dogs have had administered to them a large quantity of sugar with their animal food, sugar has been freely discoverable in the urine.

Not only have we this evidence to denote that sugar is naturally stopped on its passage through the liver, but the principle can be identified, as I will proceed to show, into which, on being detained, it is transformed.

I have already referred to amyloid substance as a material of the carbo-hydrate group which has been discovered to exist in the liver. It is a principle which possesses diametrically opposite physical properties to sugar, being a colloid, and therefore non-diffusible, instead of a crystalloid and diffusible. By micro-chemical examination it can be shown to be lodged in the hepatic cells, within which its non-diffusibility permits it to be retained for proceeding on, as it may be assumed to do, in the train of assimilative metamorphoses. Now, one of the sources of this amyloid substance is evidently saccharine matter—at least such, I think, will be conceded, on casting the eye through the following *résumé* of experimental results that I obtained, and published in the "Philosophical Transactions" for 1860. A very striking effect, it will be noticed, was produced through the medium of food on the condition of the liver, and it is to the amount of amyloid substance that it was attributable.

In the first place, an observation conducted upon eleven dogs, which had been restricted for some time to an animal diet, gives the state existing under an absence of the introduction of sugar with the food. The dogs were carefully weighed, and also the livers, and the figures furnished showed a relative weight of 1 to 30—the weight of the livers, in other words, amounted only to one-thirtieth of the body-weight.

A quantitative determination of the amyloid substance present was made in seven out of the eleven instances, and the mean amount given was 7.19 per cent.

To four other dogs animal food was given with an admixture of sugar, the quantity of sugar administered amounting to about a quarter of a pound daily. In these the results of weighing showed a remarkably increased relative weight of liver, the proportion being as 1 to 16½ of body-weight instead of as 1 to 30. The quantity of amyloid substance present amounted, as a mean for the four livers, to 14.5 per cent.

Five other dogs were kept for several days upon a purely vegetable diet, the food consisting of barley-meal and potatoes, or, where this was refused, of bread and potatoes. The weight of the livers was here found to amount to as much as one-fifteenth of the body-weight—exactly double the relative weight under purely animal food. In two of the instances no quantitative determination of the amyloid substance was made, but from the rough examination conducted it was evidently present in very large quantity. It was, in fact, these identical livers that first suggested the idea which led me to prosecute my subsequent inquiry. The three other livers were subjected to analysis, and the amyloid substance averaged the large amount of 17.23 per cent.

From these observations it appears that the ingestion of sugar and starch produces an augmentation of the size of the liver, due to an increase of the amyloid substance contained in it. The inference naturally to be drawn is that absorbed saccharine matter, on reaching the liver, is transformed by the assimilative action of the organ into amyloid substance, which is stored up in its cells for subsequent further change, preliminary to being appropriated to the purposes of life. That the saccharine matter derived from the food becomes thus transformed into amyloid substance is even more strongly exemplified by the results obtained in the following experiment performed upon rabbits.

A couple of full-grown rabbits were selected, which as closely as possible resembled each other in size and condition. To the one, starch and *grape*-sugar only were administered, and to the other, no food at all. The rabbit which had fasted was found to weigh 3 lbs. 1 oz., and its liver 1⅖ oz. The rabbit fed on starch and grape-sugar weighed 3 lbs. 4 oz., and its liver 2¼ oz., or just double the weight of the other. In the liver of the rabbit that had fasted there was practically no amyloid substance present, while the other contained 15.4 per cent.

Upon another occasion a couple of half-grown rabbits, also as closely as possible resembling each other in size and condition, were submitted to experiment. One was fed on starch and *cane*-sugar (cane-sugar being used this time instead of grape, as in the first experiment), and the other, as before, was kept fasting. The latter was found to weigh 1 lb. 14 oz., and its liver 1 oz., with no amyloid substance present. The former weighed 1 lb. 14¾ oz., and its liver 2⅜ oz., with amyloid substance present to the extent of 16.9 per cent.*

Nothing could be more simple than the conditions here dealt with, and nothing could more conclusively show that saccharine matter conduces to the production of amyloid substance. But, as has been seen, amyloid substance is also present in the liver when no saccharine matter has been supplied from without, as, for instance, in the case of an animal restricted to a purely animal diet. Under such circumstances it is probably derived from the metamorphosis of the complemental part to urea, which takes origin in the splitting up of the nitrogenous molecule. It has been, for example, already shown how the nitrogenous portion of food undergoes conversion into urea, which is eliminated, and a residue of carbon, hydrogen, and oxygen, which is retained for utilization in the system. Now, there is evidence producible which tends to show that the splitting up of the nitrogenous molecule occurs in the liver, and nothing is more probable than that the utilizable non-nitrogenous portion passes on in the same way as sugar into amyloid substance.

The view here enunciated receives support from the relation that has been observed by Dr. Sydney Ringer to exist between the urea and sugar eliminated in diabetes mellitus when either abstinence from food or restriction to a purely animal diet is enjoined. Under such circumstances

---

* Full details of the experiments upon this subject are to be found in the author's work, Researches on the Nature and Treatment of Diabetes, p. 89 et seq.

it was noticed that the urea and sugar rose and fell together in almost exactly the same ratio. Now, in diabetes mellitus it happens that there is a want of power to assimilate and make use of the carbohydrate group of principles, which occasions their escape, unutilized, with the urine; and, if the complemental part to urea of the nitrogenous molecule follows the same course in the system (and it has been suggested that it is converted in the liver into amyloid substance) as the carbohydrate, it is only natural to expect that where the defect in question exists it should pass off from the system in the same manner as a carbohydrate, and that thus, where there is only nitrogenous matter as a source for the eliminated sugar, this principle and urea—the other representative of the nitrogenous molecule—should bear a relation in amount to each other.

To amyloid substance, then, it may be considered that the carbohydrates can be followed. We now, however, reach a break in the chain of metamorphoses, and have to step over some missing links. But, if we cannot further trace the absorbed sugar in open view onward, and point out the particular changes it next undergoes, still we learn, in another way, that it leads on to the production of fat; and let us examine the grounds on which this statement is based.

A sharp controversy was carried on, some years back, between the German and the French schools, upon the point as to whether animals possess the power of forming fat. Liebig, on the one side, partly upon experimental evidence and partly by a train of reasoning, contended that in the animal system the carbohydrates were convertible into fat. Dumas and Boussingault, on the other hand, asserted that the food of animals contained preformed fat sufficient to account for that met with in the body, and thence that there was no need for a fat-forming capacity to exist.

This controversy gave rise to the performance of a number of experiments which have proved of considerable service to science, inasmuch as they have led to the matter in question being placed in a definitely settled position.

Huber's experiments on bees are the first that can be said to have afforded any substantial evidence bearing on the point. They go toward showing that from sugar the animal can produce wax, which is admitted to belong to the group of fats.

Grundlach subsequently repeated Huber's experiments, and obtained confirmatory results. Both these experimentalists, however, neglected to prove that the wax yielded during subsistence upon a saccharine diet had not been drawn from a pre-existing store in the body of the animal. Dumas and Milne-Edwards* conjointly undertook the performance of experiments to decide the point. They assigned to themselves the task of first of all determining the amount of wax existing in the bees at the commencement of the experiment, and then compared this with the wax formed into comb, and that remaining in the animals at the conclusion of the experiment. They started by restricting the animal to a diet of pure sugar, but failed in obtaining a satisfactory development of comb. They, therefore, abandoned experimenting with sugar, and substituted honey. Upon this they succeeded in getting, from one swarm out of four on which they experimented, a fair yield of wax. As the honey itself contains a minute portion of wax, this also required to be looked to as one of the items to be taken into account. It is not necessary to give here

---

* Annales de Chimie, tome xiv., p. 400. 1845.

the actual numerical results obtained. It will be sufficient to state that the amount of wax formed and the fatty matter existing in the animals at the conclusion of the experiment greatly exceeded the fat ingested with the honey and that pre-existing in the bees, a result which shows that a real *production* of wax took place. In the words of the experimentalists, the production of wax may be, therefore, said to constitute a true animal operation, and consequently the opinion entertained by the older naturalists, and by some modern chemists, among whom one of the experimentalists themselves (viz., Dumas) had previously found it necessary to range himself, must be set aside.

In the production of the *foie gras* a further proof is afforded of the formation of fatty matter within the animal system. The process of fattening geese for obtaining this article of luxury is carried on so extensively in Alsace as to form an important industrial employment in that locality. Strasburg constitutes the headquarters of the trade; and in Murray's "Handbook for Travellers on the Continent" we are told that the cellars of nearly every house in the town form the scene of *foie gras* production. Almost from time immemorial the goose has been turned to account in the manner under consideration. The Roman epicures, it is said, delighted in the enlarged liver of the goose as a delicacy at the table. In our own time the demand for the article is widely spread, and proportionately met.

The *modus operandi* for producing the fatty liver is described to be this: The geese, in a lean state to start with, are placed singly in wooden coops just large enough to admit them without allowing them to turn round. There is an opening in front for the head to project. Below stands a wooden trough, kept always full of water, in which fragments of wood charcoal are immersed, and a little salt introduced. Morning and evening, maize or Indian corn, previously soaked in water, is crammed down the bird's throat to repletion. During the day it "drinks and guzzles" in the water before it. In about a month the breathing becomes difficult, and then it is known to be necessary to kill the animal, otherwise death would occur spontaneously. The liver is now found to weigh from one to two pounds. The goose itself is fit for food for the table. On being roasted as much as from three to five pounds of fat, it is said, escape from it. The fattening process is carried on in cellars, or places where but little light is admitted, and the winter is the season selected. It is not in every case that it is successful. Some of the geese employed fail to turn out so as to allow the fattener's expectations to be realized.

Persoz,* a professor in the Faculty of Science of Strasburg, and therefore located in the midst of the operation, applied the advantage thus presented to account for investigating the question of the production of fatty matter from the carbohydrates.

It is known that maize, the article employed in fattening the geese, is charged to a greater extent with fatty matter than the generality of the cereal grains. Was this the secret of the phenomenon of *foie gras* production? Persoz undertook to determine whether the fat contained in the food sufficed to account for the accumulation of fat that occurred. Taking a number of geese, he killed one to begin with, and ascertained the amount of fat existing in the body. This served as the basis of comparison. The others were fed in the way usually adopted by the fattener, and were killed between the nineteenth and twenty-fourth days. Persoz

---

* Annales de Chimie, tome xiv., p. 408. 1845.

remarks that in his neighborhood expert fatteners assert that the process cannot be effected with profit if the goose is obliged to be killed before the eighteenth day or after the twenty-fourth. In fact, after a certain period the animal, it is stated, begins to lose instead of gain weight, and this period is known by the dejections assuming a lactescent character. An account was taken of the amount of food ingested, and the fat contained in it was estimated, and found to be altogether inadequate to explain the accumulation of fat which examination showed had taken place in the fattened animal. Persoz's results clearly convinced him that in the fattening process the goose forms a true laboratory or manufactory of fat from the starch and sugar in its food. The liver became five or six times larger than at the beginning, but the deposit in the liver occurs only as a part of a general process, fat being so accumulated as to cause the blood to assume a lactescent character, and also being correspondingly distributed through the various parts of the body. The blood, it was stated, was found to have undergone a further modification, namely, as regards its albuminous element, the serum failing to give the usual precipitate of albumen with heat and nitric acid.

Boussingault * repeated Persoz's experiments, and obtained confirmatory results. His investigations were conducted upon eleven geese, five of which were examined in the lean state, and the remaining six, after the process of fattening, which in his case was carried on for a period of thirty-one days. Boussingault estimated the fat contained in the dejections as well as in the food of the animals. This amounted to something considerable, and, therefore, correspondingly increased the amount of fat that had to be reckoned as formed within the system.

Boussingault likewise experimented, in a similar manner and with the same result, on ducks. When fed with 140 grammes (about 5 ounces) of maize *per diem*, a duck of rather over 2¼ pounds weight gained, he says, in fifteen days, 180 to 200 grammes (about 6¼ to 7 ounces) of fat.

He also tried if the same result could be obtained on substituting rice, in which fatty matter is at a minimum, for maize. In the case of two out of three ducks operated upon no marked increase of fat was observable. In the third, however, an increase appears to have occurred —assuming, that is, that the bird was not in reality fatter at the beginning of the experiment than it was estimated to be, which may be regarded as an open point.

Other ducks were fed on the same quantity of rice, to which some butter was added, and, Boussingault states, were rapidly raised to a degree of fatness truly remarkable.

A duck which had been fed only on butter died at the end of three weeks of starvation. Butter, it is said, exuded from all parts of the body, and the feathers seemed as if they had been soaked in melted butter.

It thus seems, from these observations on geese and ducks, that conclusive evidence is afforded that the carbohydrate element of food is susceptible of undergoing conversion into fat, but that, for this result to ensue, it must not be administered without a due accompaniment of the other alimentary principles.

It may here be mentioned that the practice has prevailed, it appears, in some parts of this country, of fattening fowls for the London market in a somewhat similar manner to the process resorted to with the Stras-

---

* Annales de Chimie, tome xiv., p. 401. 1845.

burg geese. Although in this case fat is added to the food, yet, doubt-less, the *modus operandi* is the same. Mavor * says: "They are put up in a dark place and crammed with a paste made of barley-meal, mutton suet, and some treacle or coarse sugar mixed with milk, and are found to be completely ripe in a fortnight. If kept longer the fever that is in-duced by this continued state of repletion renders them red and unsala-ble, and frequently kills them."

Boussingault † furthermore experimented upon pigs with reference to the point under consideration. Like in the case of his ducks fed with rice, he found that pigs would not fatten on potatoes only, as on food of a less exclusively farinaceous nature. After a time they ceased to make progress in growth, and it was estimated that the fatty matter already contained in the potatoes ingested sufficed to account for whatever fatty accumulation occurred. When, however, the pigs were fed on potatoes mixed with " wash "—a refuse liquid derived from the kitchen and dairy, and, therefore, containing nitrogenous and fatty matter—fattening was observed to ensue, and the fat which accumulated was found greatly to exceed that introduced from without with the food, and from which it was evident that a formation of fat within the system must have oc-curred.

Liebig adduces,‡ as giving support to his own view, some observa-tions of Boussingault on a milch cow, and expresses his astonishment that Boussingault, with the results that were before him, should oppose the opinion that the formation of fat occurs within the body.

It appears from these researches of Boussingault that a milch cow fed on potatoes and chopped straw upon one occasion, and on potatoes and hay upon another, gave out in the form of butter far more fatty matter than was contained in the food ingested. Nay, it even appears, accord-ing to Liebig's calculation, that the cow's egesta contained as much fatty matter (substances soluble in ether) as the ingesta, and therefore the whole of the butter of the milk, amounting in the latter observation to 6¼ pounds in six days, must be put down as having been derived from an internal pro-cess of formation.

Dr. Lyon Playfair § has likewise made investigations of a similar character, and with a like result. A cow, subjected to observation for several days, yielded about a pound, sometimes more, sometimes less, of butter *per diem* in excess of the fatty matter contained in the food.

Further, Messrs. Lawes and Gilbert, from their extensive and very searching investigations into the fattening of animals, have abundantly confirmed Liebig's view. They say, with reference to some experiments on the fattening of pigs, carried on for a period of eight and ten weeks,|| that " of the determined or estimated fat stored up in the increase, the proportion which could possibly have been derived from the ready formed fat of the food, even supposing the whole of that supplied had been assimilated, was so small as to leave no doubt whatever that a very large proportion of the stored-up fat must have been pro-duced from other constituents than the ready-formed fatty matter of the food."

---

* Agricultural Reports of Berkshire. By William Mavor, LL.D. 1813.
† Op. cit., p. 419. ‡ Animal Chemistry, 2d edition, p. 313.
§ Philosophical Magazine, vol. xxiii., p. 287. 1843.
|| Ibid., vol. xxxii., p. 448. 1866.

In the communication from which this extract has been taken they are discussing the question, not only as to whether a formation of fat can be shown to occur in the animal system, but whether it can be derived from both nitrogenous and non-nitrogenous matter; and the conclusion they arrive at from the evidence before them they sum up as follows:

" *First.*—That certainly a large proportion of the fat of the herbivora fattened for human food must be derived from other substances than fatty matter in the food.

" *Second.*—That when fattening animals are fed upon their most appropriate food much of their stored-up fat must be produced from the carbohydrates it supplies.

"*Third.*—That nitrogenous substances may also serve as a source of fat, more especially when it is in excess and the supply of available nonnitrogenous constituents is relatively defective."

In addition to this array of evidence, one more instance may be referred to, which affords a crowning proof, if such were wanted, of the truth of the view that has been advocated. MM. Lacaze-Duthiers and Riche * have shown that the fat which abounds in the larva of the cynips, an animal which is developed in the interior of the gall-nut, cannot possibly, from the composition of the nut, be directly derived from its food. In the starchy matter, however, existing around, the animal is supplied with material for its formation.

Nothing further, then, may be considered to be required to show that the carbohydrates conduce to the production of fat. From what has been already stated, however, it will be remembered that it is not when ingested alone that such production can take place. The process requires the co-operation of nitrogenous in conjunction with saline matter, and it is probably through the medium of the change excited by the metamorphosis of the former that the result is brought about. The researches that have been referred to have shown that on a diet of potatoes and of rice—alimentary articles containing but a small amount of nitrogenized matter—no accumulation of fat is to be looked for. The combination of fat with the carbohydrates, it has been seen, conduces to the accumulation of fat in the body, but this may be due to the direct appropriation of the fat ingested, and not to its having anything to do with promoting the metamorphosis of the carbo-hydrates.

Liebig has suggested the following as a representation of the chemical change that may occur. It can only be looked upon, however, as showing how, simply by the separation of carbonic acid and oxygen from the formula of a carbohydrate, the formula for fat may be left. There is no evidence that such is the actual manner in which the change occurs. Suppose, he says, that from one atom of starch ($C_{12}H_{10}O_{10}$) we take one atom of carbonic acid (CO_2) and seven atoms of oxygen, we have in the residue one of the empirical formulæ for fat, viz., $C_{11}H_{10}O$.

Without professing to be able (at present, at least) to bring forward anything in the shape of proof that the liver is the organ in which the metamorphosis of sugar, finally or almost so, into fat occurs, there are grounds for believing that such is the case, and that the formation of amyloid substance constitutes the preliminary step in the process. For some years I have been engaged in conducting researches upon this subject, and have a large mass of evidence to deal with, but it has not yet assumed a shape sufficiently definite to induce me to commit myself, at

* Annales des Sciences Natur. (Zoologie), 4me serie, tome xi., p. 81.

present, to any decided expression of opinion regarding the manner in which the final result is attained.

It now only remains for the ultimate use of the carbohydrates to be spoken of. In leading on to fat-production, nothing further need be said about their final application, the purposes subserved by fat having been fully gone into at an earlier part of this work. The question, however, confronts us, whether or not the carbohydrates contribute to force-production by undergoing direct oxidation in the system. That they do so we have nothing experimentally to show; and taking all that we know about them into account, my own opinion is that they do not.

Saccharine matter, in which form the carbohydrates are mainly, if not wholly, absorbed from the alimentary canal, is naturally detained and metamorphosed by the liver, and, whenever it happens, no matter in what way, to reach the general circulation, it is immediately drawn upon and eliminated from the system by the kidneys. This appears to me to afford a strong argument against oxidation of saccharine matter occurring, at least to any significant extent, within the circulatory system as one of the functional operations of life.

Without any facts to support it, the older chemico-physiologists believed that sugar was disposed of in this way. Mialhé, for instance, suggested that, under the influence of the alkali and oxygen of the blood, the sugar derived from the ingesta underwent oxidation, and that diabetes mellitus—a disease attended with the escape of sugar with the urine—was due to a defective oxidizing capacity, from the blood being deficient of its normal amount of alkali.

Lehmann has refuted, by direct experiment, this theoretical allegation, and has shown (as my own experiments corroborate) that sugar, introduced either with an alkali or without one (for the result is the same in the two cases), into the circulation, fails to undergo the alleged oxidation, as is evidenced by its subsequent appearance in the urine. Moreover, as regards non-oxidation from a deficient amount of alkali in the blood being the cause of the escape of sugar occurring in diabetes, this also rests only upon hypothesis, for Lehmann has found that analytical examination gives no evidence of the deficiency referred to in the amount of alkali belonging to the blood in the disease.

Whatever the series of changes undergone—whether oxidized after passing through the stage of fat or through any other line of metamorphosis—supposing complete oxidation to occur, it may be considered that the amount of force evolved will always be the same. Looking, therefore, at these compounds as force-producers, we must take them in their original state, and upon the amount of unoxidized oxidizable elementary matter they contain will depend their value in force-production.

In all of them, there being just the quantity of oxygen to represent the equivalent of the hydrogen in combination as water, their capacity for appropriating oxygen corresponds only with the carbon that is present. In fatty compounds, on the other hand, there exists a quantity of hydrogen, as well as carbon, free for oxidation; and thus these latter are of a correspondingly higher value as force-producers. Nitrogenous matter also, even although disposed of as it is within the system, where a portion of its oxidizable elementary matter escapes unconsumed under the form of urea, possesses a higher capacity for appropriating oxygen.

For further particulars concerning the application of the carbohydrates to force-production, the reader is referred to the discussion that has pre-

6

ceded under the heads of nitrogenous and fatty matters (*vide* pp. 50, 61). It will suffice to reinsert here a tabular representation of the relative value they possess.

	Amount of oxygen required to oxidize 100 parts as oxidation occurs within the body.	Units of heat produced by oxidation of 1 gramme (15.432 grs.) as oxidation occurs within the body (Frankland).
Grape-sugar, . .	106	3,277
Starch, . . .	120	3,912
Albumen, . .	150	4,263
Fat, ...	293	9,069

There are other ternary compounds consumed, which, if they do not hold the significant position as alimentary articles held by the principles already considered, are yet susceptible of oxidation within the system, and will thus contribute in some degree to force-generation, heat being probably the form of force to which they give rise.

In some of these compounds, such as pectine and the vegetable acids, the oxygen is in excess of that required to form water with the hydrogen.

Pectine forms the basis of vegetable jellies. It is met with in most fruits and many vegetables, but does not exist to an extent sufficiently large to be of much importance in an alimentary point of view. Fremy's old formula for pectine was $C_{32}H_{22}O_{22}$; under the new notation it is now given as follows: $C_{16}H_{10}O_{16},4H_2O$.

Organic acids, such as *citric acid* ($C_{12}H_5O_{11},3HO$) [$H_3C_6H_5O_7$], *tartaric acid* ($C_8H_4O_{10},2HO$) [$H_2C_4H_4O_6$], *malic acid* ($C_8H_4O_8,2HO$) [$H_2C_4H_4O_5$], and others of less extensive distribution, are met with in various vegetable juices. *Lactic acid* ($C_6H_5O_5$) [$HC_3H_5O_3$] and *acetic acid* ($C_4H_3O_3+HO$) [$HC_2H_3O_2$], although carbohydrates, appear to behave like the above-enumerated acids within the system.

Wöhler asserts, with regard to these principles, that when they are ingested in a free state they pass through the system and appear unchanged in the urine; whereas it is well known that when they are introduced in combination with alkalies—that is, as alkaline salts—they undergo oxidation, the alkali escaping with the urine in combination with carbonic acid. Within thirteen minutes after taking half an ounce of lactate of soda, Lehmann found that his urine had acquired an alkaline reaction from the presence of alkaline carbonate. Lehmann also found, in experiments on dogs, that the injection of lactate of soda into the jugular vein was followed in five, or at the most twelve minutes, by an alkaline behavior of the urine, showing, unlike what occurs with sugar, that the direct introduction into the general circulatory system is attended with the same result as introduction into the alimentary canal.

Alcohol ($C_4H_6O_2$) [C_2H_6O], looked at chemically, stands on the other side of the carbohydrates, and may be regarded as holding a position intermediate between the carbohydrates and the fats. From its composition, which is given above, it is seen to be a less oxygenated body than the carbohydrates, and more highly so than the fats.

There has been much discussion as regards the destination of alcohol in the animal economy. It was one of Liebig's propositions that it is consumed by oxidation like any other non-nitrogenous alimentary principle. "Alcohol," he says, "stands only second to fat as a respiratory material." Liebig, however, adduced no physiological evidence in support of his assertion, but based it as a generalization on chemical considerations.

That alcohol should occupy the position thus defined seemed so reasonable that Liebig's view originally met with general and unquestioned acceptance. A reaction, however, was started by the announcement of MM. Lallemand, Perrin, and Duroy, that alcohol escapes from the body in an unchanged state after being ingested. It was found, in observations both upon man and the dog, that when a moderate quantity of alcohol had been administered, it was recognizable in the pulmonary and cutaneous exhalations, and also in the urine for some hours afterward. Hence was supplied the ground for the denial that alcohol constituted a food; and in harmony therewith it was further found that it remained untransformed in the system, so as to be discoverable in the brain for a period, it is stated, of as many as thirty-six hours after its ingestion.

Dr. Edward Smith repeated these experiments of Lallemand and the others, and obtained similar results. The test that was employed consisted of one part of bichromate of potash dissolved in three hundred parts of strong, pure sulphuric acid. Chromic acid being liberated by this admixture, a cherry-red colored liquid is produced. This, in contact with alcohol, becomes changed to an emerald green from the reduction of the chromic acid to the oxide of chromium that ensues. Dr. Smith asserts that he has frequently detected alcohol in the breath for four hours after 1½ ounce had been taken. Lallemand showed its presence in the exhalation from the skin by confining a dog in a closed case, through which a current of air was made to pass and subsequently traverse the test. Dr. Smith enclosed a man's arm in an impermeable bag, and similarly, with a current of air passed through, readily obtained an indication of the escape of alcohol.

If the alcohol ingested escape from the body in an unaltered state, it cannot, of course, be looked upon as possessing any alimentary value. Dr. E. Smith sides with the French observers, whose experiments he has confirmed in taking this view. He considers that it does not increase the production of heat in the body as a chemical agent, but by the power it possesses of stimulating the activity of the vital functions. In his experiments on respiration he found that in every dose up to the usual one in taking spirits and water it increased, but only, he says, to a moderate degree, the amount of carbonic acid evolved, and this he ascribes to a similar cause.

Looking at the very large quantity of alcohol under the form of various beverages that is consumed amongst us, and consumed under the idea that it is an article capable of being turned to useful account in the system, the question before us becomes one of extensive interest and importance. Now, suppose it be conceded that evidence has been adduced sufficiently decisive to show that alcohol, after being ingested, escapes from the body through various channels; this would form all that it can be contended has been discovered. Neither of the persons whose observations have been referred to has collected the alcohol or done anything toward showing that what escapes is equivalent to that which enters.

Dr. Anstie * directs attention to the experiment of M. Baudot, and gives the results of a repetition, with modifications of his own, which throw doubt upon the soundness of the opinion of M. Lallemand and others. It is asserted that the chromic acid test is one of extreme delicacy, being affected by the presence of the minutest quantity of alcohol, and that it is only when an excessive quantity of alcohol has been administered that

---

* On Stimulants and Narcotics. Macmillan, 1864.

its escape is to be recognized by any other means. It is also contended that, through the delicacy of this test, the quantity escaping may easily be overrated—that although a reaction is distinctly obtainable with the test, in reality only a fraction of that which enters is eliminated, and, if such be the case, there is nothing to prevent us from regarding alcohol as having an alimentary value.

Considering the diffusible property which alcohol possesses, it is not inconsistent that a small portion should escape and yet that the article should form a utilizable agent in the body. It certainly may be reasonably considered that evidence of a stronger nature' than that which has been adduced should be brought forward before it would be right to look upon alcohol as devoid of alimentary value.

Dr. Parkes, in conjunction with Count Wollowicz, has recently * prosecuted an inquiry into the action of alcohol on the human body, and the question of elimination is touched upon as one of the points of consideration. Although they confirm previous observers in recognizing it, after its administration, by means of the chromic acid test, in the urine and the exhalations from the lungs and skin, and further find it to a slight extent in the alvine dejections, yet their observations were only of a qualitative nature, and did not enable them, they say, to solve the difficult problem as to whether all the alcohol passes off or whether some is retained and destroyed.

In a later communication on the action of claret wine † they state that they obtained a marked reaction with the chromic acid test from the condensed perspiration of the arm, when no alcoholic fluid had been taken for twenty-six days previously. They are, therefore, led to suggest that the perspiration may at times contain some non-alcoholic substance capable of exerting the same reducing action, and conclude that fresh experiments are necessary to determine the reliance to be placed on the test when applied to the condensed perspiration.

Communications have since been published in the "Proceedings of the Royal Society," ‡ giving the results of Dr. Dupré's experiments. Dr. Dupré agrees with Anstie and Thudichum in this country, and Schulinus and Baudot abroad, in believing that the chief portion of the alcohol ingested undergoes consumption in the body.

Dr. Dupré starts with the proposition that "obviously three results may follow the ingestion of alcohol. All the alcohol may be oxidized and none be eliminated, or a portion only may be oxidized and the rest be eliminated unaltered ; or, lastly, all may be eliminated again unaltered. Assuming the last to be the case, it would follow that if a certain quantity of alcohol were taken daily, the amount eliminated would increase from day to day, until at last the amount eliminated would equal the daily consumption, be this in five, ten, or more days. If, on the other hand, all the alcohol consumed is either oxidized or eliminated within twenty-four hours, no increase in the daily elimination would take place, in consequence of the continuance of the alcohol diet."

"Assuming, for the sake of argument, that all the alcohol is eliminated, and that such elimination takes ten days, it would follow," aptly observes Dr. Dupré, "that if a certain quantity of alcohol were taken daily,

---

* Proceedings of the Royal Society, No. 120. May, 1870.
† Ibid., No. 123. June, 1870.
‡ On the Elimination of Alcohol, by Dr. A. Dupré, Proc. Roy. Society, No. 131, p. 107, 1872, and No. 133, p. 268, 1872.

the amount eliminated would increase from day to day until, from the tenth day onward, the quantity eliminated daily would equal the daily consumption; in other words, the quantities which would be eliminated, if this theory were correct, might be measured by ounces instead of by grains, and even the most ordinary processes of analysis could not fail to yield considerable quantities of alcohol."

Now, from the results obtained in two series of experiments conducted upon himself, Dr. Dupré sums up as follows:

"The amount of alcohol eliminated per day does not increase with the continuance of the alcohol diet; therefore, all the alcohol consumed daily must of necessity be disposed of daily, and as it certainly is not eliminated within that time, it must be destroyed in the system."

"The elimination of alcohol following the ingestion of a dose, or doses, of alcohol, ceases in from nine to twenty-four hours after the last dose has been taken."

"The amount of alcohol eliminated, in both breath and urine, is a minute fraction only of the amount of alcohol taken."

In agreement with what had been noticed by Dr. Parkes and Count Wollowicz, Dr. Dupré found in the course of his experiments, that after six weeks of total abstinence from alcohol, and even in the case of a tee-totaller, a substance was eliminated in the urine, and perhaps also, it is stated, in the breath, which, though apparently not alcohol, gave all the reactions ordinarily used for the detection of traces of alcohol. "It passes over," Dr. Dupré says, "with the first portions of the distillate; it yields acetic acid on oxidation, gives the emerald-green reaction with the bichromate of potassium and strong sulphuric acid, yields iodoform, and its aqueous solution has a lower specific gravity and a higher vapor tension than pure water." Dr. Dupré further remarks that "the presence of a substance in human urine and the urine of various animals, which yields iodoform, but is not alcohol, had already been discovered by M. Lieben. The quantity present in urine is, however, so small that the precise nature of this substance has not as yet been determined."

Shortly after the publication of the first edition of this work, an article from the pen of Dr. Anstie appeared in the *Practitioner*,* entitled "Final [and the word final has received a melancholy expressiveness by Dr. Anstie's untimely death] Experiments on the Elimination of Alcohol from the Body." In harmony with what has preceded, evidence is there adduced which shows that only a fractional proportion of the alcohol in-gested is eliminated through the various channels of exit from the body. An experiment is related in which, after the administration of Bordeaux wine to six persons in sufficient quantity to produce intoxication, not more than one per cent. of the alcohol ingested could be recovered by dis-tillation from the collected samples of urine. In another experiment, af-ter the administration of brandy to the extent of one ounce daily for ten days to a dog, the animal was killed, and the alcohol obtained from its whole body determined. The quantity recoverable amounted only to about one-fourth of that contained in the dose which had been adminis-tered two hours previous to death. "These experiments," it is remarked by Dr. Anstie, "certainly furnish us with a final and conclusive demon-stration of the correctness of Dr. Dupré's arguments against the possi-bility of material *accumulation* of alcohol in the body."

From a review of the evidence as it at present stands, it may reason-

---

* Practitioner, p. 15. July, 1874.

ably be inferred that there is sufficient before us to justify the conclusion that the main portion of the alcohol ingested becomes destroyed within the system, and, if this be the case, it may be fairly assumed that the destruction is attended with oxidation and a corresponding liberation of force, unless, indeed, it should undergo metamorphosis into a principle to be temporarily retained, but nevertheless ultimately applied to force-production. The subject appears to me to be open to physiological as well as chemical investigation, and probably some additional light may be hereafter thrown upon it by an approach through the former channel.

THE INORGANIC ALIMENTARY PRINCIPLES.

Although it is to the play of changes taking place in organic matter that the manifestations of life are to be traced, yet organic matter alone, it has been found experimentally, will not suffice for supplying all that is wanting for the occurrence of living action. Inorganic matter, under the form of water and certain saline principles, constitutes an indispensable part of a living being, and hence must enter into the composition of food.

Water, besides fulfilling many other subsidiary offices, is essential for the occurrence of molecular change or mobility—the essence of the manifestations of life. In the absence of water a state of molecular rest, which means an absence of vital activity, prevails. Water does not in itself undergo any chemical alteration, and hence is not susceptible of liberating force—does not, in other words, constitute a force-producing agent; but it contributes to chemical change by supplying a necessary condition for its occurrence in other bodies.

Saline matter stands, if not to the full extent, nearly so, in the same position as water, as regards the non-possession in itself of force-producing properties. Some of the saline matter of food, it is true, may be susceptible of oxidation, and thereby give rise to the liberation of force, but this, it may be considered, is not the particular office which saline matter is designed to fulfil. It forms a necessary part of the organism, without, however, constituting the source of the manifestation of power. It exists intimately incorporated with the organic principles comprising the different component parts of the fabric, and enters as an essential element into the constitution of the secretions. It may be looked upon in the light of an integrant portion of the structure of the machine, other agents being concerned in supplying the moving power.

Mineral matter is thus required to be furnished for the growth and nutrition of the constituent parts of the organism, and also for the formation of the secretions. It is required by the plant as well as by the animal, and hence we find in all natural organic products a certain admixture of mineral matter. It hereby follows that whether the food be derived from the animal or vegetable kingdom, there exists, entering into its constitution, a definite proportion of mineral matter; and, just such as is required by the animal being has been drawn from the inorganic kingdom by the plant, whereby, without going further than the organic substance itself, the animal meets with the mineral matter that is needed.

Of the various saline principles necessary, the chief consist of combinations of lime, magnesia, potash, soda, and iron, with chlorine, phosphoric acid, carbonic acid, and, in smaller quantity, sulphuric acid. Each has its share of importance, but lime and phosphoric acid may be looked upon as occupying the highest position in this respect. From no structural element of the body is phosphate of lime, it would appear, absent, and its incorporation with the nitrogenous constituent principles is so intimate that much difficulty is experienced in effecting a complete separation without involving the destruction of the compound. Caseine is a nitrogenous principle which is conspicuous for the tenacity with which it holds a large quantity of phosphate of lime incorporated with it. From what is observed, indeed, in the relations of the organic and mineral principles to each other, it seems that in many instances an actual chemical union of the two exist.

On account of what has been mentioned, the chemist, in conducting an analysis for the determination of the mineral matter that is present in an organic product, subjects it to a preliminary process of incineration. After being thus treated, however, no knowledge is to be derived of the precise state or mode of arrangement under which the mineral matter originally existed. Even the mineral combinations found may not identically correspond with those present in the product, for in the process of incineration effects are produced which leads to new compounds being formed. There is the reducing influence of carbon, for instance, in operation upon the sulphate. There is also a production of carbonic acid from the oxidation of carbonaceous matter; and the saline principles, under the elevated temperature to which they are exposed, are likely to react to some extent upon each other.

That the various kinds of saline matter must fulfil a specific office in the economy of life may be looked upon as shown, if proof of it, indeed, were wanted, by the special manner in which it is distributed. Although so closely allied in their chemical properties, potash and soda cannot be made to replace each other in the living system, and the same is likewise noticeable in the case of lime and magnesia. In the process of vegetable alimentation a qualitative and quantitative selection is made by the organism from the soil around. Whilst in some plants one kind of mineral matter may preponderate, in others it may be another kind, and to such an extent may this preponderance reach as to have led to plants being characterized as potash plants, lime plants, siliceous plants; and so on. In the animal organism a like inequality of distribution is also observable. Thus, in the blood—and here the circumstances are of the most favorable nature for an equal distribution of saline matter, if a special appropriating action were not in operation—it is found that phosphates and potash salts predominate in the corpuscles, and chlorides and soda salts in the plasma around. Again, as regards the distribution of potash and soda, generally, it is noticeable that the former is the alkali belonging particularly to the formed tissues, the latter to the infiltrating fluids.

It is no mere indiscriminate diffusion of saline matter, therefore, that has to be dealt with. Saline matter, on the contrary, is evidently concerned as one of the factors of the formative operations carried on, and no food can satisfy the requirements of life that does not contain an appropriate amount of certain saline principles.

In the egg, and also in milk, we have articles provided by nature for the special purpose of being employed in the construction and subsequent maintenance of the animal organism. Milk is complete in itself. In it exists, besides the organic principles, all the inorganic matter, including both saline and water, that is needed. The egg, taken as a whole, stands in a similar position, but it is not so with regard to the contents exclusive of the shell. It is well known that from the egg all the constituent parts of the young animal are formed—its skeleton as well as its various soft textures. Now, for the construction of the skeleton an amount of earthy matter is required which does not exist preformed in the soft contents of the egg, but has to be drawn from the shell. During the process of incubation, with the co-operation of the atmospheric air which permeates the shell, it appears that the phosphorus present in the yolk gradually undergoes oxidation and becomes converted into phosphoric acid. This acts upon and dissolves the carbonate of lime belonging to the shell, which thus, as incubation proceeds, becomes thinner and thinner. As Liebig therefore remarks, if it be compared with milk, both the contents and the shell must be reckoned to bring them into an analogous position.

It has lately been urged by Liebig [*] that saline matter has failed to receive its due consideration as a nutritive element of food. It is perfectly true, as he has pointed out, that in the preparation of food for human consumption the natural article is often considerably depreciated in nutritive value by the abstraction that may happen to have occurred. Meat soaked or boiled in water loses more or less of its soluble portion, and, included in this, are its nutritive salts. Roasted meat, on this account, is of higher value than boiled. In the process of salting a portion (about 15 per cent., Liebig says) of the nutritive juice escapes into the brine. In the boiling of vegetable nutritive principles, and particularly the nutritive salts, are removed by the water. The separation that is effected in the dressing of flour leaves this product in an inferior position to the grain from which it is derived. Both the saline and nitrogenous matters belonging to wheat are chiefly encountered in the outer or tegumentary part of the grain, and are, therefore, more or less excluded from white bread. It is a scientific fact, Liebig remarks, which Magendie has proved by experiment, that a dog dies if fed on white bread, while its health does nor suffer at all if its food consist of brown bread, or bread made of unbolted flour. Liebig also asserts his belief that many millions more men could be daily fed in Germany if it were only possible to persuade the population of the advantage which bread made of unbolted flour has over that ordinarily eaten.

This doctrine, however, is hardly to be accepted in the precise terms that Liebig has proposed it. It must certainly be conceded that if our food consisted only of eggs, we should require, in order to satisfy the requirements of nutrition, to place ourselves in the same position as the developing chick, and consume the shell as well as its contents. Again, if corn formed our staple food, as it may happen to do in the case of the horse, etc., we should be obliged to consume the whole of the grain to obtain all the nutritive principles we require. It is a mixture of animal and vegetable food, however, which forms our natural diet, and the diet which is actually employed by the great majority of mankind. Now, if we are supplied with the nutritive salts through meat or the other articles consumed, we can spare them without detriment from our bread. Nor need there be waste involved in this proceeding. If our taste leads us to prefer bread made from white flour, and thereby to reject the outer part of the grain, it does not follow that in so doing we are committing an act of dietetic prodigality, for what we do not use ourselves may be, and in reality is, turned to account in feeding animals that are either kept to serve some useful purpose, or reared for consumption as food; and, in the latter case, the nutritive salts which we originally rejected in separating the bran from flour may actually reach us after all amongst the constituents of animal food.

---

[*] On the Nutritive Value of Different Sorts of Food, Lancet, vol. i. 1869.

ALIMENTARY SUBSTANCES.

ALIMENTARY substances comprise products of the animal and vegetable kingdoms in which the various alimentary principles are combined. It is to the consideration of these products that attention will now be directed; and first to be described will be those derived from the animal kingdom.

ANIMAL ALIMENTARY SUBSTANCES.

Animal food being identical in composition with the structures of the body, requires neither addition nor subtraction to enable it to administer to the purposes of nutrition:

The chief characteristic of animal food is the large amount of nitrogenous matter it contains. This, it is true, adapts it for the construction and maintenance of the body, but food is also required for force-production, and provided a certain amount of nitrogenous matter be supplied, the force-production is better derived from one or other of the forms of non-nitrogenous matter. Such may be effected by the presence of a certain quantity of fat with the nitrogenous matter, and with a proper combination the adjustment may be made from animal food alone, so as just to meet the requirements without incurring waste on either side. Hence the advantage of the common practice, which is doubtless due to something more than accident, of eating some kinds of food rich in fatty matter, as bacon or pork, with food such as chicken, rabbit, etc., which consists almost entirely of nitrogenous matter.

Animal food is comprised of: 1, the various parts of animals; 2, eggs; and 3, milk, with its derivatives—cream, butter, and cheese.

Honey is also enumerated by Payen amongst the articles belonging to animal food, but this substance is in reality a vegetable product, having only been collected and stored up by the animal to whose industry we owe it.

The food falling under the first head is popularly classified into meat, poultry, game, wild-fowl, fish, and shell-fish.

Like popular classifications in general, this will not bear close inspection; still, for the description about to be undertaken, it forms, upon the whole, the most convenient arrangement to follow.

MEAT.—The meats we ordinarily consume are all derived from vegetable feeders.* They consist of beef, mutton, veal, lamb, pork, bacon, and venison.

---

* The pig is, strictly speaking, an omnivorous animal, but reared for the purpose of food, it ought to be a vegetable feeder ; offal, however, is often given to it with other food.

Rabbit and hare may be conveniently considered with game. Turtle is employed for the preparation of soup. The flesh of a very large number of other animals than those yielding the meats above named is likewise eaten in various parts of the globe. A separate section will be hereafter devoted to this subject.

· The flesh, bones, internal or visceral organs, and even, as from the pig, the blood of the slaughtered animal, are all turned to account as food. They each require consideration. First, however, remarks will be made on the influence of age, sex, size, season, mode of life, nature of feeding, and mode of death, upon the flesh of animals.

The flesh of young animals is more tender than that of old, but experience shows that it is more resistant to the digestive powers. Veal and lamb, for instance, are found by the dyspeptic to tax the stomach more than beef and mutton. The flesh of an aged animal, as is well known, may be so tough as to be almost uneatable. The tissues of young animals are more gelatinous, less stimulating, and of less nutritive value than those of the adult and aged, which, instead, contain a larger amount of fibrine and of the flavoring principle, osmazome. The flesh of very young animals, indeed, contains so little fibrine and osmazome as to be almost unpleasantly soft, flabby, and insipid.

According to the information given me by an intelligent and experienced grazier, and evidently a connoisseur of meat, ox beef is in highest perfection at four years old. An ox that has been employed for working does not afford such good meat, and in grazing does not put on fat so evenly, or become so shapely, as one that has not been worked. Wether mutton is best at three years old; and in the case of both beef and mutton the meat of the female is in its prime rather earlier than that of the male. Ewe mutton undergoes deterioration by the occurrence of lambing.

Sex greatly influences the quality of the flesh, that of the female being more delicate and finely grained (the hen pheasant is very noticeably more tender and delicate eating than the male bird) than that of the entire male, which, during the time that the genital organs are in a state of functional activity, may be so coarse and rank as to render it almost uneatable. The buck, bull, and ram form examples. Castration deprives the meat of this strong flavor, and improves it altogether for edible purposes. Spaying also improves the edible qualities of the female animal. These operations, therefore, particularly that of castration, are commonly performed where the animals are destined to serve only as food. They are even practised in the case of the bird. The capon and poulard are examples; and it is well known that in this mutilated state the animal becomes larger, fatter, and more tender than where the sexual organs remain intact.

The flesh of an animal is generally coarse in proportion to its size. The difference in this respect in the flesh of the larger and smaller quadrupeds is sufficiently striking. The remark is applicable not only to different kinds of animals, but to different varieties of the same species.

In season and *out of season* are common expressions as applied to animals. Their meaning is well known, and they signify that there is a season when an animal is in a better state for consumption as food than at another. Beef and mutton are never actually out of season, but are most in season during autumn and the early part of winter, that is, just after the animal has been afforded the advantage of an abundant supply of fresh summer food. The precise period of highest perfection in flavor is just before removal from the green pasturage, viz., during the months of

·

September and October. There is a saying that the time for beef in its choicest state is whilst French beans are in. By stall-feeding on dry and artifical food, although the animal gains in fat, the meat loses in choiceness of flavor. Pork is absolutely out of season during the summer months. Buck venison is in highest season from the middle of June to the beginning of September, when the rutting period commences. Doe venison is in season during the winter. The season for young meats, as veal and lamb, is when a sufficient time has elapsed after the breeding period for the animal to have arrived at a state suitable for consumption as food. The breeding period varies somewhat in different breeds, and thus a supply of young meat may be secured for some length of time. By exposure to certain conditions, also, the period of heat in a female may be considerably advanced. In this way it is that lamb is procurable as an article of luxury for the table of the wealthy as early as December or even November. With sheep kept on a cold or poor hill pasture the lambing season is retarded.

The mode of life exerts its influence on the flesh of animals. In the wild state there is very much less fat present than in a well-fed domesticated state. In the former case the meat also is higher in color and richer in flavor and extractives.

Some kinds of food influence in a marked manner the character of the meat. Feeding oxen upon oil-cake communicates a yellow color to the fat. Oily foods also have a tendency to make soft fat. Turnips give a flavor to mutton which is distinctly recognizable by the epicure. The fragrant herbs belonging to different pastures produce their influence upon the taste of the meat. The peculiar flavor of mountain sheep is easily appreciable by all.

The art of feeding animals is directed to increasing the amount of fat: they are fattened, in other words, for the table. If this fattening process be carried only to a certrin point, the alimentary value of the meat is increased, but when carried to an extreme, as we see it in some of the animals exhibited at the Christmas Cattle Shows, the fat, as far as our requirements are concerned, is out of proportion to the nitrogenous matter, and thus an actual waste is incurred.

Violent exercise just previous to death gives increased tenderness to the flesh, hence the greater tenderness which is well known to belong to the flesh of the hunted animal.

In the process of slaughtering, the animal is drained as far as practicable of its blood. Either life is destroyed by the removal of blood, or the blood is allowed to escape immediately after resort to some other means of occasioning death. The loss of blood certainly involves a loss or waste of nutritive material. It would be thereby to be condemned if it did not possess counterbalancing advantages. Besides rendering the meat more pleasant to the eye, it enables it to keep longer, and improves the delicacy of its flavor. The Mosaic law is very strict regarding the killing of animals for food, and the regulations are such as to secure to the fullest extent the removal of the blood. Jews, as a point of religion, will not eat the flesh of any animal that has not been killed by a slaughterer of their own persuasion. They consider their meat superior to our own; and it is even eaten in preference by some Christians.

It is usual to keep an animal for a short time without food before being killed, and it is believed that the meat thereby keeps better. It is obvious, however, that the fasting must not be prolonged sufficiently to produce an unhealthy state.

To give additional whiteness to veal, which is looked upon as a desirable quality for it to possess, it was formerly a common custom to bleed the animal pretty freely a day or two before being killed. This practice appears now, however, to be almost if not entirely abandoned. Whatever may formerly have been the case, it does not appear that calves slaughtered for the London market are now ever treated in this way.

It is well known that meat is greatly improved in tenderness by being allowed to hang for some time after the animal is killed. Whilst the fibres are set by *rigor mortis*, it is much harder than before or afterward; and unless cooked before this state has supervened, which can but seldom be convenient, it should be allowed to remain until it has passed off, if not longer.

With these general remarks I will now speak in detail of the various kinds of meat and the other alimentary products derived from animals. The analyses given on the forthcoming pages, unless otherwise stated, are taken from a table contained in Dr. Letheby's work on Food.* It must be understood, however, that no fixed composition exists, and that the analyses furnished by other authorities may show figures that somewhat differ. The relative amount of fat and nitrogenous matter, for instance, varies considerably in samples of meat obtained from different animals.

The following is Ranke's analysis of cooked meat, the composition of which necessarily differs from that of fresh meat on account of the loss which occurs in cooking. For particulars regarding the loss under different modes of cooking, *vide* the section on the culinary preparation of food.

Composition of Cooked Meat (Roast), no Dripping being Lost— Boiled assumed to be the same (Ranke).

Nitrogenous matter, ...	27.6
Fat, ...	15.45·
Saline matter, ...	2.95
Water, ...	54.00
	100.00

Beef is of a firmer texture and more satisfying to the stomach than mutton. Rightly or wrongly, it is generally reputed as possessing also higher strengthening properties.

Composition of Lean Beef.

Nitrogenous matter, ...	19.3
Fat, ...	3.6
Saline matter, ...	5.1
Water, ...	72.0
	100.0

---

* On Food, p. 6. Longmans, 1870.

Composition of Fat Beef.

Nitrogenous matter, ...	14.8
Fat, ...	29.8
Saline matter, ...	4.4
Water, ...	51.0
	100.0

Mutton appears to be a meat more easy of digestion than beef. This is not appreciable by a healthy person, because the digestive power is in excess of what is required for the easy digestion of either when a proper amount only is consumed. In the dyspeptic, however, where a nice balance may exist between the digestive power possessed and that required—where, in other words, the digestive power is only just sufficient for what is wanted, the usual experience is that mutton taxes the stomach less than beef. There are many, for instance, who find that whilst mutton can be eaten without exciting discomfort, beef rests somewhat heavily upon the stomach if it do not even actually disagree.

Idiosyncrasies, however, exist for meat as well as for other kinds of food. Dr. Prout* records an instance of a person known to him on whom mutton acted as a poison. "He could not," says Prout, "eat mutton in any form. The peculiarity was supposed to be owing to caprice, and the mutton was repeatedly disguised and given unknown to the individual; but uniformly with the same result of producing violent vomiting or diarrhœa, and from the severity of the attacks, which were, in fact, those of a virulent poison, there can be little doubt that if the use of mutton had been persisted in, it would soon have destroyed the life of the individual."

Composition of Lean Mutton.

Nitrogenous matter, ...	18.3
Fat, ...	4.9
Saline matter, ...	4.8
Water, ...	72.0
	100.0

Composition of Fat Mutton.

Nitrogenous matter, ...	12.4
Fat, ...	31.1
Saline matter, ...	3.5
Water, ...	53.0
	100.0

Veal and lamb.—It has been already stated that these meats, although more tender, are more resistant to digestive action. They appear also to possess less strength-giving properties. It need scarcely be said that there is a deeply rooted belief that for sustaining the powers under great

---

* On the Nature and Treatment of Stomach and Urinary Diseases, 3d. ed., p. 30.

exertion these meats are not to be compared to beef and mutton. They are meats that it is desirable to avoid, generally speaking, in case of dyspepsia.

Composition of Veal.

Nitrogenous matter, .	16.5
Fat, .	15.8
Saline matter, .	4.7
Water, .	63.0
	100.0

Pork is of all meats the most difficult to digest. It is rich and trying to the stomach on account of the large quantity of fat it contains. The flesh of the wild hog is easier of digestion and not so fat as that of the domestic animal (Forsyth*). All fat meats contain a relatively smaller proportion of water than lean, on account of fat not being infiltrated with fluid to the same extent as the other tissues.

Composition of Fat Pork. ♦

Nitrogenous matter, .	9.8
Fat, .	48.9
Saline matter, .	2.3
Water, .	39.0
	100.0

Bacon.—Cured meats generally are less digestible than the same meat in the fresh state. Bacon, however, occupies an exceptional position in this respect. Its fat, certainly, is less likely to disagree with the stomach than the fat of pork. It contains but a small proportion of water, and, therefore, weight for weight, is an advantageous kind of food. It should not lose more than 10 to 15 per cent. in cooking (Letheby). Among the laboring classes it forms an almost universal article of diet. Its popular use, like that also of boiled pork with lean meats, such as veal, chicken, and rabbit, and also with other articles rich in nitrogenous matter, as eggs, beans, and peas, is founded upon a rational principle, serving, as it does, to establish a proper proportion in the supply of nitrogenous and carbonaceous material.

Composition of Dried Bacon.

Nitrogenous matter, .	8.8
Fat, .	73.3
Saline matter, .	2.9
Water, .	15.0
	100.0

---

* Dictionary of Diet. London, 1835.

Composition of Green Bacon.

Nitrogenous matter, ... 7.1
Fat, ... 66.8
Saline matter, ... 2.1
Water, ... 24.0
_____
100.0

Venison (the flesh of the deer only is here understood to be referred to) partakes more of the character of game than of butchers' meat. It is lean, dark colored, and savory. It constitutes one of the most digestible of meats, and would be, therefore, well suited for the dyspeptic and convalescent were it not for its rich and savory character.

Bone.—The relative amount of bone in animals varies according to their condition. Taking the whole animal, 20 per cent. may be allowed (Parkes). In lean animals it is in too large a relative proportion viewed in reference to economy. In the various joints "it is rarely less than 8 per cent. In the neck and brisket of beef it is about 10 per cent., and in shins and legs of beef it amounts to one-third, or even to half the total weight. The most economical parts are the round and thick flank, then the brisket and sticking-piece, and, lastly, the leg. In the case of mutton and pork, the leg is the most profitable, and then the shoulder" (Letheby).

Bones contain a considerable amount of nutritive matter, both nitrogenous and fatty. To extract it the bones should be broken up into small fragments and boiled for many hours. Dr. E. Smith says,* " When reporting to the Privy Council upon the dietary of the Lancashire operatives, I had special analyses made of the nutritive material which was extracted from bones, and the result showed that bones were equal in nutriment to about one-third of their weight of flesh in carbon, and one-seventh in nitrogen; and at the relative prices of bones and flesh, the use of the former rendered the dietary more economical." According to this statement, therefore, three pounds of bones represent the equivalent of one pound of meat in carbon; and seven pounds, one pound of meat in nitrogen. Gelatine, which forms the basis of soup, is the nitrogenous principle extracted by boiling from bones.

Blood.—The only animal from which the blood is saved and employed for dietetic purposes is, as a rule, the pig, but sometimes bullock's blood is also made use of. It is mixed with groats, fat, and spice, and sold under the name of " black pudding."

Liver.—The liver of the calf, lamb, and pig is largely consumed as human food. It is generally fried, and, thus prepared, forms a rich and savory dish. Its richness renders it an inappropriate food for a delicate stomach.

Composition of Calves' Liver (Payen).

Nitrogenous matter, ... 20.10
Fat, ... 5.58
Carbohydrate (amyloid matter), ... 0.45
Saline matter, ... 1.54
Water, ... 72.33
_____
100.00

* Report on Dietaries of Lunatics and Workhouses, p. 46.

The *foie gras* which is produced for the rich as an article of luxury is obtained by subjecting the goose to the process of feeding described at p. 77. The liver thereby becomes enormously enlarged and loaded with fat. Its highly fatty nature is shown by the following analysis:

Composition of Foie Gras (Payen).

Nitrogenous matter,.	13.75
Fat,.	54.57
Carbohydrate (amyloid matter),	6.40
Saline matter, .	2.58
Water, .	22.70
	100.00

Kidney.—The substance of the kidney is of a close, fleshy nature. It can never be looked upon as otherwise than an article of difficult digestibility, but as regards this quality a great deal depends upon the process of cooking. When lightly cooked it is soft, juicy, and agreeably sapid, but cooked for some time, and with the employment of a high temperature, it undergoes considerable contraction, and becomes hard, dry, comparatively tasteless, and exceedingly indigestible. The amount of fatty matter present is small.

Composition of Sheep's Kidneys (Payen).

Nitrogenous matter,	17.250
Fatty matter,.	2.125
Saline matter,	1.100
Non-azotized organic matter and loss, .	1.325
Water, .	78.200
	100.00

Heart.—The heart consists of fat and muscular tissue, like ordinary meat. The muscular tissue, however, is of a much closer texture, and this gives the greater hardness which is well known to belong to it both in the cooked and uncooked states. On account of this closeness of texture and hardness, it forms an indigestible article of food.

Tripe.—The tripe which is consumed as human food consists of the paunch or first portion of the ruminant stomach of the ox. This is the only instance of any part of the alimentary canal being applied to our own use, excepting in the case of the pig, where the chitterlings are cleansed and eaten. The muscular fibres belonging to tripe possess a different structure from those belonging to ordinary meat, and yield more readily to digestion. Tripe, indeed, is an easily digestible article of food, but the fat present renders it somewhat rich.

Composition of Tripe.

Nitrogenous matter, .	13.2
Fat, .	16.4
Saline matter,	2.4
Water, .	68.0
	100.0

Sweetbread embraces more than one organ. Stomach sweetbread and throat sweetbread are spoken of. The former constitutes the pancreas, the latter the thymus. Sweetbread is easy of digestion, and, when plainly cooked, forms a suitable food for the convalescent. When richly dressed, as it is usually served up at company dinners, it is neither suited for the dyspeptic nor invalid.

Lungs.—Pig's lights are eaten as a fry with the animal's liver. A food is prepared called " fagots," from bullock's and sheep's lights mixed with bullock's liver.

Spleen.—The milt of the bullock, sheep, and pig is sold for human food. It is usually stuffed and roasted.

UNWHOLESOME MEAT.—Meat cannot be subjected, like many alimentary articles, to adulteration or falsification, but it may be in an unwholesome state, and thereby unfit for food.

Good meat, according to Dr. Letheby,* has. the following characters:

" *First.*—It is neither of a pale pink color nor of a deep purple tint, for the former is a sign of disease, and the latter indicates that the animal has not been slaughtered, but has died with the blood in it, or has suffered from acute fever.

" *Second.*—It has a marbled appearance, from the ramifications of little veins of fat among the muscles.

" *Third.*—It should be firm and elastic to the touch, and should scarcely moisten the fingers, bad meat being wet, and sodden, and flabby, with the fat looking like jelly or wet parchment.

" *Fourth.*—It should have little or no odor, and the odor should not be disagreeable, for diseased meat has a sickly, cadaverous smell, and sometimes a smell of physic. This is very discoverable when the meat is chopped up and drenched with warm water.

"*Fifth.*—It should not shrink or waste much in cooking.

"*Sixth.*—It should not run to water or become very wet on standing for a day or so, but should, on the contrary, be dry upon the surface.

"*Seventh.*—When dried at a temperature of 212° or thereabouts, it should not lose more than 70 to 74 per cent. of its weight, whereas bad meat will often lose as much as 80 per cent."

To this it may be added, that there should be no sign of the presence of parasites. The fat also should neither be deficient nor excessive.

To assist in judging of the freshness of meat, a clean knife may be passed into it and applied to the nose on withdrawal. In this way the condition of the centre may be ascertained.

Unwholesomeness of meat may be due (1) to the condition of the animal previous to death, or (2) to the effects of decomposition afterward. Remarks will be offered under each of these heads:

1.· *Unwholesomeness of meat arising from the condition of the animal previous to death.*—The conditions productive of unwholesome meat, under this head, are:—

    a. The existence of parasites;

    b. Infectious diseases; and

    c. Contamination by some drug or other noxious agent administered or consumed during life.

---

* Lectures on Food, p. 235. 1870.

a.—Meat infested with parasites is known with absolute certainty to be liable to injuriously affect the consumer.

There is one form of parasite which is frequently met with, particularly in the flesh of the pig, here giving rise to what is known as " measly pork." It constitutes the *Cysticercus cellulosæ*, which consists of a little animal possessing a tapeworm-like head with a bladder-like tail, from which its name is derived. It lies in the flesh, surrounded by a cyst, which in the pig is about the size of a hemp-seed, and thus is easily seen. It appears to be widely spread amongst the pigs in Ireland, to the extent, it is stated,* of rendering at least 3 per cent. and probably 5 per cent. measly. The *cysticerci* of beef and veal are much smaller than those of pork, and require close inspection to discover them.

Now, when meat thus infested is eaten in the raw or imperfectly cooked state, it gives rise to the development of tapeworm in the alimentary canal. The *cysticerci*, unless they have been killed, as they can be by the meat being well cooked throughout, change their form when they reach the alimentary canal into that of tapeworms. The *cysticercus* of pig's flesh becomes the *Tænia solium*, and that of beef and veal the *Tænia medio-canellata*.

Far more serious effects are produced by meat infested with another parasite—the *Trichina spiralis*. This animal has been known and described for some years, but it has only recently been recognized as capable of exerting a mischievous action within the system. It was formerly noticed that the animal was occasionally come across, as it were accidentally, in the course of anatomical dissection, and it could not be learnt that there was anything to betray its existence in the individual during life. It was therefore looked upon as a harmless parasite, and rather simply in the light of a dissecting-room curiosity than anything else. In 1860, however, circumstances occurred which led to the discovery that this animal was not at all times the innocent or harmless guest that had been formerly supposed. Briefly stated, the circumstances that brought this to light were these:

A robust maid-servant, aged twenty-four, was admitted into the Dresden Hospital, January 12, 1860, under Prof. Zenker's care. She had been ailing since Christmas, and confined to bed since New Year's Day. Her symptoms presented some resemblance to typhoid fever, and, in the absence of other indications, were at first put down to this malady. Soon, however, a new train of symptoms became developed. The whole muscular system became the seat of great pain, which was much increased by the slightest movement. The patient was constantly moaning. •The arms and legs were drawn up, and could not be extended on account of the agony which the attempt induced. Inflammation of the lungs now supervened, and death occurred on the 27th. A *post-mortem* examination revealed the existence of vast numbers of *Trichinæ* in the muscles in the non-encysted state, and disclosed the cause of the patient's anomalous symptoms and death. Inquiry was now set on foot, and it was ascertained that, four days before the girl was first taken ill, two pigs and an ox had been slaughtered at the house of her master. Some smoked ham and sausage were fortunately obtained by Prof. Zenker, which had been derived from one of the pigs that had been killed, and an examination showed that the flesh was infested with *Trichinæ* in an encysted state.

---

*Prof. Gamgee's communication in the " Fifth Report of the Medical Officer to the Privy Council," 1863.

Since this case occurred others have been noticed, more particularly in Germany, in which the effects of the *Trichinæ* were recognized in their true light. In 1863 a catastrophe happened at Helstädt, in Prussia, which aroused universal attention, and excited a great deal of uneasiness in England as well as abroad. One hundred and three persons, mostly men in the prime of life, sat down to a festive dinner ordered at an hotel. Within a month more than twenty, it is stated, had died, and most of the others were suffering from the effects of the parasite. The result was traced to some smoked sausages, which had been made from a pig that had been noticed to be out of condition, and happened to be slaughtered for food by mistake. The *Trichinæ* were discovered in the muscles of those affected, and the sausages that remained, and the meat from which they had been prepared, were found to be swarming with the parasite. After this, people naturally became frightened to eat German sausages, and inspectors were appointed to examine the meat before being used.

The whole progress of the affection is now thoroughly known. When meat is eaten containing *Trichinæ*, if the heat employed in cooking be not sufficient to destroy the life of the animal, symptoms begin to show themselves in a few days' time. The first effect noticeable is irritation of the alimentary canal, manifested under the form of vomiting and diarrhœa. On reaching the stomach, the capsule in which the parasite is contained becomes dissolved. Thus liberated from its previously imprisoned condition, and finding in the intestine a favorable locality for its growth, the animal increases in size, and in two or three days attains three or four times its original dimensions. It may now be discerned by the naked eye, looking like a small piece of fine thread. The sexes are distinct, and the female gives rise to a large progeny—from three to five hundred, it is said—of little ones. These at once begin to migrate from the alimentary canal. They straightway pierce the walls of the intestine, pass through the peritoneal cavity, and spread themselves throughout the body. Now it is that febrile symptoms become established, and that they produce the terrible affection of the muscular system which forms so striking a feature of the sufferer's complaint. From the state induced, the strongest person may be carried off in the course of a few weeks' time. But should the patient survive the first effects of the parasite, a cyst is developed around it, and this, in the course of time, becomes calcareous. Thus imprisoned, the animal seems to be perfectly harmless, and, apparently, may remain for years without further betraying any evidence of its existence. It is only, indeed, on reaching the alimentary canal of another animal that it occasions any further mischief, and then occurs a repetition of what has been described.

Trichinæ have been discovered in the flesh of a variety of animals—birds, and frogs, as well as mammals; but the pig is the animal that is most frequently found to be infested. Whilst in a free state within the muscle they may be scarcely susceptible, or even unsusceptible of detection without the aid of a microscope. When first encysted, also, from the transparency of the cyst they are not easily seen, but when calcification of the cyst has occurred they are readily recognizable, and appear as white specks, or like little nits, lying amongst the muscular fibres. Within the cyst the minute thread-like worm lies coiled up after a spiral fashion; hence the qualifying adjunct (*spiralis*) applied to the generic name.

As a point of practical importance, it may be stated that neither salting, smoking, nor moderately heating, affords any security against the development of the trichinous disease from infested meat. Exposure, however, to the temperature of boiling water effectively kills the animal, but it is obvious that the temperature must be raised throughout every particle of the meat to ensure that it is rendered harmless.

Other parasites are encountered in the visceral organs of animals, but the *Cysticerci* and *Trichinæ* are the only ones, as far as is known, of a hurtful nature, in an alimentary point of view, that infest their *flesh*.

b. There are various diseases of an acute infectious nature and malignant type, such, particularly, as rinderpest, anthrax, and pleuro-pneumonia, to which animals are subject. Can the meat of animals that have been thus affected be eaten without producing injurious consequences? The idea of it is repulsive, and, strangely, the answer to the question cannot be given in such a manner as our preconceived notions would lead us to expect. The conflicting opinions of various persons on this point show the amount of uncertainty that exists with regard to it.

The diseases of live stock in relation to the public supply of meat for alimentary purposes, formed the subject of investigation by Professor Gamgee for the Fifth Report of the Medical Officer to the Privy Council, published in 1863. From the evidence before him, Professor Gamgee, unpleasant as it may sound, arrived at the conclusion that as much as one-fifth of the common meat of the country was then derived from animals killed in a state of disease. It is difficult to obtain complete and precise data on such a point, but whether the estimate be correct or not, it may be taken as showing that a large amount of diseased meat was consumed by the public. This, however, included all diseases, and it is positively known that some need not be regarded as depriving the meat of wholesomeness as food.

Animals killed in the early stage of the simple inflammatory affections may be safely eaten, and also, of course, those killed by or as the result of some accidental injury. But what is the evidence for and against the deleteriousness of meat when a contagious poison has existed in the system?

On the one hand, it is stated, as an authentic fact, that during the prevalence of the cattle plague, or *rinderpest*, in England in 1865, large quantities of the meat of animals killed in all stages of the disease were eaten without being followed by any ill effect. The same absence of ill effect is also stated to have been observed after the consumption of meat derived from animals affected with anthrax and epidemic pleuro-pneumonia—other virulent contagious diseases. It is even asserted that when the *steppe murrain* was prevalent in Bohemia some years ago, the carcases of infected animals that had been killed and buried by order of the Government were dug up and eaten by the poor without any injury being sustained.

On the other hand, instances have been placed on record where the most serious consequences have arisen from the employment of meat of this kind. A marked case in point is cited by Mr. Simon in his report to the Privy Council above alluded to.* He adduces it as conclusively showing that under some circumstances human life may be endangered by the use of cooked meat derived from an animal affected with anthrax, and states that the account of it was communicated to him by Mr. Keith, Senior Surgeon to the Aberdeen Royal Infirmary. Subjoined are the main particulars.

---

* Fifth Report of the Medical Officer to the Privy Council, p. 28. 1863.

During the first week of November, 1840, a two-year-old heifer, at a farm in Aberdeenshire, was observed to be unwell, and was slaughtered by the ploughman, aided by a neighboring blacksmith. A portion of the animal was salted down, and another appropriated to immediate use. A piece of the latter, which appeared quite fresh, and about which there was nothing wrong to be seen, was cooked next day in a pot of broth for the dinner of the family, which consisted of eleven persons. Of the eleven, two did not partake of it, and these remained well, whilst the nine who did partake of it were soon seized with such alarming symptoms of poisoning that a medical man was at once called in. Two died and the others recovered. On the 12th of November both the ploughman and the blacksmith were admitted into the Aberdeen Royal Infirmary, suffering from phlegmonous erysipelas of the arm. The offal of the animal was cast upon a dung-heap, to which two swine had access. They ate it freely, and were both taken ill and died.

The data in this case stand quite complete, the ill effects having been traced to the infected animal. More frequently it is only the ill effects that are observed, without information being procurable regarding the animal from which the meat was derived. For example, instances have been from time to time noticed, and some few have been placed on record, where a number of persons have suffered from symptoms of irritant poisoning after partaking of meat that has been purchased in a casual way, meat, it may be, that has presented no visible signs of unwholesomeness. Pork is known to be more likely to produce such ill effects than other kinds of meat, but perhaps something in this case may be due to the unwholesome food on which the animals are often fed.

It has been suggested that the prevalence of boils and carbuncles may be sometimes attributable to the unconscious consumption of meat from diseased animals, and some statistics have been adduced in support of this view. The flesh of animals affected with a certain disorder is specifically stated to have the effect of producing carbuncles. Dr. (now Sir Robert) Christison asserts * that the solids and fluids of animals suffering from a gangrenous carbuncular disorder, denominated *Milzbrand* in Germany, and analogous to the *Pustule maligne* of the French, are rendered so poisonous, that not only those who handle but those who eat the flesh are apt to suffer severely—the affection thus produced in man being sometimes ordinary inflammation of the alimentary canal, but most commonly an eruption of one or more large carbuncles, resembling those of the original disease of the animal. Dr. Livingstone, in his "Missionary Travels and Researches in South Africa," p. 136, 1857, speaks of the occurrence of malignant carbuncle, called *Knatsi* or *Selonda*, as a result of eating the flesh of diseased animals.

Looking, therefore, at the evidence before us regarding the effects of consuming meat derived from animals suffering from infectious disease, it appears that diametrically opposite results have been observed. It may be concluded that some kind of subtle poison exists, and that this may become neutralized or destroyed by the process of cooking and digestion, but why such an event should occur in some cases and not in others, is indeed difficult to understand. Practically, however, seeing that serious consequences *may* ensue, it is only right to look upon all such meat as unsafe and unfit for human food.

---

* On Poisons, p. 633. Edinburgh, 1845.

c. Meat may be rendered unwholesome by contamination with some drug or noxious agent administered or consumed during life. Many examples of this have been known. The following is a striking one, bearing on contamination by a drug administered as a remedial agent previous to slaughtering. It is quoted by Professor Gamgee and related by Dr. Kreutzer in the *Central Zeitung für die gesammte Veterinärmedizin für* 1854. "Three hundred and one persons partook of the flesh of an ox that had been treated during life with the potassio-tartrate of antimony. Of these, one hundred and seven suffered from violent vomiting, purging, etc., and mothers that were suckling children noticed violent effects on their babies. One of the affected persons died, and the cause of the attack was demonstrated by chemical analysis of the flesh, and of the contents of the stomach and intestine of the person that succumbed. This person had eaten only half a pound of the meat. Pigs, dogs, and cats that partook of the meat also suffered. Some of the meat was given to a magpie and it died."

The flesh of cattle is sometimes rendered poisonous by the food consumed, without the animals themselves being affected. For instance, it is known that cattle fed in some of the districts of North America cannot be eaten without giving rise to violent symptoms of poisoning. The flesh of hares, also, which have fed upon the *Rhododendron chrysanthemum* is considered to be poisonous.

2. *Unwholesomeness of meat arising from decomposition.*—Dr. Christison says: "the tendency of putrefaction to impart deleterious qualities to animal matters originally wholesome has long been known, and is quite unequivocal. To those who are not accustomed to the use of tainted meat, the mere commencement of decay is sufficient to render meat insupportable and noxious. Game, only decayed enough to please the palate of the epicure, has caused severe cholera in persons not accustomed to eat it in that state."* It cannot be said, however, that even putrid meat is poisonous to all, although it may prove so to many. The effect of habit would appear to confer some sort of immunity, judging from the accounts that are given of the state in which meat is eaten in some countries. "The American Indians," says Wilkes, "all prefer their meat putrid, and frequently keep it until it smells so strong as to be disgusting. Parts of the salmon they bury underground for two or three months to putrefy, and the more it is decayed the greater delicacy they consider it."† Simmonds also states, with reference to the food of the Greenlanders, that "the head and fins of the seal are preserved under the grass in summer, and in winter the whole seal is frequently buried in the snow. The flesh, half frozen, half putrid, in which state the Greenlanders term it mikiak, is eaten with the keenest appetite."‡ Rotten fish, we are also told, is used by the Burmese, Siamese, and Chinese as a sort of condiment, without any bad effect being produced.

Cooking doubtless neutralizes, to some extent, the effect of decomposition; and the secretion of the stomach (gastric juice), with the strongly antiseptic properties it possesses, will tend to prevent any further advance of ordinary decomposition as soon as the food reaches the stomach. Notwithstanding these salutary influences, however, experience shows

---

* On Poisons, p. 635. Edinburgh, 1845.
† U. S. Exploring Expedition, vol. iv., p. 452.
‡ Curiosities of Food, p. 32. 1859.

that the resisting power enjoyed by those accustomed to our mode of life is not sufficient to allow meat tainted with decomposition to be consumed without incurring a risk of more or less severe gastro-intestinal derangement, if nothing more, being set up.

In addition to meat being rendered unwholesome by ordinary putrefaction, it sometimes becomes so from undergoing, during the process of curing, another kind of decomposition. Meat rendered noxious by this modified and peculiar form of decomposition may present no marked external signs of being unwholesome, and thus is produced a very serious source of danger. The change has been especially found to occur in the sausages cured by drying and smoking in Germany, and many fatal results have been occasioned therefrom. Bacon, cheese, and other kinds of animal food have been also noticed in a similar manner to become deleterious. The nature of the poisonous principle is not precisely known, but it is generally believed to consist of an acrid fatty acid. The symptoms produced are those of severe gastro-intestinal irritation, followed by nervous depression and collapse. Dr. Christison's work on "Poisons" contains a collection of particulars bearing on this matter.

POULTRY, GAME, AND WILD-FOWL.—Next to mammals, birds are of the most importance to us in an alimentary point of view. As far as is known, there is no bird, and no part of any bird, nor any bird's egg, which may not be safely used as food. It must be stated, however, that some birds are rendered poisonous by the food which they have eaten. The pheasant, for instance, which feeds on the buds of the *Calmia latifolia* in North America, is deemed poisonous during the winter and spring. It is also well known that the American partridges sent over here have been sometimes found to possess poisonous properties.

The flesh of birds differs from that of mammals in never being marbled or having fat mixed with the muscular fibres.

Domesticated or tame birds, such as the common fowl, turkey, guinea-fowl, duck, and goose, fall under the denomination of poultry. Under the head of game a limited number of wild birds are included, and particularly the pheasant, partridge, and grouse. Wild-fowl comprise untamed aquatic birds. There are many other edible birds, including especially the smaller ones, which cannot be grouped under either of these heads.

The flesh belonging to different birds presents considerable variation —in some being white, and in others quite dark-colored. It also varies in different parts of the same animal, that on the wings and breast being whiter, drier, and of a more delicate taste than that on the legs. On account of the legs being higher flavored, they are preferred by many. In the blackcock the layer of muscles forming the outer part of the breast is of a dark brown color, whilst the deeper part is white. To a less extent a similar difference is also observed in many other birds.

The fowl, turkey, and guinea-fowl amongst poultry, which form white-fleshed birds, stand in a very different position from ducks and geese. The flesh of the former is delicate-flavored, tender, and easy of digestion. It also possesses less stimulating properties than ordinary meat, and is thus well adapted for the delicate stomach of the dyspeptic and invalid. The flesh of the latter, on the other hand, is harder, richer, or stronger tasted, and far more difficult of digestion. It is therefore to be avoided where weakness of stomach exists.

The fattening of poultry for the table forms in some parts of the country an extensive branch of industry, and the improvement that is effected in the quality, equally as regards tenderness and flavor as size, of the bird is exceedingly striking. Exercise is unfavorable to fatty deposit, and wild birds, unless it should happen that they keep at rest, are not likely to become fat. Domesticated birds, also, that are allowed to run about do not become fat to the same extent as those confined at rest. The art of fattening consists in keeping the animal at rest, and supplying it with an abundance of an appropriate fattening food, and it is subjected to this process for a few weeks before it is required. It is found that the animal in a sexless state grows to a larger size, fattens better, is more tender eating, and finer flavored than one in which the sexual organs exist (*vide* p. 90). Improvement for the use of the table is thus effected by castration and spaying. For the proper effect it is necessary that the operation should be performed at an early age. The capon and poulard are the result, and their superior qualities are well known.

The flesh of game contains a smaller amount of fat than that of poultry, and is regarded as possessing more strengthening properties. It is also tender and easy of digestion, and possesses a marked but delicate flavor, which increases by keeping. The aromatic bitter taste, for instance, of the grouse is more pronounced after the bird has been hung a little time than when eaten in a fresh state. The flesh about the back possesses this flavor in a higher degree than that elsewhere, and hence this part is often selected as a *bonne bouche* by epicures. Each kind of bird has its special flavor, and thus considerable variety is presented. The flavor of the partridge and quail is exceedingly delicate, and so also is that of the snipe and woodcock, but these latter birds are richer. From the qualities possessed by it, game is tempting to the appetite of the invalid. Its easy digestibility renders it further well suited for a weak stomach. It therefore forms a valuable article of food for the sick room, and is often found to be better borne than poultry or meat. It may, however, prove too rich; and to obviate this, as far as possible, the bird should be kept long enough to secure tenderness, and the breast only should be eaten.

Wild-fowl requires strong digestive power to dispose of it. Its flesh is close and firm. Its taste also is strong, and often of a fishy nature—a character which becomes more pronounced by keeping, so that the bird is at its best when in a fresh state for eating.

The pigeon and many other birds are eaten which do not fall under the head of either poultry, game, or wild-fowl. The flesh is usually tender in proportion to the smallness of the animal.

The flesh of the rabbit and the hare more resembles that of poultry and game than butcher's meat. It is characterized in each case by the small quantity of fat it contains. That of the hare possesses to a marked extent savory and stimulating properties, of which the flesh of the rabbit is comparatively void. So far the rabbit would form suitable food for a delicate stomach; but, although tender, its fibres are close, and it cannot be regarded as possessing the digestibility belonging to many other kinds of animal food.

FISH.—Fish is an important article of nourishment. A very large number of different kinds of it, both fresh water and salt water, are consumed, giving great variety to this kind of food. The amount that must exist in the vast waters of the ocean may also be regarded as rendering the supply inexhaustible. In some places it constitutes by necessity the chief or sole sustenance of the people, who are hence styled *Ichthyophagi*. The inhabitants of the most northern parts of Europe, Asia, and America, where it is too cold for any of the higher forms of vegetation to grow, are mainly dependent upon food of which the chief portion consists of fish derived from the sea. In Siberia, fish after being dried, is ground into powder, and formed into a substance which is used instead of bread. Putrid fish, we are told, is even the favorite and ordinary food of some tribes.

Although from time immemorial fish has formed an article of food more or less consumed by most people, yet many prejudices used to exist with regard to it. The Egyptian priests were forbidden to eat fish of any kind, under the idea that it increased the sexual appetite, or that it was the cause of leprosy. For the latter reason the people also were forbidden to eat fish not covered with scales. In the writings of Moses it is stated: " Whatsoever hath fins and scales in the waters, in the seas, and the rivers, them shall ye eat. . . . Whatsoever hath no fins or scales in the waters, that shall be an abomination unto you." * Rightly or wrongly, English history says that Henry I. got a surfeit, and died from eating too heartily of lampreys, a food against which he had been often cautioned. There does not appear to be any substantial foundation, however, for the belief that formerly prevailed; for the lamprey and the sturgeon also—another fish without scales—are now extensively eaten by some communities without any bad effects.

If present experience does not permit any basis of selection being given, it does show that fish is not invariably free from poisonous properties. It is especially in tropical climates where poisonous fish are encountered. Some are poisonous at all times, others only at certain seasons. Individuals of certain species may be poisonous, whilst others of the same species, that are not to be distinguished by any external characters, are free, it is stated, from deleterious properties—a circumstance which renders the eating of fish in such countries not without danger. Some persons, it is also said, escape, whilst others are injuriously affected. The symptoms produced† are sometimes allied to those of cholera. Sometimes an eruption, often resembling nettle-rash, is occasioned, and, it may be, various nervous disorders, as trembling or convulsive twitches of the limbs, paralysis, and stupor.

It is not definitely known to what the deleterious effects of the poisonous fish are to be ascribed. They have been variously referred to the aliment on which the animals have fed, to their being in a diseased state, to decomposition, and to idiosyncrasy on the part of the person affected. A fish is said to justify suspicion " if it has attained an unusually large size, or is destitute of the natural fishy smell, or has black teeth, or if silver or an onion boiled along with it becomes black; but all these tests are unreliable."

As an article of nourishment, fish does not possess the satisfying and stimulating properties that belong to the flesh of quadrupeds and birds. Still the health and vigor of the inhabitants of fishing towns, where fish may form the only kind of animal food consumed, show that it is capable of contributing, in an effective manner, to the maintenance of the body under active conditions of life. On account of its being less satisfying than meat, the appetite returns at shorter intervals, and a larger quantity. is required to be consumed.

---

* Leviticus xi. 9–12.　　　　† Pereira on Food and Diet, p. 284. 1843.

Dr. Davy says: "If we give our attention to classed people—classed as to the quality of food they principally subsist on—we shall find that the ichthyophagous class are especially strong, healthy, and prolific. In no other class than in that of fishers do we see larger families, handsomer women, or more robust and active men." *

As a less stimulating article of food than meat, fish possesses valuable properties in a therapeutic point of view, and is constantly being advantageously employed when the powers are too weak for the stronger kinds of animal food to be borne.

The flesh of some fish is white, and that of others more or less red. The former is less stimulating and lighter to the stomach or more easy of digestion than the latter.

Amongst the fish having white flesh are the whiting, haddock, cod, sole, turbot, brill, plaice, flounder, etc. The flesh contains but little fat, as the following analysis will show. The fat existing in the animal is especially accumulated in the liver, and in the cod-fish, particularly when in season, the liver is enormously gorged with oil.

Composition of White Fish.

Nitrogenous matter,	18.1
Fat,	2.9
Saline matter,	1.0
Water,	78.0
	100.0

The flesh of the salmon, particularly, presents a strong contrast in color to that of the fish above enumerated. It approaches meat in redness, and is regarded as approaching it also more closely than other fish in sustaining properties. Fatty matter is incorporated with the muscular fibres, and there is also a layer of superficial fat beneath the skin. This is more abundant in the abdominal or thinner than in the dorsal or thicker part of the animal—hence the richer flavor, and thereby the preference given to the former for eating.

Composition of Salmon.

Nitrogenous matter,	16.1
Fat,	5.5
Saline matter,	1.4
Water,	77.0
	100.0

The mackerel, eel, herring, sprat, and pilchard are other fish characterized by the presence of fatty matter incorporated with the flesh. Thus it is that these fish are richer and less suited to a delicate stomach than the white fish. The eel especially is rich in fat, as is shown by the following analysis from Letheby's table:

---

* The Angler and His Friend, by John Davy, M.D., F.R.S., p. 114. London, 1855.

Composition of Eels.

Nitrogenous matter,	. . . .	9.9
Fat,	. . . .	13.8
Saline matter,	. . . .	1.3
Water,	. . . .	75.0

100.0

Payen's analysis gives a still considerably larger quantity of fat, thus:

Composition of Eels Deprived of the Non-edible Portions (Payen).

Nitrogenous matter,	. . . . .	13.00
Fatty matter,	. . . .	23.86
Mineral matter,	. . . . . .	0.77
Non-nitrogenous matter and loss,	. . . .	0.30
Water,	. . . .	62.07

100.00

Of all fish the whiting may be regarded as the most delicate, tender, easy of digestion, and least likely to disagree with a weak stomach. It is sometimes styled the chicken of the fish tride. The haddock is somewhat closely allied but has a firmer texture, and is inferior in flavor and digestibility. The sole is a tender and digestible fish. It also has a delicate flavor, and deservedly enjoys a high reputation as an article of food for the invalid. The flounder is light and easy of digestion, but insipid. In all cases where fish is required for a weak stomach, either boiling or broiling should constitute the process of cooking. Frying is objectionable on account of the fatty matter used rendering the fish rich and more indigestible.

The cod-fish is far from possessing the digestibility that is enjoyed by most other white fish. It varies in quality a great deal, but some of it is exceedingly hard, tough, stringy or woolly, and indigestible. I believe it to be a more trying article of food to the stomach than is generally credited. When reputed to be in good condition, or in season, the flesh, which is arranged in flakes, becomes opaque on boiling. The juice between the flakes also undergoes alteration, and produces a layer of white curdy matter, apparently consisting of coagulated albumen. When out of season, this white curdy matter is absent, and the flesh remains, after being boiled, semi-transparent and bluish. In this state it is evidently not so nourishing, but being more watery and soft, I believe it is more easy of digestion. Indeed, some few instances have fallen under my notice where eating what would be called cod-fish in a state of high perfection—that is, cod-fish in a firm, flaky, and opaque state after being boiled—has been followed by an attack of indigestion.

Crimping increases the firmness of the flesh, and is often employed in the case of cod-fish. It must be effected whilst the muscular fibres retain their vitality, or before *rigor mortis* has set in. The fish when caught is struck on the head, and afterward a number of transverse incisions are made. It is then immersed in cold water, which occasions a strong contraction of the muscular fibres, and causes the flesh to assume a firmer state than would otherwise be the case. It is considered that crimped cod is not only firmer, but keeps longer, and has a better flavor than that which has not been crimped. Rigidity or firmness of flesh being due to *rigor mortis*, which passes off in the course of time, its existence in all fish affords a sign of freshness.

The turbot for flavor is deservedly held in high estimation. It is firmer and richer, but less digestible than other kinds of flat fish, as the sole, flounder, and plaice.

Brill is also an excellent fish, but is inferior in flavor to the turbot, for which it is sometimes substituted.

In both turbot and brill, the skin, on boiling, swells and assumes a gelatinous character. This is eaten as a choice part. Its appearance would lead to the supposition of its being easily digestible, but, whether on account of its rich flavor or not, it appears to be more apt than the flesh to disagree with the stomach.

The sturgeon is a fish that is not much eaten in this country. Its flesh is looked upon as presenting some resemblance in taste and character to veal.

The quality of fish as an article of food is influenced by the act of spawning, and presents considerable variation at different periods. It is just previous to spawning that the animal is in its highest state of perfection. Its condition altogether is then at its best point. The animal is fatter than at any other period, and of a richer flavor for eating. During the process of spawning its store of fatty matter is drawn upon, and it becomes poor, thin, and watery or flabby. It is now said to be "out of season," and requires time to arrive in condition again. In fish like the cod, where the fatty matter accumulates specially in the liver, this organ presents a most striking difference in volume and condition before and after spawning; whilst in such as the salmon, herring, etc., where the fat is dispersed amongst the flesh, it is the body which affords the chief evidence of change. As the salmon enters the rivers from the sea, for the purpose of ascending them and depositing its spawn, it is plump and well provided with fat. On its return the contrast in its condition is very great. It is now so exhausted and thin as to be looked upon as unfit for food.

Young fish which have not arrived at an age for spawning do not present any variation, but are always " in season."

After the operation of castration and spaying, it has been found also that fish maintain a uniform condition. The operation has never been practised to any extent, but an account of it has been given by Mr. Tull in the " Philosophical Transactions " for 1754. The object of its original performance appears to have been to prevent the excessive increase of fish in some ponds where the numbers did not permit any of them to grow to an advantageous size. Not only, it is stated, was the desired result attained, but the fish that had undergone the operation grew much larger than their usual size, were more fat, and remained always "in season."

The flavor of fish is much influenced by the nature of their food. In general, sea-fish are better that have been caught in deep water off rocky headlands where the current is strong, than in estuaries and bays where the water is shallow and the current weak. As regards fresh-water fish, those which have been obtained from deep lakes or ponds with clear water and a rocky or gravelly bottom are far superior in flavor to those obtained from shallow water on a muddy bottom. The earthy taste of the latter, indeed, may be so strong as to render them also uneatable, but fish bred in such water may be deprived of their unpleasant flavor by being kept for some time, before being killed, in ponds of clear water with a gravelly bottom.

With reference to the edible qualities of fish, Dr. Davy says: "As to individual species, whether of sea or fresh-water fish, there are notable differences and peculiarities, some depending on the species, some on the qualities of the feed. Of the first we have instances almost without number, inasmuch as almost each kind has some distinctive peculiarity. The delicate smelt has the odor of the cucumber ; the grayling of thyme ; some of those of the *Scomber* family abound in blood, have a comparatively high temperature, and dark-colored muscles; others, as those of the *Galidæ*, of which group the whiting is one, have little blood, at least few red corpuscles, have white muscles, and are delicately tasted; some, as the common ray, and most of the order of cartilaginous fish, have a muscular fibre of much firmness and power of resistance, yielding and becoming tender from keeping, and consequently, contrary to the general rule applicable to fish, they should not be dressed fresh; and other differences might be pointed out: one kind abounding in oil, as the pilchard, herring, and eel—the eel especially, and so luscious in consequence—other kinds containing little or no oil, as the sole and ray.

"Of the influence of feed on the same kind of fish we have striking examples, both in many salt-water and fresh-water species. Of the former, how different in quality is the herring caught off different parts of the coast; so too, of the common haddock. What herring is equal to that of Loch Fine; what haddock equal to that of the Bay of Dublin ? Of fresh-water fish, what a contrast there is between the lake-trout and the brook-trout !—the one well fed, well flavored, of the color of the salmon; the other small, colorless, and insipid. What a contrast between either of these and the trout of bog-water; the latter black, ill-formed, and ill-tasted. What a contrast, again, between the trout inhabiting a stream in a fertile limestone district fed by springs, fluctuating little, and the in-dwellers of the mountain-stream of a primitive country, subject to great fluctuations—one day a raging torrent, in a brief space run out and all but dried up. As with other animals, whether beast or bird, domestic or wild, much, we know, as to their quality depends on their feed, its kind, and quantity, and so with fish. Of these the paradoxical sturgeon may be mentioned as another and very striking example; by the Norwegians, we are informed by Block, it is even designated after the fish on which, from its flavor, it is supposed to have fed, as the mackerel-sturgeon, herring-sturgeon, etc.

"Other circumstances besides food, no doubt, have likewise an effect —all which anywise influence the health, such as climate, air, water, etc. ; nor amongst these should age be omitted. This last, in the instance of fish, and of fish only, is little thought of at home; and it may be because, in our well-fished seas, rivers, and lakes, few fish are allowed to reach a very advanced age; but not so in the tropical seas, where there is not the same activity practised in the capture of fish; there it is not uncommon to be helped at table to an old fish, and to have its hardness and toughness explained by one's experienced host by reference to age." *

The turbot is a fish which improves in flavor and tenderness by keeping for a little time before being dressed. Trout and salmon cannot be sent to table too soon after being caught. Eaten immediately after being killed, they possess a delicate sweet flavor which quickly disappears on keeping. It is thus impossible to have trout, in particular, in the same state of perfection at a distance from the stream where they are caught as on the spot itself.

---

* The Angler and His Friend, by John Davy, M.D., F.R.S., p. 117. London, 1855.

What is called the roe of fish constitutes the reproductive secreting organs, which attain a very large size, and render the animals exceedingly prolific. The hard roe belongs to the female, and is formed by the ovary. The soft roe or milt belongs to the male, and is formed by the spermatic organ. Both are eaten. The parts belonging to the male cod are used as a garnish to the fish when served.

Caviare is the hard roe of the sturgeon preserved by salting. It is pretty extensively employed as a common food in Russia, but in this country is consumed only as a relish at the table of the rich, the mode of serving it being on dry toast.

Cod sounds represent the swimming-bladder of the animal. They are dried and eaten separately. The swimming-bladder of the sturgeon, in particular, also yields the well-known article, isinglass.

The processes of drying, salting, smoking, and pickling are employed for the preservation of fish. Each process considerably lessens the digestibility of the article, and fish so prepared are, therefore, unsuited for the dyspeptic and invalid.

SHELL-FISH.—Shell-fish are derived from both the crustacean and molluscous tribes of animals. They yield a less nutritive kind of food than that which has been already considered, but must nevertheless be looked upon as holding a position of considerable importance in an alimentary point of view.

Shell-fish, taken altogether, are more indigestible and apt to upset the stomach than other kinds of animal food. Whether from idiosyncrasy on the part of the person affected, as is doubtless often the case, or from noxious properties in the particular animals eaten, shell-fish not unfrequently produce urgent symptoms of derangement. Sometimes the symptoms are those of gastro-intestinal irritation, as, for instance, nausea, vomiting, colic, cramps, and purging. Sometimes an eruptive disorder of the skin, and more particularly nettle-rash, is induced. So strong, indeed, is the tendency in some for such affection of the skin to be developed, that it is occasionally found necessary to scrupulously exclude shell-fish from the diet. At other times giddiness and other symptoms of disorder of the nervous system, as paralysis, coma, and convulsions, have been noticed, and instances of death have been known to occur.

The crustaceans commonly eaten consist of the lobster, crab, crawfish, shrimp, and prawn. They are all regarded as choice articles of food. The flesh belonging to them is white and firm.

Composition of the Edible Portions of the Lobster (Payen).

	Flesh.	Soft internal substance.	Spawn.
Nitrogenous matter, ...	19.170	12.140	21.892
Fatty matter, ...	1.170	1.444	8.234
Mineral matter, ...	1.823	1.749	1.998
Non-nitrogenous matter and loss, . .	1.219	0.354	4.893
Water, ... : . .	76.618	84.313	62,983
	100.000	100.000	100.000

The lobster occupies a higher position in public estimation than the crab. The flesh of the two is much alike, but the flavor is different, that of the lobster being the more delicate, and apparently the least likely to disagree.

The female, or hen-lobster as it is called, is in special request for making sauce, for the sake of the spawn or eggs belonging to it. These are attached beneath the tail, and consist of little round bodies. They are black in their natural state, but become of a bright red on boiling. They are pounded and mixed with the sauce, and thus give it after boiling the desired red color, as well as some amount of flavor. There is another part inside the animal which becomes of a bright red color on boiling. This is called the coral. It consists of the ovary, and is used for garnishing.

The flesh of the lobster is mainly found in the tail and claws. That of the claws is more tender, delicate, and digestible than that of the tail, which is firmer and closer.

The thorny or spiny lobster, or sea-crawfish, is sometimes substituted for the ordinary lobster. It eats much like it, but is, perhaps, rather inferior in flavor and tenderness.

The flesh belonging to the claws of the crab is far less likely to disagree with the stomach than the soft part contained within the shell. This is rich, and somewhat of the consistence of brain-matter, a name that is often popularly applied to it, although it really consists of liver.

The branchiæ, or gills, sometimes called "dead men's fingers," are in the case of both the lobster and the crab carefully avoided, but there is no foundation for the notion that they possess any deleterious properties.

Although an agreeable article of food to many, the lobster and crab are not fit, on account of their difficult digestibility, for the stomach of the invalid and dyspeptic. They also disagree with some persons possessing an ordinary amount of digestive power: producing a sense of weight in the epigastrium, nausea, and, it may be, vomiting. A cutaneous eruption, and other urgent symptoms, have occasionally been produced by these as well as other shell-fish.

Popular usages generally rest upon some substantial foundation, and the almost universal employment of vinegar and pepper as an adjunct to the kind of food under consideration has doubtless arisen from the advantage shown by experience to accrue therefrom. Indeed, the use of these condiments is almost looked upon as a matter of course, and they will have the effect—the one of stimulating an increased flow of digestive secretion, and the other of furnishing a certain amount of additional acid, and thereby augmenting the energy of the natural secretion. Thus increased power will be provided, by the agency of these adjuncts, to meet the difficult digestibility of the crustaceans in question.

The river or fresh-water crawfish is obtained from brooks and streams in certain localities. It is an animal of only moderate dimensions. Its flesh is softer and more digestible than that of the lobster. When eaten it is rather as a relish than for the actual amount of nourishment yielded. It enters as an ingredient into Bisque soup, and sometimes it is used simply as a garnish.

Shrimps and prawns are a favorite article of food with all classes of society. Although they cannot be reputed as easy of digestion, or adapted for a weak stomach, yet they are not so likely to disagree as the lobster and crab.

Of the shell-fish belonging to the molluscous tribe consumed in this country some are bivalve, such as the oyster, mussel, scallop and cockle, whilst others are univalve, as the periwinkle, whelk, and limpet.

Oysters have always held a high rank amongst the *deliciæ gulosorum*. They are found on various parts of our coast, and are caught by dredging, but instead of being consumed at once they are transferred to oyster-beds in creeks along the shore for the purpose of being "fattened." Here they quickly undergo a marked increase in size, become more plump, and improve in flavor. Colchester is the head-quarters as a feeding-ground for the metropolis. Arrived in London, some of the salesmen keep them for a few days and place some oatmeal in the water with the view of still further improving their whiteness and plumpness. The small "native" has the greatest delicacy of taste, and possesses the highest market value.

Oysters are a nutritious kind of food. Different opinions have prevailed regarding their digestibility. Seeing, however, how often they can be borne without inconvenience by a delicate stomach, it may be concluded that they are not difficult to dispose of, and especially when it is considered that from the manner in which they are usually eaten, viz., without being subjected to mastication, they are rarely swallowed in as favorable a state for digestion as other kinds of food. By many the whole animal is eaten, whilst those who are dainty over them remove the outer fringed part, or beard, which constitutes the gills. Of the remainder there is a soft and a somewhat hard portion. The former consists mainly of liver, which in this animal is a very bulky organ. The latter is composed of the adductor muscle, which serves to connect the two shells together. It forms by far the most indigestible part of the oyster, and should be carefully rejected where any weakness of stomach exists.

Oysters are more digestible in the raw than in the cooked state. Cooking, whether by grilling, scalloping, or stewing, coagulates and hardens them, and thereby renders them more difficult of solution in the stomach.

Composition of Oysters (Payen).

	Mean of two series of analyses.
Nitrogenous matter,	14.010
Fatty matter,	1.515
Saline matter,	2.695
Non-nitrogenous matter and loss,	1.395
Water,	80.385
	100.000

Though generally wholesome, oysters have been sometimes known to possess noxious properties, and to have given rise to symptoms of poisoning. At the time of spawning they lose their good condition, and are reckoned "out of season." It is in the month of May that they cast their spawn, which the dredgers call the spat. They are now in a poor and sickly state. During the months of June and July they pick up, and in August regain their former condition. There is an old saying that an oyster is only good when there is an "r" in the name of the month.

Mussels are consumed pretty largely, but they do not reach the table of the higher classes in the same way as the oyster. They are subjected to a preparatory process of cooking, usually by stewing in their own liquor. There is a little tongue-like, hardish, dark-colored mass belonging to them which is generally picked out, under the supposition that it is deleterious. No proof of this, however, exists, as many persons consume the mussel whole without experiencing any injurious consequences.

Composition of Mussels (Payen).

Nitrogenous matter, ... 11.72
Fatty matter, ... 2.42
Saline matter, ... 2.73
Non-nitrogenous matter and loss, ... 7.39
Water, ... 75.74
                                                    ———
                                                   100.00

Of all kinds of shell-fish most frequently found to exert deleterious effects, the mussel stands pre-eminent. It is well known to the public that it is liable to act in this way. Sometimes all who partake of a prepared dish suffer, whilst at other times some may be affected and others escape. Dr. Christison, in his work on "Poisons," refers to an instance which occurred at Leith in 1827, in which no fewer than thirty people were severely affected and two persons died. As in other cases, it has not been clearly ascertained to what the poisonous effects are attributable.

Scallops, cockles, periwinkles, limpets, and whelks are not of sufficient importance as articles of food to require any further notice here. They are principally sold in the streets, and eaten only by a limited class of people.

EGGS.—Eggs necessarily contain all that is required for the construction of the body, as the young animal is developed from it, but, as Liebig has pointed out, the shell must be taken into account as well as its contents. During the process of incubation, in fact, the earthy matter of the shell becomes gradually dissolved and applied to the purposes of growth. Phosphoric acid, formed by the gradual oxidation of phosphorus, constitutes the solvent agent, and the shell is found to become progressively thinner and thinner, until at last it is no thicker than a sheet of letter paper.

Various eggs are eaten, including those of reptiles—as, for instance, the turtle—as well as birds; but it is especially the egg of the fowl which is employed as a general article of food, and to this the succeeding remarks are intended to refer.

The average weight of an egg is about two ounces avoirdupois, and the quantity of dry solid matter contained in it amounts to about two hundred grains. It is composed of shell, white, and yolk, and in one hundred parts about ten consist of shell, sixty of white, and thirty of yolk.

Composition of the Entire Contents of the Egg.

Nitrogenous matter, ... 14.0
Fatty matter, ... 10.5
Saline matter, ... 1.5
Water, ... 74.0
                                              ———
                                             100.0

8

Composition of the White of Egg.

Nitrogenous matter, ...	20.4
Fatty matter, ...	—
Saline matter, ...	1.6
Water, ...	78.0
	100.0

Composition of the Yolk of Egg.

Nitrogenous matter, ...	16.0
Fatty matter, ...	30.7
Saline matter, ...	1.3
Water, ...	52.0
	100.0

The *white of the egg*, as shown by the above analysis, contains a considerably larger proportion of water than the yolk. It contains no fatty matter, but consists mainly of albumen in a dissolved state, and enclosed within very thin-walled cells. It is this arrangement which gives to the white of egg its ropy, gelatinous state. Thoroughly shaking or beating it up with water breaks the cells and removes the ropy state.

The *yolk of the egg* forms a kind of yellow emulsion. All the fatty matter of the egg is accumulated in this portion of it, and it here amounts to as much as 30 per cent. The fat is held in suspension or emulsified by the albuminous matter of the yolk, which constitutes a slight modification of that of the white, and is called vitelline. The yolk contains relatively a less proportion of nitrogenous matter than the white. The proportion of solid matter, on account of the fat, is considerably greater. An enveloping membrane or bag surrounds the yolk, and keeps the fluid matter of which it is composed together. Being lighter than the white, it floats to that portion of the egg which is uppermost, but is kept in position between the two extremities by two processes of inspissated albumen, called chalazæ, which pass and are attached one to either end of the egg.

The quality of eggs varies according to the food upon which the fowl is kept. Certain articles of food communicate a distinct flavor to the egg.

In an alimentary point of view, therefore, the white and yolk differ markedly from each other, the one being mainly a simple solution of albumen, the other a solution of a modified form of albumen associated with a considerable quantity of fat.

Reckoning the weight of an egg at two ounces, and that one-tenth of this consists of shell, the contents will furnish the following amounts of dry constituents, the percentage composition given above being taken as the basis of calculation:

Dry Constituents of the Contents of an Egg.

	Grains.
Nitrogenous matter, ... \.	110
Fatty matter, ...	82
Saline matter, ...	11
Total solid matter, . . .	203

Raw and lightly boiled eggs are easy of digestion. The hard-boiled egg offers considerable resistance to gastric solution, and exerts a constipating action on the bowels.

The egg changes by keeping, and certain devices are practised to preserve its freshness. The shell, being porous, allows of the evaporation of fluid, and air accumulates in its place at one of the extremities. Thus, an egg under exposure to the air loses weight from day to day, and the diminution in density indicates the length of time it has been kept. For example, a solution of salt in the proportion of about 10 per cent.—that is, one ounce of salt in ten ounces of water—will just allow a fresh egg to sink, whilst one which has been kept several days will swim. Bad eggs become sufficiently light to float even in pure water.

The air which finds its way through the pores of the shell into the egg causes gradual decomposition, until ultimately a state of putrescence is attained. With the view of excluding the air, eggs are sometimes placed and kept in lime-water. The shell is also sometimes covered with a layer of wax and oil, or some other kind of fatty matter, and sometimes with gum. By packing in bran, salt, or some such material, they keep longer than they otherwise would do, but it must be remembered that eggs easily acquire a taste from that which surrounds them. Immersed for some hours in a solution of salt, some of the saline matter penetrates and tends to preserve the egg under subsequent exposure to the air.

Fresh eggs are easily known by their translucency when held up to the light. By keeping they become cloudy, and when decidedly stale a distinct, dark, cloud-like appearance is discernible opposite some portion of the shell. A little instrument is sold as an egg-tester. It consists of a small square box, with a hole at the top to receive the egg, and another at one side to look into. By an arrangement of mirrors within, the state of the egg is seen when a strong light is thrown in such a manner as to be transmitted through it. If the egg be fresh, the image seen in the mirror is almost transparent, whilst if stale it is more or less dark.

Eggs are sometimes noticed to break spontaneously on being boiled. This occurs when the egg is suddenly plunged into a considerable amount of boiling water. The sudden expansion of the contents produced by the heat causes the shell to give way. Immersed in a small quantity of water only, the temperature is lowered sufficiently to prevent any immediate extensive expansion, and then, with the subsequent gradual elevation of the temperature, time is given for a little fluid to be forced through the pores of the shell from the pressure within, and perhaps, for the shell itself to undergo some expansion. A stale egg is less likely to become broken in this way than a fresh one, on account of the air which has replaced the evaporated fluid admitting easily of compression.

MILK.—Milk, an article furnished and intended by nature as the sole food for the young of a certain class of animals, necessarily contains, like eggs, all the elements that are required for the growth and maintenance of the body. Holding the position it does, it may be justly regarded as the type of an alimentary substance.

Good milk is a homogeneous, opaquely white, or very faintly buff-tinted liquid, which is entirely free from any viscidity, and undergoes no change on being heated. It has a sweet taste, and a slightly perceptible, agreeable odor. Its reaction, although formerly described as faintly acid, has been more recently ascertained to be slightly alkaline, or else neutral, when in a natural state and at the moment of removal. A little later an acid character becomes perceptible, and is evidently due to the effect of change after removal. Its density varies, but 1030 may be looked upon as about the average in the case of cow's milk. Although appearing homogeneous to the naked eye, it in reality consists, as is shown by microscopic examination, of a clear liquid holding in suspension a multitude of little particles or globules, which constitute the cause of its opacity. These globules are of a fatty nature, and, being lighter than the surrounding liquid, gradually rise to the surface, and form the cream which collects at the top of milk that is allowed to repose.

The ingredients of milk consist of nitrogenous matter, fatty matter, lactine, or sugar of milk, mineral matter, and water.

The *nitrogenous matter* is chiefly composed of caseine, a principle which, unlike albumen, is not coagulated by heat, but is coagulable by acids, organic as well as mineral, and also by a neutral organic substance obtainable from the stomach, viz., pepsine, which forms the active principle of rennet. It is caseine which constitutes curd and the basis of cheese. It is thrown down, carrying with it in an entangled state the suspended fatty globules, not only by the addition of the agents mentioned, but as a result of the spontaneous change which milk undergoes under exposure to air. The cause of this spontaneous coagulation is the development of lactic acid by a fermentative transformation of the lactine. As is well known, warmth greatly favors this change, and it does so to such an extent, that during the hot weather of summer, milk very quickly passes into a coagulated or curdled state. Contact with the smallest quantity of milk that has undergone the change also rapidly induces curdling throughout the whole bulk. Hence arises the necessity, as has been found by experience, of exercising the most scrupulous care in securing the utmost cleanliness of the vessels used for the purpose of storage. It may further be mentioned that, at the commencement of the change, an amount of lactic acid may have been generated insufficient to curdle the milk at the ordinary temperature, but sufficient to do so at a greater heat, because the action of the acid is then more energetic. This accounts for the circumstance frequently noticed in household economy, that milk may be liquid, and apparently fresh, at the ordinary temperature, and yet shall curdle upon being boiled.

Besides caseine, milk contains a little albumen, and a third nitrogenous principle in a small amount, which has been named lacto-proteine.

The *fatty matter* constitutes butter. Whilst existing in milk it is suspended, as has been already mentioned, under the form of microscopic globules. These globules appear to be surrounded by an envelope of caseine or albuminoid matter, which becomes broken in the process of churning for the production of butter, so allowing the incorporation of the fatty matter to occur. It is seemingly on account of this envelope that ether fails to dissolve out the fat when simply shaken up with milk; for if a small quantity of an alkali, as, for instance, potash, which may be presumed to dissolve the envelopes, be previously added, then ether immediately takes up the fat, leaving a clear watery liquid, consisting of the caseine, etc., lactine, and salts.

Lactine forms one of the varieties of sugar, and remains dissolved in the liquid from which both the curd and butter may have been separated. It has a less sweet taste, and is less soluble in water than ordinary sugar, is nearly insoluble in alcohol and ether, readily crystallizes, and reduces the cupro-potassic solution like grape-sugar, but is not *directly* susceptible of alcoholic fermentation. Alone it forms a stable

compound, but in contact with decomposing nitrogenous matter it undergoes conversion into lactic acid, which accounts for the sourness that
milk acquires on keeping.

The *mineral matter* and *water* comprise the inorganic principles required for the purposes of life.

According to the analysis given in Dr. Letheby's table, cow's milk
contains 14 per cent. of solid matter, which is distributed as follows:

Composition of Cow's Milk.

Nitrogenous matter,	4.1
Fatty matter,	3.9
Lactine,	5.2
Saline matter,	0.8
Water,	86.0
	100.0

One pint of milk of the above composition, reckoned at a sp. gr. of
1030 which will give 9,012 grains as its weight, will contain the following
amounts of the several solid constituents represented in grains and
ounces:

Solid Constituents in One Pint of Milk.

	Grains.	Ozs.
Nitrogenous matter,	369	0.843
Fatty matter,	351	0.802
Lactine,	468	1.069
Saline matter,	72	0.164
Total solid matter,	1,260	2.878

The proportion of the several constituents of milk varies in different
animals, and also under different circumstances in the same animal.

First, as regards the composition of the milk of different animals.
As it does not happen that a fixed or invariable composition exists, it is
not surprising that the analyses of different authorities should be found
to vary to some extent. They so far agree, however, as to give marked
distinctive features to the milk of certain animals. The following table
is furnished by Payen as affording a mean representation:

Mean Composition of the Milk of Various Animals (Payen).

	Woman.	Cow.	Goat.	Sheep.	Ass.	Mare.
Nitrogenous matter and in- soluble salts,	3.35	4.55	4.50	8.00	1.70	1.62
Butter,	3.34	3.70	4.10	6.50	1.40	0.20
Lactine and soluble salts,	3.77	5.35	5.80	4.50	6.40	8.75
Water,	89.54	86.40	85.60	82.00	90.50	89.33
	100.00	100.00	100.00	100.00*	100.00	100.00*

* The correct additions here do not quite correspond with the figures given, a deviation to the extent of 1.0 existing in the one case and 0.1 in the other. The soluble
salts, which in the above table are grouped with the lactine, are in Payen's table put

The milk of the cow, according to the above analysis, the most closely approximates to that of woman, but it is rather more highly charged with each kind of solid constituent. Next follows the milk of the goat, which, taken altogether, is again rather richer. That of the sheep is characterized by its marked richness in nitrogenous matter and butter. The milk of the ass and mare presents a striking difference from the rest. The peculiarity consists of the small amounts of nitrogenous matter and butter, and the large amount of lactine or sugar. The milk of the mare forms the higher representative of this peculiarity of the two, and so large is the amount of sugar contained in it, that in Tartary it is fermented and converted into an extensively consumed spirituous liquor, which is known by the name of *koumiss*. Ass's milk is well known to form a most useful aliment for persons too delicate in health to bear cow's milk. Its prominent characters as an article of food are sweetness of taste and facility of digestion; and a glance at its composition suffices to account for the possession of these qualities. It is said to have the objection of being sometimes apt to occasion diarrhœa.

I have selected and introduced Payen's analysis, but it must be stated that somewhat different results are furnished by other analysts, and particularly as regards woman's milk, in which the proportion of sugar is given as considerably larger, and that of caseine smaller, thus bringing it in respect of these constituents closer to the milk of the ass.

With reference to the caseine, it is stated that the coagulum or curd of woman's milk is "in general somewhat gelatinous, and not so dense or solid as that of cow's milk, and, therefore, more easily digested by the child's stomach" (Lehmann).

The quality of milk further varies in different breeds of animals. The milk of the Alderney cow, for example, is well known for its great richness in fat, and that of the breed of long-horns is reputed to contain a larger proportion of caseine than exists in the milk of other cows. It is also a popular belief that dark-complexioned women possess superior qualifications for nursing than fair-complexioned women, and this view is supported by the results of a comparative analysis made by L'Heritier* of the milk of two nursing mothers, aged twenty years, one of whom was dark and the other fair, it having been found that the secretion of the *brunette* was richer in each of the organic constituents than that of the *blonde*.

Besides these variations in the milk of individual animals, variations of a certain nature are noticeable in the milk of the same individual. The fluid which is first secreted after parturition, is in a very different condition from ordinary milk. It goes by the name of *colostrum*, and is of a somewhat viscid or stringy consistence, something like soap and water, with a turbid and yellowish appearance, and a strongly alkaline reaction. It contains more albumen than caseine, and hence undergoes coagulation on boiling. Examined microscopically, a number of large, irregular bodies are seen, which consist of conglomerations of small fat-globules held together by an amorphous, somewhat granular substance. These are called *colostrum-corpuscles*. The secretion of the cow remains in this state for several days—it may be for a month after calving. Pos-

---

down at 1.06 per cent. for woman's milk. This is obviously an error, and it may be concluded that 0.06 is meant. These figures have been taken above and bring the addition correct.

* Traité de Chimie pathologique, p. 638. Paris, 1842.

sessing during this time a somewhat sickly odor and purgative properties, it must be regarded as in an unfit state for human food.

A marked difference exists in the quality of the milk as regards the amount of cream which is obtained at the commencement and at the end of milking. It has been ascertained by direct observation, both on the Continent and in England, that the latter, especially when intervals of some duration are allowed to elapse between the periods of milking, contains more than double, and it may be as much as four times, the amount of cream in a given quantity of milk. This appears to be due to the fatty matter rising upward whilst the milk is contained within the gland, just as it is known to do after removal. In this way the last removed portion, consisting of that which occupied the highest position, will contain the largest amount of fatty matter, and may consist, in fact, of a species of thin cream. It is important that this should be known by those who obtain the measure of milk they require in a separate vessel direct from the cow. Of course, if a whole milking is received into one vessel, a uniform admixture will occur and an average quality be yielded.

According to results obtained in a series of observations conducted by Dr. Hassall, it appears that the afternoon milk of the cow is richer both in cream and curd (butter and caseine) than the morning.

Evidence is not wanting to show, as might be anticipated, that the quality of the milk is influenced by the nature of the food. Our knowledge is still imperfect regarding the precise effect exerted by different alimentary articles on the amount of the respective constituent principles of milk; but this much has been clearly ascertained, that an insufficient diet quickly leads to its impoverishment in solid material. It is nothing more than might be expected that, to maintain the milk in good condition, a proper and sufficient diet must be supplied; and in the case of the cow, no food can be considered equal to that which is yielded by the fresh pasture of country fields, the plants of which give a richness, sweetness, and agreeable aroma, which cannot be supplied by any other mode of feeding.

That milk is susceptible of being in a marked degree influenced by special ingesta, is a fact with which most people are acquainted, and many familiar illustrations of it can be adduced. It is known, for instance, that the color may be modified by mixing saffron or madder with the food; the odor, by the consumption of plants belonging to the cabbage and onion tribes; and the taste, by the ingestion of a bitter article such as wormwood. Milk also is known to acquire poisonous properties from the nature of the herbage in certain localities, without the animals themselves (cows, goats, etc.) being poisoned, just as has been previously mentioned may happen in the case of meat. This is noticed to occur abroad, and especially in Malta and in some of the districts of North America. A further illustration of the influence exerted by food is afforded by the fact that the milk of meadow-fed cows, and likewise the cream which rises from it, is liable to acquire a marked unpleasant flavor in the autumn from the fallen and decayed leaves which may happen to be consumed by the animal.

Suckling mothers have to practice self-denial in eating and drinking for the sake of the ease and comfort of their infants. Experience teaches them that by partaking of fruit and green vegetables, or anything of a sour or acid nature, their milk is apt to acquire griping and purging properties.

The medical practitioner is likewise well aware that medicinal agents produce their effect upon the milk. Infants may be salivated, purged, and narcotized by mercury, drastic purgatives, and opiates respectively, administered to the mother. Sometimes, also, medicines are purposely given to influence the child through the medium of the milk, instead of being administered directly to the infantile patient.

Lastly, it may be mentioned that violent exercise and certain mental states are known to communicate pernicious properties to the milk. An instance is quoted by Payen in which the milk of a woman, the subject of nervous attacks, became, in less than two hours after each paroxysm, mucilaginous like the white of egg.

Milk appears, also, sometimes to acquire specially deleterious properties from a peculiar change taking place, attended with the development of a low form of vegetable growth. Dr. Parkes observes that "Professor Mosler has directed attention to the poisonous effects of 'blue milk,' that is to say, milk covered with a layer of blue substance, which is, in fact, a fungus, either the *Didium lactis* or *Penicillium*, which seems to have the power, under certain conditions, of causing the appearance in the milk of an aniline-like substance. The existence of this form of fungus was noted by Fuchs as long ago as 1861. Milk of this kind gives rise to gastric irritation (first noted by Steinhof); and, in four cases noted by Mosler, it produced severe febrile gastritis.

"Milk which is not blue, but which contains large quantities of *Didium*, appears from Hessling's observations to produce many dyspeptic symptoms, and even cholera-like attacks, as well as possibly to give rise to some aphthous affections of the mouth in children." [*]

In a foot-note, it is stated that "blue milk is given by feeding cows with some vegetable substances, as *Myosotis palustris, Polygonum aviculare* and *Fagopyrum, Mercurialis perennis*, and other plants (Mosler), but this is different from the blue color referred to above." [†]

There are certain derivatives from and modifications of milk, viz., cream, skimmed milk, buttermilk, curds, whey, condensed milk, butter, and cheese, which will now receive consideration.

Cream.—Cream consists mainly of the fatty matter of milk, which, by virtue of its lightness, rises to the surface, the milk being allowed to repose for some time for the purpose. It contains some of the watery liquid part of the milk which holds in solution the other constituents. The composition of cream will necessarily vary a great deal according to its purity, or the manner in which its collection by skimming is effected. The following is the composition given in Dr. Letheby's table:

Composition of Cream.

Nitrogenous matter,	2.7
Fatty matter,	26.7
Lactine,	2.8
Saline matter,	1.8
Water,	66.0
	100.0

---

[*] Practical Hygiene, third edition, p. 239.

[†] Although not strictly falling within the scope of this work, it may here be mentioned that some recent outbreaks of typhoid fever have been very distinctly traced to the milk consumed. It does not appear that the milk has originally possessed noxious properties, but has acquired them by admixture with polluted water before distribution to the consumer.

In the six analyses made by Mr. Wanklyn, and introduced into his work on "Milk Analysis," the amount of fat varied from 14.1 to 43.90 per cent.

Devonshire, or clotted cream, differs from ordinary cream in being of a solid consistence. The difference is produced by its being collected from milk which has been previously heated just to the point of simmering. A scum forms, and is associated with the fatty matter that subsequently rises.

Skimmed milk.—Skimmed milk is the residue of milk from which cream has been collected. It is simply milk deprived of a certain amount of its fatty constituent. Being less rich than ordinary milk, it sometimes forms a useful aliment for a weak stomach.

Composition of Skimmed Milk.

Nitrogenous matter, ...	4.0
Fatty matter, ...	1.8
Lactine, ...	5.4
Saline matter, ...	0.8
Water, ...	88.0
	100.0

Buttermilk.—When butter is prepared directly from milk, a thin residuary liquid is yielded, which is known by the name of buttermilk. It contains a less amount of fatty matter than skimmed milk. Mixed with other food it is by no means an insignificant article of nourishment, containing, as it does, the nitrogenous matter, sugar, saline matter, and a small portion of the fatty matter of the milk. It is extensively used by the peasantry in some localities, and when not so employed is turned to account for feeding swine.

Composition of Buttermilk.

Nitrogenous matter, ...	4.1
Fatty matter, ...	0.7
Lactine, ...	6.4
Saline matter, ...	0.8
Water, ...	88.0
	100.00

Curd.—The essential basis of curd is caseine; but, as this principle undergoes coagulation during the transformation of milk into curds and whey, it entangles and carries with it the suspended milk-globules. Curd, therefore, consists of the nitrogenous portion of milk mixed with the chief part of its fatty element. It constitutes the basis of cheese.

Whey.—This forms the opalescent liquid left from the separation of the curd; it contains the lactine and salts of the milk, and likewise retains a little caseine and fatty matter. It is of some value, but not much, in an alimentary point of view. It is frequently, however, used to advantage in the sick room as a drink in febrile and inflammatory diseases, and possesses sudorific and diuretic properties. It is prepared by the addition of various agents to milk, and is designated according to the agent employed, as, for instance, rennet whey, white-wine whey, cream of tartar whey, tamarind whey, alum whey, etc.

Condensed milk.—Milk is now to be obtained in a condensed and preserved state. It is sold in hermetically sealed tins, and thus circumstanced may be kept ready for use, whenever required, for years. It is found in a syrupy or semi-liquid state, miscible with water, and will remain good for some days after the tin is opened. The process of preservation, it appears, was first successfully carried out in America, and there the "plain condensed milk," or milk simply reduced from four volumes to one, and subjected to a process of superheating, is sold as well as condensed milk to which cane-sugar has been added to assist in its preservation. In England there are three kinds of condensed milk supplied to the public—that of the Anglo-Swiss Company, which is prepared at Cham, in Switzerland (London office, 38 Leadenhall street); that of the Aylesbury Company, which is prepared at Aylesbury, Buckinghamshire (London office, 96 Leadenhall street); and that of Messrs. Crosse & Blackwell. Each contains, according to a report in *Food, Water, and Air* for October, 1872, genuine condensed milk in a perfect state of preservation, with the addition only of cane-sugar. * The following are the results furnished in the " Report " alluded to of the respective analyses of the three:

Condensed Milk.

	Anglo-Swiss.	Aylesbury.	Crosse & Blackwell's.
Caseine,	18.52	17.20	16.30
Fatty matter,	10.80	11.30	9.50
Sugar of milk,	16.50	12.00	17.54
Cane-sugar,	27.11	29.59	27.06
Ash,	2.12	2.24	2.39
Phosphoric acid,	.649	.67	.708
Water,	24.30	27.00	26.50
	100.000	100.00	100.000

Liebig's food for infants.—This constitutes a food, devised upon chemical principles, to form an appropriate substitute for woman's milk. The name of the originator has been sufficient to carry it into extensive use in Germany, and it has also been made widely known in England. It is composed of malt-flour, wheat-flour, cow's milk, bicarbonate of potash, and water, in such proportions as to give a representation of woman's milk as regards the relation of nitrogenous and non-nitrogenous principles. The following is described as the easiest and most simple way of making the food:

Take half an ounce of wheat-flour, half an ounce of malt-flour, and

---

* Amongst the correspondence contained in the Lancet for November 2 and 9, 1872, some remarks are to be found regarding the employment of condensed milk as an article of food for infants brought up by hand. Whilst it is admitted that infants take it readily on account of its sweetness, grow plump, and appear to thrive remarkably well upon it, it is alleged that the appearance, which depends simply upon an accumulation of fat, is delusive, and that they in reality possess so little power that they become prostrated by diarrhœa and other affections, and rapidly sink in a manner that is not observed under other modes of feeding. The evidence at present adduced can only be looked upon as suggestive, but the matter is an important one, and worthy the consideration of those whose field of observation affords them an opportunity of obtaining and furnishing trustworthy information on the point.

seven and a quarter grains of crystallized bicarbonate of potash, and after well mixing them add one ounce of water, and lastly five ounces of cow's milk. Warm the mixture, continually stirring, over a very slow fire till it becomes thick. Then remove the vessel from the fire, stir again for five minutes, put it back on the fire, take it off as soon as it gets thick, and, finally, let it boil well. It is necessary that the food should form a thin and sweet liquid previous to its final boiling. Before use it requires to be strained through a muslin- or fine hair-sieve, to separate fragments of husks that may be present.

To avoid the trouble of weighing, it is mentioned that as much wheat flour as will lie on a table-spoon corresponds with an ounce, and that a moderate table-spoon of malt-flour corresponds with half an ounce.

It is malt made from barley that is to be used, and a common coffee-mill answers the purpose of grinding it into flour, which is to be cleaned from the husk by a coarse sieve.

The bicarbonate of potash is added to neutralize the acid reaction of the two kinds of flour, and also to raise the amount of alkali in the food to the equivalent of that in woman's milk.

The ferment contained in the malt leads, during the exposure to the warmth employed in the process of preparation, to the conversion of the starch of both the flours into dextrine and sugar, the latter of which gives the sweet taste that is acquired. The newly formed products, also, being soluble, accounts for the mixture being thin, and it is a point contended for by Liebig, that principles in this state tax the digestive and assimilative powers of the infant much less than starch.

ESTIMATION OF THE QUALITY OF MILK.—The quality of milk may be judged of by its specific gravity and the amount of cream contained in it. No special skill is required for the determination of these points, and hence the examination may be conducted by any one possessing an ordinary amount of intelligence. The results given, if placed together, will enable a pretty accurate conclusion to be drawn, but should something more precise than this be required, recourse must be had to chemical analysis, which can only be performed by skilled hands.

Specific gravity.—The specific gravity is ascertained by weighing, or more readily by means of an instrument known as the hydrometer, which when applied to the examination of milk falls under the name of lactometer. The ordinary sp. gr. of good genuine cow's milk may be said to be about 1030 at 60° Fahr. It varies, however, within a range usually of two or three degree over and about four degrees under, and is more frequently under than over.

The addition of water lowers the sp. gr., and thus is afforded one means of detecting this adulteration. An excess of cream also lowers the sp. gr., on account of the lightness of the fatty matter, so that caution is necessary in dealing with the evidence afforded by the sp. gr. In a sample of milk examined by Dr. Hassall, containing 26 per cent. of cream (the usual quantity is from 5 to 10 per cent.), the sp. gr. was found to be 1019, and in another, containing 80 per cent., as low even as 1008; and that this was due to the cream, was proved by the fact that the same samples, when skimmed, showed a sp. gr. of 1027 and 1026 respectively. These form extreme and exceptional cases, but it often occurs that milk which is only fairly rich in cream will show a sp. gr. of 1026 or 1027 before being skimmed, and 1030 or 1031 afterward. It is better, therefore, to get rid of this modifying element, and to submit the milk, after being skimmed, to examination, and if there be then a lower sp. gr. than about 1027 or 1028, it may be fairly surmised that water has been added.

Dr. Hassall even recommends that the influence of all the fatty matter, and the caseine as well, should be eliminated, and that the whey should form the liquid submitted to examination, a few drops of acetic acid being used to effect the separation. He gives the result of the examination of the whey derived from forty-two samples of genuine milk, and, whilst considerable variation was noticeable in the sp. gr. of the milk itself, only a slight variation was observed in that of the whey, the limits of the range being 1025 and 1028.

Effect Produced on the Sp. Gr. of Milk by Dilution with Water (Hassall).

	Sp. gr.
Pure milk, ...	1030
Milk diluted with about 15 per cent. of water, . .	1026
" " 20 " " . .	1023
" " 35 " " . .	1018
" " 45 " " . .	1015
Skimmed milk, ...	1031
Skimmed milk diluted with 10 per cent. of water, .	1027
" " 20 " " .	1025
" " 30 " " .	1021
" " 40 " " .	1019
" " 50 " " .	1016
Whey, ...	1029
Whey diluted with 10 per cent. of water, . . .	1025
" " 20 " " . . .	1022
" " 30 " " . . .	1020
" " 40 " " . . .	1017
" " 50 " " . . .	1014

In an examination conducted in my own laboratory, the following are the specific gravities that were given by admixtures of definite proportions of milk of a sp. gr. of 1030 and water:

Milk.	Water.	Sp. gr. of specimen.	Sp. gr. of the whey.
100	+ 0	1030	1027.4
95	+ 5	1027.5	1025.8
90	+ 10	1026	1024
85	+ 15	1024	1022.5
80	+ 20	1022.4	1020.6
75	+ 25	1021.4	1019
70	+ 30	1019.6	1017.8
65	+ 35	1018.4	1016
60	+ 40	1017	1014.6
55	+ 45	1015.2	1013.3
50	+ 50	1014	1012
40	+ 60	1011	1009

For estimating the amount of cream, the appliances known as the *creamometer* and the *lactoscope* have been devised.

The *creamometer*, or, as it is often badly named, *lactometer*, consists of a long glass tubo or vessel graduated into 100 measures. The vessel is filled to 0° at the top of the graduated scale and placed aside for the cream to rise. The thickness of the layer can then be read off in *percentages*. The amount of cream varies considerably in different samples of genuine milk, and no precise limits can be given. It may be said, however, that if found below 5 per cent., a suspicion of adulteration with water may be reasonably entertained. The average appears to be about 8 or 9 per cent., but it may amount to and even considerably exceed 20 per cent.

A popular notion is entertained that the addition of a small quantity of warm water to milk increases the amount of cream yielded. The notion, however, has been shown by observation to be entirely erroneous. It evidently arose from the circumstance that the addition of water, by diminishing the sp. gr. of the milk, facilitates and expedites the ascent, but ultimately the product is even less.

Lactoscope.—A more scientific and precise way of estimating the amount of fat in milk is by the use of an instrument called the *lactoscope* This measures the degree of opacity of the liquid, and, as the opacity of milk is due to the fatty matter, it affords an indication of the amount that is present. The lactoscope of Donné, the original inventor of the instrument, consisted of an arrangement for increasing or diminishing the thickness of the layer of milk placed between two glass plates; and according to the thickness required to obscure the light of a candle, looked at through the apparatus, a measure was furnished of the amount of fat, which could be read off from an index adjusted for the purpose.

The lactoscope of Donné has been improved upon by Vogel, whose very simple contrivance affords an easy and speedy means for closely determining the amount of fatty matter suspended in any given specimen of milk. The apparatus consists of a half-moon-shaped trough, with two parallel sides formed of flat glass plates, one-fifth of an inch distant from each other; a glass cylinder on a foot and with a spout, graduated to 100 c.c.; and a small pipette, graduated in cubic centimetres divided into halves. In conducting the examination the measure is filled to 100 c.c., with water, and then a few cubic centimetres, say 3, of milk are dropped in from the graduated pipette. The mixture is well shaken, and the trough afterward filled with it. A candle is placed about three feet from the trough, and the flame looked at through the diluted milk, the back of the observer being directed toward the window of the room. If the candle-flame is clearly seen, the mixture is to be returned to the measure, and more milk added to it from the pipette, and then to be tried again in the trough. This is to be repeated, adding each time either one or half a c.c., until the candle-flame becomes obscured. From the quantity of milk required to be added to the 100 c.c., of water to produce this effect, the amount of fatty matter can be calculated, the following formula having been found, by comparing the results obtained with those yielded by chemical analysis, to give the information required. Let 23.2 be divided by the number of cubic centimetres of milk employed, and 0.23 be added, and the product will give the percentage amount of fat. Suppose, for instance, 6 c.c., of milk to have been required, then the fat will amount to 4.09 per cent. Thus:

$$\frac{23.2}{6} + 0.23 = 4.09$$

The following table gives the results worked out, and will enable the percentage of fat to be at once read off:—

C.C. of milk employed.	Percentage of fat in the milk.	C.C. of milk employed.	Percentage of fat in the milk.
1	23.43	14	1.88
1.5	15.46	15	1.78
2	11.83	16	1.68
2.5	9.51	17	1.60
3	7.96	18	1.52
3.5	6.86	19	1.45
4	6.03	20	1.39
4.5	5.38	22	1.28
5	4.87	24	1.19
5.5	4.45	26	1.12
6	4.09	28	1.06
6.5	3.80	30	1.00
7	3.54	35	0.89
7.5	3.32	40	0.81
8	3.13	45	0.74
8.5	2 96	50	0.69
9	2.80	55	0.65
9.5	2.77	60	0.61
10	2.55	70	0.56
11	2.43	80	0.52
12	2.16	90	0.48
13	2.01	100	0.46

BUTTER.—Butter is the fatty portion of milk, and is obtained by the process of churning, either cream or the milk itself being subjected to the operation. The effect of churning is to cause the milk-globules to run together or coalesce, and thus to become incorporated into a solid mass. This is supposed to be brought about by the mechanical rupture, in the first place, of the envelopes of the globules, the contents of which are then permitted to become agglomerated; and, it is found by experience that the process is facilitated by being conducted at a temperature of about 60° Fahr. When the butter is formed, it is removed from the churn and well kneaded and washed with water, to remove as much as possible of adhering caseine and other ingredients of the milk; and the more completely this is effected the better will the butter afterward keep. More or less salt is added to promote still further its power of keeping, and the quantity is regulated according as the butter is to be eaten fresh or to be preserved for future consumption.

The pure fatty matter of butter is composed of a mixture of several fatty principles. Six have been enumerated by Chevreul, viz.: Margarine (palmitine), oleine (butyroleine), capryline, butyrine, caprine, caproine (capronine).

These are neutral fats, and are resolvable into glycerine and margaric (palmitic), oleic, caprylic, butyric, capric, and caproic acids respectively: the first two acids being of a fixed, and the last four of a volatile nature. It is to the latter agents that the characteristic taste and smell of butter are due, although they are present only in small amount. According to Bromeis, 98 per cent. of butter (the pure fat) is composed of margarine (palmitine) and oleine (68 per cent. of the former and 30 per cent of the latter), and the remainder of the volatile fatty acid compounds.

Such is the composition of the pure fatty matter of butter. Butter, however, as it is obtained and furnished for consumption, contains a certain quantity of other matter, but the fat ought to amount to from 86 to 92 per cent. Caseine is present to the extent of from 3 to 5 per cent. only in good specimens. In a bad sample there may be considerably more. Some of the watery portion of the milk is retained, and with it the constituents that are held in solution. The water should not amount to more than from about 5 to 10 per cent., but it is sometimes found in considerably larger quantity. The practice of beating up the butter with water before being put into the scales forms a process which tells in favor of the retail dealer. A description of butter known as " Bosh " has been found to contain a proportion of water amounting in some cases to more than a third of the article (Hassall). Salt is present as an admixture in all butters. In fresh butter the average amount ranges from 0.5 to 2 per cent. In salt butter the quantity should not exceed 8 per cent.

Butter may be separated from the above-mentioned adventitious ingredients by applying heat so as to melt it. The fatty matter rises in a pure state to the surface, leaving a watery liquid containing the other principles present below. Its flavor, however, is much deteriorated by the process, for the agreeable taste belonging to fresh butter is in great part due to the natural accessory matter present. It is true butter has a peculiar odor and flavor which are given to it by its volatile fatty acid compounds, and these will be retained in the melted article; but there are, besides, sapid qualities belonging to fresh butter which are due to other ingredients derived from the milk which yielded it. It is well known that the taste of butter is much influenced by the nature of the food upon which the cow is kept, and that a delicate and agreeable aroma is given by some pastures which is not afforded by others. A decidedly unpleasant flavor (which, as previously mentioned, may be likewise perceptible in the milk and cream) is also sometimes noticeable in the butter made in the autumn, and at other times of the year, arising from the fallen and decayed leaves which the cow may happen to have consumed with its food.

Fresh butter, especially in hot weather, is very prone to undergo change, and in the course of a short time to become rancid. This arises from the nitrogenous matter of the milk with which the butter is impregnated acting as a ferment and leading to the liberation of the fatty acids. The more completely butter is deprived of this adventitious matter by washing, the better is it found afterward to keep; and, if it be completely deprived of it by melting and agitation with boiling water it will bear preservation for a considerable period, but the process involves a loss of the agreeable flavor which belongs to the article in the fresh state. When butter has become rancid it may also be rendered again eatable by melting it and shaking it repeatedly with boiling water for the purpose of removing the free fatty acids; and, if the melted butter be then poured into ice-cold water, it is stated to assume the appearance of fresh butter. The addition of salt to butter checks the decomposition of the caseine that may be present, and thence, also, the change of the butter itself. It is upon this principle that salt is used as a preservative agent, and sugar enjoys a similar capacity. Butter laid in syrup is said to keep even better than salted butter. Exclusion from air affords another means of preserving butter, and simply covering it with water renewed every day will suffice to keep it good for a week and upward. Instead of water a weak solution of tartaric acid has been recommended by Bréon, and, according to Payen, is far more efficacious. Payen states that some butter upon which the process was tried with a view of testing its efficacy was found to have retained its freshness at the end of two months under the existence of a temperature of from 60° to 68° Fahr.

Butter is a form of fatty matter less likely than most others to disagree with the stomach. This applies to butter in a perfectly fresh or unchanged state; when rancid or when the fatty acids have been liberated by exposure to heat, like all fatty matter in a similar state, it is very apt to occasion gastric derangement.

CHEESE.—Cheese consists of the caseine of milk with a varying admixture of butter, according to the manner in which it has been prepared. The caseine is coagulated usually by the employment of rennet (an article obtained from the fourth or digesting stomach of the calf), but sometimes by the agency of an acid. In being precipitated the caseine entangles and carries with it the suspended fat-globules (butter) of the milk. After coagulation has been effected the curd is collected and subjected to pressure in a mold, of the future form of the cheese, to deprive it as far as possible of the liquid portion of the milk, or whey. It is kept in the mould until it has acquired sufficient consistence to hold together, and is then removed and exposed on shelves in a cool and airy situation. Here it is kept for a considerable time for the process of ripening to occur. Salt is applied to the surface, and frequent turning has to be performed. Changes occur attended with the development of various volatile fatty acids, and the cheese passes from a comparatively odorless and insipid state to the condition well known to belong to the ripened article. The larger the quantity of fatty matter, or butter, present, the larger is the capacity for the production of the volatile fatty acids, and the more strongly marked do the odor and flavor become. The caseine, however, appears also to undergo change, and to contribute to the production of these characters. If circumstances exist which permit the change still further to proceed, an advance to ordinary putrefaction occurs, accompanied with the evolution of ammonia. In this pronounced state of decay the taste and smell may be such as to be actually offensive, and the article may acquire a highly irritating, and even, as experience has shown, poisonous properties.

Various qualities of cheese are met with, and they are generally known in commerce by the names of the localities producing them. The quality depends upon the amount of fatty matter present in the milk from which the cheese is made. In the richest cheeses, as Stilton and double Gloucester, cream is added to the milk. Cheshire cheese is made from unskimmed milk; single Gloucester, Chester, and American, from milk with a little cream removed; and Dutch, Parmesan, Suffolk, and Somersetshire, from skimmed milk. Cream cheese consists of the fresh curd which has been moderately pressed. It is eaten without being allowed to ripen.

Fatty matter gives softness and richness to the cheese, but, at the same time, renders it more prone to change and decay on keeping. It is the poor and close cheese, such as is made from skimmed milk, as the Dutch, Parmesan, etc., which is found to keep the best. Parmesan, particularly, is characterized by its power of keeping; and after having been kept for some time it becomes of a hard and somewhat horny consistence, and requires grating to place it in a suitable condition for consumption.

Composition of Cheese (from Parkes *).

Nitrogenous matter, ...	. 33.5
Fatty matter, ...	. 24.3
Saline matter, ...	. 5.4
Water, ...	. 36.8
	100.0

Composition of Cheddar Cheese (from Letheby).

Nitrogenous matter, . . .	. . 28.4
Fatty matter, ...	. . 31.1
Saline matter, ...	. . 4.5
Water, ...	. . 36.0
	100.0

Composition of Skim Cheese (from Letheby).

Nitrogenous matter, ...	. . 44.8
Fatty matter, ...	. . 6.3
Saline matter, ...	. . 4.9
Water, ...	. . 44.0
	100.0

Composition of Various Kinds of Cheese (Payen †).

	Roquefort.	Gruyère.	Dutch.	Neufchatel (fresh).	Neufchatel (matured).
Nitrogenous matter, ...	26.52	31.5	29.43	8.00	13.03
Fatty matter, ...	30.14	24.0	27.54	40.71	41.91
Saline matter, ...	5.07	3.0	—	0.51	3.63
Non-nitrogenous matter and loss,	3.72	1.5	6.93	15.80	6.96
Water, ...	34.55	40.0	36.10	36.58	34.47
	100.00	100.00	100.00	100.00‡	100.00

	Camembert.	Brie.	Chester.	Parmesan.
Nitrogenous matter, ...	18.90	18.48	25 99	44.08
Fatty matter, ...	21.05	25.73	26.34	15.95
Saline matter, ...	4.71	5.61	4.16	5.72
Non-nitrogenous matter and loss,	4.40	4.93	7.59	6.69
Water, ...	51.94	45.25	35.92	27.56
	100.00 §	100.00	100.00	100.00

* Practical Hygiene, 3d ed., p. 165.
† Substances Alimentaires, p. 197 *et seq.* Paris, 1865.
‡ Total according to the figures given, 101.60.
§ Total according to the figures given, 101.00.

9

On account of its richness in nitrogenous matter cheese constitutes
an article of considerable dietetic value. Amongst the poorer inhabitants
of rural districts it enters as an important aliment into the daily diet,
serving to supply the nitrogen which is deficient in the bread or other
kind of vegetable food which is employed as the staple article of subsistence. By the less indigent classes, where the meat consumed suffices
to supply the nitrogen required, cheese is rather employed as a condiment, or relish, than as a direct article of nourishment, and for this purpose it is the more tasty kind of cheese that is selected, of which only a
small quantity is eaten, and this at the end of the repast.

The digestibility of cheese varies much according to its nature. The
poorer and closer kinds of cheese, those which contain the largest proportion of caseine, require strong digestive power for their solution. The
softer, stronger-tasted, and more friable kind of cheese, however, is by
no means similarly difficult of digestion, and it may, indeed, taken in
small quantity, aid the digestion of other food by its stimulant action on
the stomach. Toasted cheese, no matter of what kind, for in all the consistence becomes close by toasting—is one of the most indigestible articles
that can be eaten.

Cheese, especially the richer kinds, is very liable to form the seat of
growth of certain animal and vegetable organisms. The larvæ, or mag-
gots, of a fly (*Piophila casei*), constituting what are known as hoppers or
jumpers, flourish upon it. Another animal frequently met with is the
cheese mite or *Acarus domesticus*. It exists in great numbers, and is so
small that its form is only distinctly to be perceived by the microscope.
The mould of cheese is composed of minute vegetable organisms belonging to the tribe of fungi, blue mould being formed by the *Aspergillus
glaucus*, and red mould by the *Sporendonema casei*.

Cheese is also liable, as has been mentioned to occur likewise with
meat, to undergo a modified form of decay, attended with the development of poisonous properties. Instances of cheese-poisoning have been
chiefly observed in Germany, but some cases have also been recorded as
having been met with in Cheshire. The symptoms produced have very
much resembled those arising from sausage-poisoning, viz., gastro-intestinal irritation with great depression, and have shown themselves within
half an hour or a few hours after the cheese has been eaten. According
to Westrumb, poisonous cheese presents no peculiarity in its appearance,
taste, or smell; but Hünefeld says that it is yellowish and tough, with
harder and darker lumps interspersed, and that it has a disagreeable
taste, reddens litmus, and becomes flesh-red instead of yellow under the
action of nitric acid.*

ANIMAL FOODS SOMETIMES BUT NOT ORDINARILY EATEN.

The information contained in the following pages has been gathered
from numerous sources, chiefly works on travels, and placed together in a
collected and systematic form. It shows that an almost endless variety
of animals are eaten in different parts of the globe, and supplies what I
have been able to learn has been said regarding their edible qualities. In
the case of some of them, their consumption occurs upon a sufficiently extensive scale to give them a position of considerable importance in an

---

* Christison on Poisons, 4th edition, p. 642.

alimentary point of view. In that of others, however, the fact of their consumption cannot be looked upon as anything beyond a point of curiosity in dietetics. The statements furnished are authenticated by reference to the works from which they have been taken; but instead of introducing and repeating the names of the works amongst the text, numbers are employed and a key to them supplied at the end of the section, vide pp. 142, 143. Where the page and volume of a work are given, these are placed after the reference number within a parenthesis.

CANNIBALISM.—There is reason to believe the practice of eating human flesh has not at all times been confined to the lowest savages, but it is difficult to obtain much satisfactory information respecting it.

There is little doubt that our ancestors, the ancient inhabitants of Britain, were guilty of eating human flesh, and St. Jerome specially charges the Attacotti, a people of ancient Scotland, with preferring the shepherd to his flock [9] (vol. i., p. 688).

There have been numerous instances of cannibalism among people suffering from starvation in sieges and from shipwreck, and the evidence is tolerably strong that some men belonging to civilized races, living in wild places, have occasionally decoyed persons to their dens and eaten them. Andrew Wyntoun, in his rhyming chronicle, charges a man who lived early in the fourteenth century with this crime [10] (vol. ii., p. 236).

Lindsay, of Pitscottie, also relates that a man and his wife and family were all burnt on the east coast of Scotland for the crime of eating children that they had stolen away [10] (p. 163). During the horrors of the great French Revolution, the heart of the Princess Lamballe was plucked out of her body by one of the mob, taken by him to a restaurant, and there cooked and eaten [12] (vol. ii., p. 564).

Statements are given, to the effect that there is something attractive in the taste of human flesh to those who have been addicted to the revolting practice of cannibalism.

In the account mentioned by Lindsay that has been just referred to, it is stated that one of the daughters of the man, when going to the place of execution, cried out, " Wherefore chide ye with me, as if I had committed ane unworthy act ? Give me credence and trow me, if ye had experience of eating men and women's flesh ye wold think it so delicious that ye wold never forbear it again " [11] (vol. i., p. 688).

In the present day the Polynesian islands are the chief home of such cannibalism as still exists in the world. The Tannese say to any one condemning their anthropophagous habits—" Pig's flesh is very good for you, but this is the thing for us." They distribute human flesh in little bits far and near among their friends as delicate morsels. Cannibal connoisseurs, it is asserted, prefer a black man to a white one, as the latter, they say, tastes salt [16] (p. 83).

Monkeys are eaten by the Chinese,[1] the natives of Ceylon,[3] the Indians, the negroes and whites in Trinidad,[3] the Dyaks of Borneo,[3] the Africans of the Gold Coast,[3] the aborigines of the Amazon [2] (p. 485), and the Indians of Spanish Guiana.[4] The flesh is said to be palatable.[5]

The Kalong, or edible roussette (a species of bat), is abundant in Java, and valued as food by the natives. The flesh is white, delicate, and tender, but generally imbued with a smell of musk.[6]

For the names of the works which the reference numbers in the above pages represent, vide the key supplied at pp. 142, 143.

The *Lion* is sometimes eaten in Africa, but its flesh is not good[4] (p. 304).

The Canadian *Lynx* is eaten by the Indians, and its flesh is said to be white, tender, and to resemble that of the American hare.[4]

Wolves are forbidden among the African Arabs, but are not unfrequently eaten by sick persons from the belief that their flesh is medicinal[7] (p. 51). The mountaineers of the American Sahara eat the small prairie wolf (*canis latrans*)[8] (p. 80).

The Hudson's Bay *Skunk* is eaten by the Indians, who esteem its flesh a great dainty.[4]

The *Otter* is eaten by Laplanders and Esquimaux, but its flesh has a fishy taste.[8]

Cats are eaten by the Chinese[9] (vol. iii., p. 761), and in the Island of Savu are preferred to sheep and goats[9] (vol. iii., p. 688). Five thousand cats are said to have been eaten in Paris during the late siege[19] (p. 299). According to the same authority, the cat is downright good eating. A young one, well cooked, is better than hare or rabbit. It tastes something like the American gray squirrel, but is even tenderer and sweeter[16] (p. 219).

Although cats, like wolves and dogs, are forbidden among the African Arabs, they are not unfrequently eaten by sick persons from the belief that their flesh is medicinal[7] (p. 52).

Dogs are eaten by the Chinese,[1][8] the New Zealanders[11] (vol. ii., p. 17), the South Sea Islanders,[8] and some African tribes.[9] One thousand two hundred dogs, it is stated, were eaten in Paris during the late siege,[19] and the flesh fetched from two to three francs per pound[20] (February 11, 1871).

According to Pliny, puppies were regarded as a great delicacy by the Roman gourmands. Young dogs, like cats, are not to be eaten by the African Arabs, but they are not unfrequently given to sick persons from the belief that their flesh is medicinal.[7]

Wild dogs are eaten by the natives of Australia[12] (vol. ii., p. 250), but in New Zealand[11] and the South Sea Islands[8] (vol. ii, p. 196) the dogs are specially fed and fattened, and European dogs are considered unpalatable.[11] Captain Cook looked upon a South Sea dog as little inferior to an English lamb[8] (vol. ii., p. 196). Fattened dog's flesh is a favorite food of the Warori, an African tribe[13] (vol. ii., p. 273).

The *Bear* supplies food to several nations of Europe, and its hams are considered excellent.[8] The flesh of the brown or black bear, which is eaten by the common people of Norway, Russia, and Poland, is difficult of digestion, and is generally salted and dried before it is used.[19] Two bears were eaten in Paris during the siege,[10] and the flesh was supposed to taste like pig[14] (February 1, 1871). The Indian tribes of the interior of Oregon eat bears[15] (vol. iv., p. 452). The Polar bear is stated by Sir John Ross to be particularly unwholesome, although the Esquimaux fed upon it, and apparently without inconvenience.[8]

The *Hedgehog* is considered a princely dish in Barbary, and is eaten in Spain[8] and Germany.[10] It is frequently eaten by the sick among the African Arabs from the belief that its flesh is medicinal[7] (p. 62).

Kangaroos are eaten by the aborigines of Australia[12] (vol. ii., p. 250)[14] (p. 67), and their flesh is considered excellent.[4] Soup made from the tail is reputed to be far superior to ox-tail soup.[4] It is imported into Eng-

----

For the names of the works which the reference numbers

land with the Australian meat in sealed tins. Three kangaroos were eaten in Paris during the siege.[10] The *Wombat* is eaten by the natives of Australia,[11] and its flesh is said to be preferable to that of all other animals of Australia.[4] *Wallabies* are eaten by the natives of Australia.[5]

The *Opossum* is eaten.in America,[6] Australia,[10] [12] [6] and the Indian islands. Young ones are reared for the table, and the flesh is white and well tasted.[5] They are considered by the natives of South America equally as good for food as the flesh of the hare or rabbit, especially the Virginian opossum.[10]

The *Bandicoot* is eaten by the aborigines of Australia[14] and by the lowest caste of Hindoos.[4]

The *Seal* is all in all to the Greenlander and Esquimaux.[4] It is eaten by Kamtschatkadales,[4] the inhabitants of the coast of Labrador[17] (vol. i., p. 4), Vancouver's Island[18] (p. 485), etc. Its flesh is coarse and oily; nevertheless, it was formerly served up at feasts in England, together with the porpoise.[5] The liver, when fried, is esteemed by sailors as an agreeable dish.[4] A seal eaten during the siege of Paris was said to taste like lamb[14] (February 1, 1871).

The *Walrus* is eaten by the Esquimaux[19] (p. 485), and highly appreciated by Arctic explorers[20] (vol. ii., p. 15).

The *Whale* is eaten largely by the natives of Western Australia, New Zealand,[3] the poorer sort of Japanese[21] (vol. iv., p. 35), the rude littoral tribes of Northern Asia and America,[3] the natives of Vancouver's Island[18] (pp. 53, 61), and the Esquimaux.[3] Blubber is used as food in Vancouver's Island,[18] and by the Esquimaux[22] (vol. i., p. 243).

The blubber and flesh of the *Narwhal*, or sea-unicorn, is considered a great delicacy by the Greenlander.[4]

The flesh of the *Porpoise* was formerly considered a delicacy, and receipts for dressing it are to be found in old cookery books. The Greenlander esteems the flesh a great dainty, and quaffs the oil as the most delicious of draughts.[4]

The *Manatee*, sea-cow, or woman-fish, a native of the seas of the West Indies and South America, is said to be excellent eating.[4] Dr. Vogel found the flesh very well flavored, and the fat like pork[14] (vol. i.). Payen states that the flesh is whitish and good to eat, and that the animal's milk has an agreeable flavor.[17]

The Indian *Dugong* is considered good eating.[4]

Mice and *Rats* are eaten in Asia, Africa,[5] Australia[12] (vol. ii., p. 250), and New Zealand[14] (vol. ii., p. 17), and considered delicate morsels. The taste of rats is pronounced to be somewhat like that of birds[10] (p. 219). The Chinese eat them,[1] and to the Esquimaux epicures the mouse is a real *bonne bouche*.[3] Rats and mice were eaten in Paris during the siege.[10] The *Porcupine* is reckoned delicious food in America and India, and resembles sucking-pig.[5] The Dutch and the Hottentots are fond of it,[3] and it is frequently brought to table at the Cape of Good Hope.[10] It is eaten in Sicily and Malta,[10] and sold in the markets in Rome.[5]

The *Agoutis*, natives of the West Indies, Guiana, and Brazil, at the first settling in the West India Islands were exceedingly numerous, and constituted a great part of the food of the Indian. The flesh is white and tender, and much esteemed by the natives when well cooked.[4]

The *Squirrel* is eaten by the natives of Australia[12] (vol. ii., p. 250), the North American Indians[22] (vol. ii., p. 250), and is a favorite dish in Sweden

in the above pages represent, *vide* the key supplied at pp. 142, 143.

and Norway.' The flesh is tender, and is said to resemble that of a barn-door fowl.⁶⁰ It is sometimes eaten by the lower classes in England' and in the United States, and is said to make excellent pies.

Several species of *Cavia* are used as food in Great Britain, Brazil, and other parts of South America, especially the guinea-pig, the spotted cavy, the long-nosed cavy, and the rock-cavy.⁶⁰

The common *Jerboa* (*Dipus Egyptius*) is eaten by the Arabs, who esteem its flesh among their greatest dainties.⁶⁰ The Alagtaga (*Dipus Jaculus*) is larger than the common jerboa, and called by the Arabs the lamb of the Israelites. Many authors consider it to be the coney of the Scriptures and the mouse of Isaiah.'

The *Marmot* of the Alps affords nourishment to the poorer inhabitants of Tyrol, Savoy, and other parts. Three other species are also eaten, namely, the Maryland Marmot, Bobath, and the Cassin or Earless Marmot.⁶⁰

The flesh of the *Beaver* is much prized by the Indians and Canadian traders especially when it is roasted in the skin after the hair has been singed off.' It is also used in South America, and said to be excellent eating.⁶⁰

The flesh of the *Bison* is the support of many Indian tribes; it nearly resembles ox-beef, but is said to be of finer flavor and easier digestion. The hump is baked, and eaten as a great delicacy.'

The flesh of the *Buffalo* is eaten by the North American Indians²⁴ (p. 122), the Sumatrans²⁵ (p. 56), and the islanders of Savu⁹ (vol. iii., p. 688). Catlin calculates that about 250,000 North American Indians subsist almost exclusively on this animal through every part of the year²⁶ (vol. i., p. 122). The beef is tough, dark-colored, and occasionally of a musky flavor. The chine is esteemed good, and is eaten by the common Italians.'

The *Camel* is eaten with relish in Africa, and its milk is believed to neutralize the injurious qualities of the date' (p. 308). The flesh is alleged to produce serious derangement of the stomach among the Arabs²⁷ (vol. i., p. 76, note). A camel eaten during the siege of Paris is said to have tasted like veal¹⁴ (Feb. 1, 1871). Camel's hump, which is spoken of as furnishing in the desert a savory dish, is to be procured in a preserved state at some of the dried provision establishments at the west end of London.

The flesh of the *Llama* is said to resemble mutton.⁶⁰

Captain Ross considered the flesh of the *Musk-Ox* excellent, and free from any particular musky flavor, though the skin has a strong smell.' When lean, however, some complain of the flesh as smelling strong.'

The *Elk* is eaten in Norway, Lapland, and Sweden, where its flesh is much esteemed.⁶⁰ The young are said to be particularly delicious.' The tongue and nose are considered great delicacies.'

The *Reindeer* is eaten in Siberia²⁸ (p. 75), and is the favorite food of the Esquimaux¹⁹ (p. 485). It is the principal nourishment of the Laplanders. The tongues are excellent when salted, and the milk is sweet and nourishing.⁶⁰

The sinewy parts of stags are highly prized by the wealthy Chinese¹⁸ (p. 551).

The flesh of the *Horse* is eaten largely by various nations. The Indian horsemen of the Pampas live entirely on the flesh of their mares, and eat neither bread, fruit, nor vegetables³¹ (p. 120). Horse-flesh is eaten by the Jakuts of Northern Siberia³⁰ (p. 23), the Tartars and natives of South America,' and by the islanders of Savu⁹ (vol. i., p. 688). Mr. Bicknell, in his paper on "The Horse as Food for Man"³² (vol. xvi., p. 349), mentions

For the names of the works which the reference numbers

fifteen European states, besides France, where horse-flesh is eaten. The Icelanders have practised hippophagy since the eighth century. The Russians have always eaten horses, and in Denmark the people returned to the custom of their forefathers in 1807. Wurtemburg was the first of the German States to adopt the practice, and commenced it in 1841. Bavaria, Baden, Hanover, Bohemia, Saxony, Austria, and Prussia followed in subsequent years.

A Berlin newspaper states that there are at the present time (1863) "seven markets for horse-flesh in that city, in which, during the first ten months of 1862, there were seven hundred and fifty horses slaughtered. No horse is allowed to be slaughtered and sold without the certificate of a veterinary surgeon" [12] (1863, p. 142).

Hippophagy was first advocated in France, in 1786, by Géraud, the distinguished physician.

A meeting was held in 1864, at the Acclimatization Garden in Paris, for the purpose of promoting the greater consumption of horse-flesh as an article of food[22] (1864, p. 472), and a grand hippophagic banquet was celebrated with great éclat at the Grand Hotel, Paris, at the commencement of 1865, under the patronage of the French Humane and Acclimatization Societies[22] (1865, p. 176).

In 1866 the first horse-butcher's shop was opened in Paris[10] (vol. xvi., p. 349).

A correspondent of the *Medical Times and Gazette* (Sept. 26, 1867) stated: "In passing along the quays on my way to the Marseilles Railway Station, I was struck by the number of stalls bearing the title 'Boucherie Hippophagique,' 'Boucherie de Viande de Cheval,' at La Villette, Paris. The attendants were very civil, and told me that they usually sold at the rate of two horses a day. Some of the customers assured me that the meat was better than beef."

Sixty-five thousand horses, it is asserted, were eaten in Paris during the siege, and the flesh was facetiously called "siege venison."

Mr. Bicknell says: "I believe the only European countries where horses are not used for food with the open sanction of the law are Holland, Portugal, Turkey, Greece, Spain, Italy, and the United Kingdom. Concerning the four first I have no information, but in Spain horses killed in bull-fights were eaten till quite recently, and during the Peninsular War the Spaniards commonly were hippophagists. The southern Italians also in several districts preserve strips of the meat by drying them in the sun."

On the 6th February, 1868, a memorable "Banquet Hippophagique" was given at the Langham Hotel, under the auspices of Mr. Bicknell. The *menu* began with

"Le consommé de cheval à l'A, B, C,"

and after comprising in appropriate order a full list of choice-sounding dishes, derived from various parts of the horse, or prepared with " huile hippophagique," ended with

"BUFFET."

" Collared horse-head.   Baron of horse.   Boiled withers."

Notwithstanding this example, horse-flesh must still be spoken of as constituting in England only canine food.

According to Pliny, the Romans at one time ate the *Ass.* The wild ass is still in much esteem among the Persians, who consider it as equal to venison.[5] One thousand donkeys and two thousand mules are reported to have been eaten in Paris during the siege.[16] The flesh of the latter is delicious, and far superior to beef; roast mule is, in fact, an exquisite dish[37] (p. 140). Ass's flesh forms the basis of the renowned sausages of Bologna[37] (p. 36).

At a banquet given by an Academician in Paris, having MM. Velpeau, Tardieu, Latour, and other notabilities as guests, the "bifticks" and " filets " prepared from the flesh of an old she-ass were unanimously pronounced, it is stated, to be more tender, succulent, and delicate than similar plats prepared, for comparison, from the horse[37] (April 8, 1865).

The *Collared Pecari,* or *Tajacu* (*Dicotyles torquatus*), an inhabitant of South America, is considered good eating, and its flesh greatly resembles pork. *Dicotyles labiatus* is also hunted by the natives of South America for food,[4] but the aborigines of the Amazon, who eat *Dicotyles torquatus,* will not touch *Dicotyles labiatus*[3] (p. 485).

The *Elephant* is eaten in Abyssinia and other parts of Africa, also in Sumatra.[5] Some steaks that were cut off Chunee, the elephant that was shot at Exeter Change, on being cooked were declared to be "pleasant meat."[6] The three elephants that were eaten in Paris during the siege were pronounced a great success. The liver was considered finer than that of any goose or duck[14] (February 1, 1871). Dr. Livingstone writes: "We had the foot cooked for breakfast next morning, and found it delicious. It is a whitish mass, slightly gelatinous and sweet, like marrow. A long march, to prevent biliousness, is a wise precaution after a meal of elephant's foot. Elephant's trunk and tongue are also good, and after long simmering much resemble the hump of a buffalo and the tongue of an ox; but all the other meat is tough, and from its peculiar flavor only to be eaten by a hungry man"[34] (p. 169).

Rhinoceros is eaten in Abyssinia, and by some of the Dutch settlers in the Cape Colony, and is in high esteem[4] (p. 92).

The *Tapir.*—The North American Indian compares the flesh of the tapir to beef.[5] Although much esteemed it is considered by the inhabitants of South America to be inferior to beef.[60]

The flesh of the *Hippopotamus* supplies a substantial meal to the African, and when young is delicate, but when old is coarse, fat and strong, being inferior to beef.[5] The young meat is much esteemed by the Hottentots and natives of Abyssinia.[4] Dr. Livingstone writes: "The hippopotamus-hunters form a separate people, called Akombwi or Mapodzo, and rarely—the women, it is said, never—intermarry with any other tribe. The reason for their keeping aloof from certain of the natives on the Zambesi is obvious enough, some having as great an abhorrence of hippopotamus-meat as Mahommedans have of swine's flesh"[34] (p. 39). The hippopotamus that was killed and partly burnt in the fire at the Crystal Palace, a few years back, was eaten by Dr. Crisp and some of his friends, who reported that the flavor of the flesh was excellent, and its color whiter than any veal[14] (vol. i., p. 240).

The *Earth Hog* (*Orycteropus Capensis*) is a native of the Cape of Good Hope. Although its food (ants) gives its flesh a strong taste of formic acid, it is relished both by the Hottentots and Europeans. The hind quarter is especially esteemed when cured as ham.[4]

The *Armadillo* is eaten in South America, and its flesh is fat and excellent.* The hunters roast it in its shell.*

Sloths are eaten by the natives of Australia¹² (vol. ii., p. 250).

The *entrails* of animals are consumed by the natives of Australia¹⁶ (p. 67), and the Hottentots consider them to be most exquisite eating¹⁵ (pp. 47, 200). Dr. Livingstone writes: "It is curious that this is the part that wild animals always begin with, and that it is also the first choice of our men"¹⁴ (p. 194).

The *Zulus* are so fond of *carrion*, or decomposed flesh with worms in it, that, according to a letter of Bishop Colenso, published in the *Times*, they use their word (ubomi) representing it as a synonym for their highest notion of happiness¹⁶ (p. 424. October, 1872).

The *Cuckoo* is not an uncommon dish on the Continent, and the Arabs consider it a great delicacy.*

Parrots and *Cockatoos* are eaten by the natives of Australia¹² (vol. ii., p. 250), and the flesh of parrots, when young, is delicate and largely eaten in Brazil.* *Toucans* are eaten by the aborigines of the Amazon* (p. 485), and in Brazil.*

The *Ostrich* affords an abundant banquet to many savage nations of Africa, where it is sometimes kept in a tame state for breeding.* Dr. Livingstone writes that the flesh is white and coarse. When in good condition it in some degree resembles that of a turkey⁴⁰ (p. 156), but the flesh is only good when young, for when it is full-grown the bird is very fat.* Three ostriches were eaten in Paris during the siege.¹⁰

The *Spotted Crake*, or speckled water-hen, is highly esteemed in France for the flavor of its flesh, and few birds can match it in autumn as a rich morsel for the table.*

The *Crane* was eaten by the Romans (Horace, Epod. ii.), and it is mentioned in England as being served up as a sumptuous dish at splendid entertainments as early as the Norman Conquest, and as late as the reign of Henry VIII. At the Enthronization Feast of George Nevil, Archbishop of York, 6 Edward IV., there were 204 cranes, 204 bitterns, and 400 heronshaws¹⁵ (vol. ii., p. 171).

The *Bustard* is good eating, and much esteemed in some places.*

The *Albatross* is eaten by the aborigines of New Zealand* (vol. iii., p. 447); its eggs are considered excellent.*

The *Cormorant.*—The Manx, like the Scotch, make a rich soup out of the blood of this bird¹² (vol. ii., p. 220).

The flesh of the *Gull* is indifferent eating, but it is often brought to market in Roman Catholic countries during Lent.* The eggs of the *Xema ridibunda* are well flavored, and the young birds were at one time in high repute in this country at the tables of the wealthy.*

The *Pea-fowl* is occasionally eaten, and its flesh is reputed to be good, but the beauty of the peacock's plumage renders it too valuable a bird to form an ordinary article of food. In olden times the peacock occupied its place at the table as one of the dishes in the second course at every great feast.

The *Pelican* is eaten by the natives of Australia¹² (vol. ii., p. 251).

Penguins are eaten by the aborigines of New Zealand* (vol. iii., p. 447).

Swans were eaten by the ancients, and often appeared of old at great banquets in England. They are eaten by the natives of Australia¹² (vol.

---

ii., p. 251), and the flesh of the cygnet, which is said to have a flavor resembling both the goose and the hare, is still considered a delicacy in
Europe.'

Birds' Nests of a special kind are an article of food much prized in
China, on account of the nutritive properties which they are supposed to
possess. They are of a gelatinous nature, and chiefly used for making
soup. They are furnished by several species of swallow, and are found
in the caverns on the sea-shore of the Eastern Archipelago. It has been
ascertained that they in great part consist of a peculiar mucus which this
bird secretes and discharges from its mouth in great abundance. The
nests adhere to the rock, and are collected after the young are fledged,
with the help of ladders or ropes. The cleansing of the nests for the
markets is a long and tedious process, and a number of persons are employed at Canton in conducting the operation" (p. 162). The prepared
article, which has the appearance of dried gelatinous-looking fragments,
is to be purchased in some of the London shops.

Lizards are eaten by the Chinese' (vol. iii., p. 761), the Bushmen' (p.
38), and the natives of Australia" (vol. ii., p. 250).

The *Iguana* inhabits South America and the West Indies, where it
is esteemed a delicate food,' although it has been usually considered
unwholesome" (vol. ix., p. 724). Its eggs are nutritious and agreeable." *Amblyrhynchus*, a genus of lizard resembling the iguana, found
in the Galapagos Islands, is esteemed by the natives a delicate kind of
food.'

The crested *Basilisk*, which is upwards of three feet in length, is eaten
by the inhabitants of Amboyna and the islands of the Indian Archipelago.
Its flesh is as white and delicate as that of a chicken.'

Snakes are eaten by the Chinese,' the natives of Australia" (vol. ii., p.
250), and by those of many other countries, but the flesh is reckoned
unwholesome, and liable to occasion leprosy' (p. 197). A nutritious
broth for invalids is made, in some places, from the flesh of the poisonous
viper" (vol. ix., p. 724).

Land *Tortoises* are eaten by the natives of the Amazon' (p. 485), of
India,' of South Africa," and by the North American Indians" (part 1,
p. 65). Payen considers the flesh of the tortoise a wholesome food," and
Dr. Livingstone found it a very agreeable dish" (p. 135). It is said to
resemble veal."

The flesh of the Marine *Turtle* is largely eaten and highly esteemed
where the animal is captured, besides yielding in this country the choicest
of soups.

The Fresh Water *Turtle* abounds in the marshes of Provence, on the
shores of the Rhone, and in Sardinia," and is eaten by the inhabitants,
as it is by the natives of Australia" (vol. ii., p. 250). The flesh of the
Trionyx Ferox is considered very delicate food, and on the coasts of
North America it is angled for with a hook and line baited with small
fish.'

The *Crocodile* is eaten and relished by the natives of parts of Africa'
(p. 379) and Australia.' Dr. Livingstone writes: "To us the idea of
tasting the musky-scented, fishy-looking flesh carried the idea of cannibalism." " (p. 452). The eggs are dug out of the ground and devoured
by the natives. Dr. Livingstone says of them: "In taste they resemble
hens' eggs, with perhaps a smack of custard, and would be as highly rel-

ished by whites as by blacks, were it not for their unsavory origin in men-eaters" " (p. 443).

Frogs are eaten by the Chinese" (vol. iii., p. 761), the natives of Australia[12] (vol. ii., p. 250), and many other countries. The *Rana esculenta* is highly prized in France for its hind legs, which form the part eaten, and these may be seen sometimes skewered together in the windows of some of the provision establishments in Paris.

Attempts have been made at different times to acclimatize the *Rana esculenta* in England, and apparently with some success in Cambridgeshire, where it is said their very remarkable and sonorous croak has procured for them the name of the " Cambridgeshire nightingales" [21] (vol. x., pp. 483, 520). The *Rana taurina*, or bull-frog, is a native of North America, and is thought by the Americans to rival turtle" (vol. ix., p. 724). This large eatable frog has been recently introduced into France by the Société d'Acclimatisation.[37] A large frog called *Matlamětlo* is eaten by the South Africans, which, when cooked, looks like a chicken[46] (p. 42).

The *Toad* is eaten by the negroes" (p. 439), and a species called *Rana bombina* is eaten in some places like a fish" (vol. ix.).

The *Axolotl* of Mexico is esteemed an agreeable article of food, dressed like stewed eels.[4]

The *Mud Eel* (Lepidosiren) is eaten by the natives of the river Gambia. It has a rich, oily flavor, and when fried tastes like an eel.[5]

The flesh of the *Sword-fish* (*Ziphias platypterus* of Shaw) was known in early times as an article of food, and its fame is not undeserved. The flesh near the vertebræ is pale salmon-colored, and any epicure of fish might be recommended to try a cutlet from it. Lower down it is red and like coarse beef" (new series, vol. vii., 1873, p. 32).

A species of *Scarus*, or parrot-fish, was highly esteemed by the Roman epicures, and the Greeks still consider it to be a fish of exquisite flavor. [4]

Sharks are eaten by the Gold Coast negroes" (pp. 220, 224) and the natives of New Zealand[11] (vol. ii., p. 43), but not by the natives of Western Australia.[5] The natives of the Polynesian Islands feast on them in a raw state, and gorge themselves so as to occasion vomiting.[5]

Dr. Hector writes as follows of edible sharks: "The Maoris are large consumers of sharks, or mango, as they term them, of various species, but chiefly the Smooth-hound (*Mustellus antarcticus*), Dog-fish of two species (*Scyllium laticeps* and *Acanthias vulgaris*), and the Tope (*Galeus canis*). All of these may be seen at certain seasons, at any Maori settlement by the sea-side, hanging on poles to dry in thousands, and rendering the neighborhood extremely unpleasant. The species most valued is, however, the smooth-hound, which is the only shark that is properly edible, as it lives on shell-fish and crabs, and has the same clean-feeding habits as the skate. In the Hebrides and north of Scotland the flesh of this harmless little shark is considered to be a great delicacy, but I have never heard of its being eaten by the white settlers in the colony" [46] (p. 120). The fins of sharks are highly prized by the wealthy Chinese" (p. 551).

Spiders are eaten by the Bushmen, and by the inhabitants of New Caledonia[5] (p. 315).

Several species of *Beetles* are eaten by women of different nations, in the belief that they will cause them to grow fat and become prolific in childbearing.

The *Blaps sulcata* is eaten, cooked with butter, by the Egyptian women,' who also eat the *Scarabæus sacer* to make themselves become prolific" (vol. iii., p. 129). The women of Arabia and Turkey eat a species of tenebrio fried in butter, to make themselves plump" (vol. iii.).

Grasshoppers are eaten by the Bushmen' (p. 38).

Locusts are eaten in great quantities, both fresh and salted" (vol. ix., p. 727). They have a strongly vegetable taste, the flavor varying with the plants on which they feed. Dr. Livingstone considered them palatable when roasted" (p. 42). They are eaten by the Persians, Egyptians, and Arabians," the Bushmen,' and North American Indians" (part 1, p. 65), and by many others. Diodorus Siculus and Ludolphus both refer to a race of people in Æthiopia supporting themselves upon locusts." Ludolphus remarks: " For it is a very sweet and wholesome sort of dyet, by means of which a certain Portuguez garrison in India, that was ready to yield for want of provision, held out till it was relieved another way." Madden states in his " Travels ": " The Arabs make a sort of bread of locusts. They dry them and grind them to powder, then mix this powder with water, forming them into round cakes, which serve for bread."

White Ants are eaten by the natives of Australia" (vol. ii., p. 250), and by those on the banks of the Zonga, where they are highly appreciated" (p. 465).

Bees are eaten by various peoples " (vol. iii.), and the Moors in West Barbary esteem the honeycomb, with young bees in it, as delicious; but by one witness it has been spoken of as insipid to his palate, and as having sometimes given him heartburn" (vol. ix., p. 727).

Moths of several varieties are eaten by the natives of Australia" (vol. ii., p. 250); one species, called *Bugong*, is said to be more prized by the Australian than any other sort of food. The bodies of these insects, it is stated, are large, and contain a quantity of oil; they are sought after as a luscious and fattening food." "

The *Cicada*, an insect of the homopterous group, was eaten by the Greeks,' and Pinto mentions a people who used *Flies* as an article of food."

The *Larvæ of Ants* are eaten by the Bushmen' (p. 38). Scopoli speaks of the larvæ of the *Musca putris* as a dainty." Ælian mentions the circumstance of an Indian king treating some of his Grecian guests with the larvæ of an insect instead of food." The larvæ of the *Cerambyx heros* is believed to be the Cossus of the ancients, by whom it was considered a great dainty.'

Caterpillars were eaten by the ancient Romans, and are in high estimation among the natives of South Africa" " (p. 42).

Grubs of all kinds are eaten by the natives of Australia" " (p. 67), and the *chrysalis* of the *Silkworm* is eaten by the Chinese."

The *Cuttlefish* is used as food in some parts of Europe;' and a bivalve allied to the oyster, called *Anomia ephippium*, which is found on the coasts of the Mediterranean, is considered not inferior to the common oyster."

The *Vineyard Snail* (*Helix pomatia*) is used as food in many parts of

Europe during Lent.⁴ It is reared and fattened with great care in some cantons in Switzerland as an article of luxury, and exported in a pickled state. Many other snails are eaten by the poor, and none are known to be hurtful³⁹ (vol. ix., p. 727). The common *Garden Snail* (*Helix aspersa*) is used in some parts as a cure for diseases of the chest.⁴ Snails on the Continent, and even slugs in China, have a reputation for delicacy of eating and nutritive power.⁴⁰

The common *Sea-Urchin*, or sea-egg (*Echinus sphœra*), is much sought after as food in some parts of Europe during the latter part of summer, at which time it is almost filled with eggs.⁴ It is also eaten by the inhabitants of Otaheite⁴ (vol. ii., p. 154).

Holothuriœ (sea-cucumbers) are eaten largely by the Chinese,⁴ the natives of the Indian Archipelago,⁴ the Australian⁴ and South Sea Islands⁴⁷ (vol. ii., p. 568). They are also taken on the coast of Naples and eaten by the poorer inhabitants.⁴

Earth-eating may be appropriately referred to here, as some kinds of earth used as food in certain localities have been found to consist in part of the remains of minute animal organisms.

Humboldt, on his return from the Rio Negro, saw a tribe of Ottomacs who lived principally during the rainy season upon a fat, unctuous clay which they found in their district⁴⁴ (pp. 143–4). This appears to have consisted of a red, earthy matter (hydrous silicate of alumina) called *bole*. It is also eaten by the Japanese after being made into thin cakes called *tanaampo*, which are exposed for sale, and bought by the women to give themselves slenderness of form.⁴ Ehrenberg found that this earth consisted for the most part of the remains of microscopic animals and plants which had been deposited from fresh water.

A kind of earth known as *bread-meal*, which consists, for the most part, of the empty shells of minute infusorial animalcules, is still largely eaten in Northern Europe; and a similar substance, called *mountain-meal*, has been used in Northern Germany in times of famine as a means of staying hunger. The Wanyamwezi, a tribe living in Central Africa, eat clay in the intervals between meals, and prefer the clay of ant-hills¹³ (vol. ii., p. 28). The colored inhabitants of Sierra Leone also devour the red earth of which the ant-hills are composed⁴⁴ (vol. xix., p. 72). Johnston asserts that the African earth did not injure the negroes, but that when they were carried as slaves to the West India Islands they were found to suffer in their health from the clay they there used as a substitute⁴⁴ (vol. ii., p. 201).

It has been found that much of the clay eaten by many of the inhabitants of the torrid zone is mere dirt, and has no alimentary value. The Agmara Indians eat a whitish clay, which is rather gritty, and has been shown by careful analysis to be destitute of any organic matter which might afford nutriment⁴⁴ (vol. i., p. 370). One of the earliest notices of the practice of dirt-eating is given by Sir Samuel Argoll, with respect to Virginia, in 1613. "In this journie," he says, "I likewise found a myne, of which I have sent a triall into England; and likewise a strange kind of earth, the virtue whereof I know not, but the Indians eate it for Physicke, alleging that it cureth the sicknesse and paine of the belly." ⁴⁷ In Guinea the negroes eat a yellowish earth called *cavuac*. In the West Indies a white clay like tobacco-pipe clay is eaten, and this the eaters prefer to spirits or tobacco⁴⁸ (vol. vii., p. 550). In 1751 a species of red earth, or yellowish tufa, is reported to have been still secretly sold in the markets of Martinique.[14]

So widely spread is the depraved appetite for dirt-eating, or "geophagie," that it is alleged to be one of the chief endemic disorders of all tropical America. The victims of the practice never appear to be able to free themselves from the habit. Children, it is said, acquire it almost from the breast, and "women, as they lie in bed sleepless and restless, will pull out pieces of mud from the adjoining walls of their rooms to gratify their strange appetite, or will soothe a squalling brat by tempting it with a lump of the same material."[80] Officers who have Indian or half-bred children in their employ as servants sometimes have to use wire masks to keep them from putting the clay into their mouths.[81] A negro addicted to this propensity is considered to be irrevocably lost for any useful purpose, and seldom lives long[88] (vol. vii., p. 550). It is impossible to keep the victim from obtaining the injurious substance. Children who commence the practice early frequently decline and die in two or three years, and dropsy usually appears to be the prominent cause of dissolution. In other cases they may live to middle age, but sooner or later dysentery supervenes, and proves fatal. Dr. Galt speaks of having himself seen a Mestize soldier sinking from dysentery with a lump of clay stuffed in his sunken cheeks half an hour before his death.[82]

KEY TO THE REFERENCE NUMBERS CONTAINED IN THE PRECEDING PAGES ON EXCEPTIONAL ANIMAL FOODS.

[1] Bowring (Sir John), The Population of China. (Statistical Society's Journal, vol. xx., pp. 41–53.)
[2] Wallace (A. R.), Narrative of Travels on the Amazon and Rio Negro. London, 1843.
[3] Simmonds (P. L.), The Curiosities of Food ; or, the Dainties and Delicacies of Different Nations obtained from the Animal Kingdom. London, 1859.
[4] Baird (W.), Cyclopædia of the Natural Sciences. London, 1858.
[5] Webster (T.), An Encyclopædia of Domestic Economy. London, 1844.
[6] Daumas (General), The Horses of the Sahara and the Manners of the Desert. Translated by James Hutton. London, 1863.
[7] Lyon (G. F.), A Narrative of Travels in North Africa in 1818–20. London, 1821.
[8] Burton (R. F.), The City of the Saints, and Across the Rocky Mountains to California. London, 1861.
[9] Cook's (Captain) First Voyage. (Hawkesworth's Voyages, 3 vols. London, 1773.)
[10] Sheppard (N.), Shut up in Paris. London, 1871.
[11] Dieffenbach (E.), Travels in New Zealand. 2 vols. London, 1843.
[12] Eyre (E. J.), Journal of Expeditions of Discovery into Central Australia in 1840–41. 2 vols. London, 1845.
[13] Burton (R. F.), The Lake Regions of Central Africa : a Picture of Exploration. 2 vols. London, 1860.
[14] Food Journal. London.
[15] Wilkes (C.), Narrative of the United States Exploring Expedition, 1838–42. 5 vols. London, 1845.
[16] Dawson, (R.), Present State of Australia. 1830.
[17] Hind (H. Y.), Explorations in the Interior of the Labrador Peninsula. 2 vols. London, 1863.
[18] Sproat (G. M.), Scenes and Studies of Savage Life. London, 1868.
[19] Lubbock (Sir John), Prehistoric Times, as Illustrated by Ancient Remains, and the Manners and Customs of Modern Savages. London, 1869.
[20] Kane (E. K.), Arctic Explorations: the Second Grinnell Expedition in Search of Sir John Franklin, 1853–55. 2 vols. Philadelphia, 1856.
[21] Thunberg (C. P.), Travels in Europe, Africa, and Asia, 1770–79. 4 vols. London, 1795.
[22] Richardson (Sir John), Arctic Searching Expedition. 2 vols. London, 1851.

[23] Schoolcraft (H. R.), Historical and Statistical Information Respecting the History, Condition, and Prospects of Indian Tribes of the United States. 3 vols. Philadelphia, 1851–53.

[24] Sullivan (E.), Rambles and Scrambles in North and South America. London, 1852.

[25] Marsden (W.), The History of Sumatra. London.

[26] Catlin (G.), Letters on North American Indians. 2 vols. 1842.

[27] Tennent (Sir Emerson), Ceylon: an Account of the Island, Physical, Historical, and Topographical. 2 vols. London, 1859.

[28] Wrangell (F. von), Narrative of an Expedition to the Polar Sea in 1820–23. Edited by Lieut.-Col. Edward Sabine. London, 1844.

[29] Barrow (Sir John), Travels in China. London, 1806.

[30] Journal of the Society of Arts. London.

[31] Head (Sir F. B.), Journeys across the Pampas. 1828.

[32] Medical Times and Gazette. London.

[33] Sarcey (F.), Paris during the Siege. London, 1871.

[34] Livingstone (Dr.), Narrative of an Expedition to the Zambesi and its Tributaries, 1858–64. London, 1865.

[35] Kolben (P.), Present State of the Cape of Good Hope. London, 1731.

[36] Quarterly Review. London.

[37] Payen (A.), Précis Théorique et Pratique des Substances Alimentaires. Paris, 1865.

[38] The Lancet. London.

[39] Encyclopædia Britannica. Seventh Edition. 21 vols. Edinburgh. 1842.

[40] Livingstone (Dr.), Missionary Travels and Researches in South Africa. London, 1857.

[41] Archæologia. Published by the Society of Antiquaries. London.

[42] Teignmouth (Lord), Sketches of the Coasts and Islands of Scotland and the Isle of Man. 2 vols. London, 1836.

[43] Loskiel (G. H.), History of the Mission of the United Brethren among the Indians in North America. 3 parts. London, 1794.

[44] Simpson (Sir George), Narrative of a Journey Round the World during the Years 1841 and 1842. 2 vols. London, 1847.

[45] Fishes of New Zealand : Notes on the Edible Fishes. By James Hector, Geological Survey Department. Wellington, 1872.

[46] Letheby (Dr.), On Food : Cantor Lectures. London, 1870.

[47] Scherzer (K.), Narrative of the Circumnavigation of the Globe in the Austrian Frigate " Novara" in 1857–59. 3 vols. London, 1861–63.

[48] Transactions of the Entomological Society. London.

[49] Andrews of Wyntown.—The Orygynal Cronykil of Scotland. With Notes by David Macpherson. 2 vols. London, 1795.

[50] Robert Lindsay of Pitscottie.—The Chronicles of Scotland. Edited by J. G. Dalyell. Edinburgh, 1814.

[51] Chambers (R.), The Book of Days. 2 vols. Edinburgh.

[52] Chambers' Encyclopædia. 10 vols. London, 1868.

[53] Turner (Rev. George), Nineteen Years in Polynesia. London, 1861.

[54] Humboldt (Alexander von), Views of Nature. Translated by E. C. Otté and H. G. Bohn. London, 1850.

[55] Journal of the Statistical Society. London.

[56] Johnston (J. F. W.), Chemistry of Common Life. Revised by G. H. Lewes. 2 vols. London, 1859.

[57] Argoll (Sir Samuel), Touching his Voyage to Virginia, 1613. (Purchas his Pilgrimes, vol. iv., p. 1765.)

[58] Encyclopædia Metropolitana. 25 vols. London, 1845.

[59] Galt (Dr.), Medical Notes of the Upper Amazon. Published in the American Journal of the Medical Sciences, and quoted in the Lancet, December 14, 1872.

[60] Forsyth (J. S.), Dictionary of Diet. London, 1835.

[61] Nature. A Weekly Periodical. London.

[62] Transactions of Royal Society of Arts and Sciences. Mauritius.

VEGETABLE ALIMENTARY SUBSTANCES.

Although vegetable substances differ so much physically, and in some respects, also, chemically, from the components of animal beings, they are susceptible of conversion into these components, and, alone, contain all that is absolutely requisite for the support of animal life. A more complex elaborating system, however, is required to fit them for appropriation than is the case with animal substances, and accordingly it is found that the digestive organs of the herbivora are developed upon a larger and higher scale than those of the carnivora.

The vegetable products that form even common articles of food are exceedingly varied and numerous. To attempt to arrange them under any strict classification would only lead to embarrassment, and often involve practical inconvenience. It will be sufficient for the purposes of description to distribute them into the following general group: farinaceous seeds; oleaginous seeds; tubers and roots; herbaceous articles; saccharine and farinaceous preparations.

FARINACEOUS SEEDS.

These rank first in importance amongst vegetable alimentary products. They are alike plentifully yielded, of easy digestion, and of high nutritive value. It is not surprising, therefore, to find that the farinaceous seeds form the largest and the most widely consumed portion of our vegetable food. Of the farinaceous seeds, those, as wheat, oats, barley, rye, rice, maize or Indian corn, etc., derived from the *Cerealia*—a tribe of grasses— take the first place as articles of food; and next follow those derived from the *Leguminosæ*, or pulse tribe, as, for instance, peas, beans, and lentils. Some other farinaceous seeds will be mentioned as employed, but they are of far less significance in an alimentary point of view.

THE CEREALIA.

The various cereal grains agree in their genera. composition, but differences exist in the relative amounts of the constituent principles, which give them different degrees of alimentary value.

The principles enumerated are:

First.—Nitrogenous compounds, consisting of glutine, albumen, caseine, and fibrine, with an active principle, chiefly encountered in the cortical part of the grain, which, like diastase, possesses the power of converting starch into sugar. The material known as gluten, as will be more particularly mentioned farther on, comprises a mixture of glutine, caseine, and fibrine.

Second.—Non-nitrogenous substances, as starch, dextrine, sugar, and cellulose.

Third.—Fatty matter, including a volatile oil, which constitutes the source of the odorous quality possessed by the grain.

Fourth.—Mineral substances, comprising phosphates of lime and magnesia, salts of potash and soda, and silica.

The following table represents the relative amounts of the constituent principles contained in various kinds of grain in a dry state, according to the analyses of Payen: *

---

* Substances Alimentaires, p. 265. Paris, 1865.

Composition of Various Cereal Grains in a Dry State * (Payen).

	Hard wheat. Venezuela.	Hard wheat. Africa.	Hard wheat. Taganrog.	Semi-hard wheat. Brie.	White or soft wheat. Tuzelle.
Nitrogenous matter, . . .	22.75	19.50	20.00	15.25	12.65
Starch, ...	58.62	65.07	63.80	70.05	76.51
Dextrine, etc., ...	9.50	7.60	8.00	7.00	6.05
Cellulose, ...	3.50	3.00	3.10	3.00	2.80
Fatty matter, ...	2.61	2.12	2.25	1.95	1.87
Mineral matter, . . .	3.02	2.71	2.85	2.75	2.12
	100.00	100.00	100.00	100.00	100.00 †

	Rye.	Barley.	Oats.	Maize.	Rice.
Nitrogenous matter, . . .	12.50	12.96	14.39	12.50	7.55
Starch, ...	64.65	66.43	60.59	67.55	88.65
Dextrine, etc., ...	14.90	10.00	9.25	4.00	1.00
Cellulose, ...	3.10	4.75	7.06	5.90	1.10
Fatty matter, ...	2.25	2.76	5.50	8.80	0.80
Mineral matter, . . .	2.60	3.10	3.25	1.25	0.90
	100.00	100.00	100.00 ‡	100.00	100.00

It will be seen from the preceding table that different kinds of wheat differ considerably in composition, and particularly so in the amount of nitrogenous matter and starch they contain, the two standing in an inverse ratio to each other. But more will be said regarding this farther on. Oats are rich in nitrogenous matter, fat, and salts. Maize contains a fair amount of nitrogenous matter, but is poor in salts. It further stands out from all the rest by virtue of the large amount of fatty matter present. Barley occupies a mean position with reference to all the constituents. Rice is characterized by richness in starch and poorness in nitrogenous matter, fatty matter, and salts. The knowledge thus supplied is of considerable value in relation to the employment of the several kinds of grain as articles of food.

WHEAT.—Wheat may be said to form the most useful article of vegetable food, and hence it is one of the most extensively and widely cultivated of the cereal grains.

As supplied for use, wheat consists of the grain deprived of the husk with which it was originally invested. Each grain is composed of a hard, colored, tegumentary portion, and a central, easily pulverizable, white substance, which yields the product constituting flour.

---

* In an ordinary state grain contains from 11 to 18 per cent. of water.
† Deviation from the correct total of + 2.0. Possibly an error in the amount of the starch.
‡ Deviation from the correct total of + 0.04.
10

The tegumentary portion consists, externally, of an exceedingly hard layer, which is of a dense, ligneous nature, and so coherent that it presents itself under the form of scales when wheat is subjected to the ordinary process of grinding. This constitutes the greater bulk of bran, and is of a perfectly indigestible nature, and, therefore, useless as an article of nutrition. Moreover, it acts, to some extent, as an irritant to the alimentary canal, and thus, whilst of service, retained with the flour, in cases where constipation exists, it should be avoided in irritable states of the bowel, and also by those who work hard, for with these it is liable to hurry the food too quickly through the alimentary tract, and occasion waste by promoting its escape without undergoing digestion and absorption.

Farther in, the cortex is softer and more friable. This part goes with the pollard obtained in the process of dressing flour. It forms the portion of the grain which is the richest in nitrogenous matter, fat, and salts. It possesses, therefore, a high alimentary value. Amongst the nitrogenous matter in this situation, a peculiar soluble, active principle is contained, called *cerealine*, which resembles diastase in being endowed with the power of converting starch into sugar.

Cerealine has been represented as leading, by a metamorphosing influence exerted during the occurrence of fermentation, to the development of the dark color and marked taste belonging to brown bread; and it is said that if the bread be made in such a way that the cerealine is not afforded the opportunity of exerting this action, the product, although derived from the external as well as the central part of the grain, has neither the high color nor the strong taste of ordinary brown bread.

The central white substance of the grain is chiefly composed of starch; but nitrogenous, fatty, and saline matters are also all present to some extent. The nitrogenous matter consists of several principles. There is albumen, mucine or caseine, fibrine, and glutine. What is called gluten—the ductile, tenacious, raw material left when flour is kneaded with water, and afterwards washed to remove the starch—does not represent a simple or pure nitrogenous principle. It is called *crude gluten*, and is resolvable into Liebig's vegetable fibrine, mucine, and glutine. The albumen of the flour is not present in it. This latter principle, being soluble in water, is carried away with the starch in the process of washing.

It has been said that the external part of the grain is richer than the central in nitrogenous matter. This remark, however, is not to be taken as applying to gluten. Gluten, indeed, preponderates in the central farinaceous part, the nitrogenous matter of the exterior being principally composed of vegetable fibrine.

It is to gluten—and this exists to a special extent in wheat—that wheaten flour owes its aptitude for being made into bread. This substance, by virtue of its tenacity, and its susceptibility of solidification by heat, is capable of entangling gas generated or incorporated amongst it, and then becoming fixed in such a manner as to furnish a light, spongy, or porous article like well-made bread.

As regards sugar as a constituent of wheaten flour, Payen remarks that, whilst some authorities have affirmed that it is present, others have declared that they have been unable to discover it. On both sides, he says, truth exists, and that it depends on the harvesting, grinding, and keeping of the wheat and flour, whether sugar is present or not. It arises from the action of the diastase-like principle contained in the grain on the starch and dextrine; and according as the circumstances are favorable or unfavorable for the change, so will be the analytical result obtained.

There are several kinds of wheat met with in commerce, and the table given at p. 145 shows that a considerable difference may exist in the chemical composition of the article. The difference depends upon the variety of the plant that has yielded the grain, and also upon the climate and soil where it has grown. What is called hard wheat is the richest in gluten. It is produced in the warm countries of the south, and upon the most fertile soils. The grain is characterized by a horny, semi-transparent appearance and hardness throughout. It is drier, keeps better, and gives a larger amount of product in the mill, but a less white flour, than other kinds of wheat. It is this form of wheat that is employed for making macaroni, vermicelli, and such-like preparations. White or soft wheat presents a more farinaceous condition; it is more easily ground and yields a whiter and finer flour. With less gluten, it contains a larger proportion of starch, and, therefore, forms the most suitable kind of wheat for the extraction of this latter principle as an article for domestic use. It is the intermediate, or semi-hard wheat, which is the best for the use of the baker. In Payen's table the nitrogenous matter in dried wheat ranges, it may be seen, from 12 to 22, and the starch from 58 to 76 per cent.

Wheat is but very rarely used in the entire state as an article of food. It forms, however, a constituent of what is called *frumenty*, which consists of wheat-grains boiled in milk. There is also a Yorkshire dish made with wheat and raisins boiled in milk (Forsyth). For ordinary alimentary purposes wheat is subjected to grinding, and usually afterward separated into flour, pollard, and bran, the flour being appropriated to our use, and the other products employed as food for the lower animals.

Meal is the simple product of grinding, and, therefore, contains all the elements of the grain. It is from this that brown bread is made. If not used in this way (and, as is well known, it is only exceptionally that it is) it is submitted by the miller to bolting, sifting, or dressing, to separate the flour from the coarser particles—forming pollard and sharps; and these, again, from the coarsest of all—forming bran. Flour, also, is produced or "dressed" of different degrees of fineness, to meet the demand of the consumer. The finer the flour is dressed, the whiter the bread that it produces. In fine flour, however, there is an exclusion of everything except the strictly farinaceous central part of the grain; and as this contains the least amount of nitrogenous matter, the eye is gratified at the sacrifice of this material. A coarser flour, although yielding a less white bread, contains a larger proportion of nitrogenous matter, and thus is better adapted to meet our requirements; for, even under all circumstances, the farinaceous element is out of proportion to the nitrogenous, looked at in relation to the demand existing in the case of each for the purposes of life. Processes have been proposed for converting more of the grain into flour than by the ordinary plan of grinding. They are referred to in connection with the subject of bread at p. 149.

Medium wheat usually yields from 72 to 80 per cent. of good flour (Payen), and from about 5 to 10 per cent. of bran. The miller sometimes tries to increase the yield of flour by grinding with the stones set closely, but it is at the expense of the quality of the flour, for the starch-granule becomes thereby bruised and damaged, and it is found to be deteriorated for the purpose of bread-making. Bakers prefer a flour which feels a little harsh between the finger and thumb, instead of soft and smooth.

Composition of Flour.

	From Letheby's table of analyses.	Payen.
Nitrogenous matter, . . .	10.8	14.45
Carbohydrates, ...	70.5	68.48
Fatty matter, ...	2.0	1.25
Mineral matter, ...	1.7	1.60
Water, ...	15.0	14.22
	100.0	100.00

The amount of gluten in wheaten flour, according to Dr. Letheby, ranges from 8 to 15 per cent., the average being about 11.

Cones, or *cones flour,* is the name applied to the flour of a particular species of wheat called *"revet."* It is used by bakers for dusting the dough and the boards upon which the loaves are made, to facilitate the manipulation by preventing adhesion. It appears, from the analyses of Dr. Hassall, to be extensively adulterated with the flour of rice and other cereals, and sometimes even not to contain a particle of wheaten flour. Thus adulterated, it can be sold at a lower price than ordinary flour, and it is not surprising, therefore, that, besides being used for the purpose named, it frequently finds its way into the constitution of the loaf, while it affords an opportunity of adulterating without appearing upon the face of it to do so.

Flour is one of the most useful alimentary materials at our disposal, and is turned to account in a variety of ways. It is not consumed in the raw state. Puddings, pastry, cakes, bread, biscuits, and other variously named articles of less note, are made from it. Bread and biscuits, about which more will be said farther on, are both nutritive and digestible. Cakes, besides flour, contain butter, eggs, sugar, and sometimes other adjuncts. They are rich, and apt to upset the stomach. Pastry, on account of the effect of the oven on the fatty matter present, is also apt to give rise to stomach derangement. Puddings (flour-puddings only are here spoken of) are not objectionable in the same way, but are, nevertheless trying to the digestive powers. Being of a more or less close consistence, they offer considerable resistance to the penetration and action of the gastric juice, and thus may engage the stomach for some time in the process of digestion, and give rise during the while to the sensation which is well known to be occasioned by an indigestible substance, and which is described as a sense of weight or heaviness at the stomach.

Baked flour.—Flour, after exposure to heat, is more digestible than when in the raw state. The starch-granules become ruptured, and a portion of the starch transformed into dextrine. The albumen is acted upon, and converted into the coagulated form. It is hence advantageous that flour should be consumed (as it only is) after having been subjected in some way or other to the influence of heat. It is sometimes prepared for use by simply putting it into a basin, introducing it into an oven, and baking. Another process, acting in a similar way, is to place it in a basin, tie it over with a cloth, and immerse it in a saucepan of water kept boiling for some time. The water does not penetrate, but from the effect of the heat the flour collects into a hard, solid mass, which requires to be scraped or grated for use. Thus prepared, it is often employed as an article of food for infants.

Bread.—Of all articles of vegetable food, bread must be considered as the most important to us. It constitutes a product of art, and amongst all civilized people the process of manufacture is known and put into practice, evidently on account of the favorable state in which the elements of food are placed for undergoing digestion. It is only from some kinds of grain that bread can be made, and no bread is equal to that prepared from wheaten grain. The amount of gluten present, for which this kind of grain is distinguished, gives it the property required for yielding a light and spongy form of bread, and it is to this lightness or sponginess that bread owes its easy digestibility; for, according to its porosity so is the facility with which it is penetrated and acted upon by the secretion of the stomach.

The first requisite toward the manufacture of bread is that the grain should be reduced to a pulverized condition. By the ordinary process it is ground in a whole state and converted into meal. This may be used for making bread—as is the case in what we call " brown bread "—but, as a rule, the flour is separated and this only employed. Other processes have been proposed, with the view of obtaining a larger yield of flour. To some extent the plan has been adopted of decorticating the grain and then reducing the remainder into flour. By such a method some of the inner layers of the tegumentary portion are retained with the farinaceous substance of the centre. There is also " whole-wheat flour " to be obtained. The bran, after separation, is ground and then mixed with the flour, for it does not answer to attempt to thoroughly reduce the whole together. It seems that the starch-granules ought not to be broken up, and that by too much crushing or friction they become damaged, thereby leading to a bad flour for bread-making purposes being produced. When too closely ground, bakers speak of the flour as " killed," from its virtue being found to be partially destroyed. The avowed object of deviating from the old-fashioned plan is to give the flour, and consequently the bread made from it, a higher nutritive value, the outside part of the grain being that which, as previously stated, is richest in nitrogenous, fatty, and mineral matters. Liebig expatiates strongly—particularly on account of the loss of phosphates—upon the ill-judged custom of preferring white bread. It is true, if bread were our sole article of sustenance, the rejection of the principles contained in the outer part of the grain would be a serious error in dietetics; but if other food be taken which furnishes a free supply of them, as is actually the case with a mixed diet, there is nothing to condemn as erroneous. It must not be considered, because we do not consume the bran and pollard of the meal ourselves, that their constituents are thereby wasted or lost to us. Employed, as such articles are, as food for other animals, we may in reality, although indirectly, get their elements in association with other matter. Looked at in this way, it being granted that animal food is taken, we are at liberty, if our inclination so dispose us, without incurring any charge of wastefulness, to select one part of the grain for ourselves and allow the other to pass to the lower animals. Whether the result of habit or not, it must certainly be owned that, with the generality of persons, bread made from ordinary flour is more pleasing to the eye and agreeable to the palate than bread made from the whole constituents of the grain.

Bread is a firm and porous substance, which is easy of mastication, and which, whilst preserving a certain amount of moisture, is not wet or clammy. To convert flour or meal into a substance of this kind constitutes the art of bread-making. A paste or dough is made by manipulation, either by kneading with the hands or by machinery, with the requisite quantity of water. Porosity is given by intimate incorporation with carbonic acid gas—either generated within, as by fermentation, or the use of one or other form of "baking-powder;" or supplied from without, as by Dr. Dauglish's process. The gluten present, by virtue of its tenacity, holds the vesicles of gas and allows a spongy mass to be formed. Whilst in this state, solidification is effected by the aid of heat applied in the process of baking, and thus is formed a permanently vesiculated or porous article. Such, in a few words, constitutes the rationale of the process of bread-making.

When the carbonic acid gas is generated by fermentation, the product is called "leavened bread," but there is no material difference between bread formed in this way and that produced by the other processes. Various kinds of ferment are employed, as, for instance, brewer's yeast or barm; German yeast; baker's or patent yeast, which is prepared from an infusion of malt and hops set into fermentation by a little brewer's or German yeast, and added to some boiled and mashed potatoes mixed with flour, to feed the growth of the ferment and increase the product; or leaven, which is old dough in a state of fermentation. In each case the active agent of the ferment—that is, the growing vegetable cells forming the yeast-fungus, or *Torula cerevisiæ*—effects the conversion of sugar into alcohol and carbonic acid gas. This takes place at the expense of the sugar contained in, and derived from, the starch of the flour, but in baker's yeast the potato introduced furnishes additional material for the growth of the *Torula*. Used in this way, the potato is not to be looked upon in the light of an adulterant.

The usual practice in making bread by fermentation is to mix a certain quantity of the flour with the ferment, some salt, and lukewarm water. These are kneaded into a stiff paste or dough, which is placed aside in a warm situation for an hour or two. The mass gradually swells up from the evolution of carbonic acid gas, or, as the baker terms it, the *sponge* rises. When the sponge is in active fermentation it is thoroughly kneaded with the remainder of the flour, salt, and water, and again set aside for a few hours in a warm situation. Fermentation extends throughout the whole, and at the proper moment the dough is made into loaves and introduced into the oven. Herein constitutes some of the chief points in the baker's art. Unless fermentation has been allowed to proceed far enough, a heavy loaf is the result; and if allowed to proceed too far, an objectionable quality is given to the bread by the commencement of another, viz., the acid fermentation. Time also must not be allowed for the dough to sink before being made into loaves and baked. Under the influence of the heat of the oven an expansion of the entangled vesicles of gas ensues, and occasions a considerable further rising of the dough; and with the subsequent setting of the substance of the loaf a permanently vesiculated mass is formed.

A special aroma or flavor is communicated to the bread by the different kinds of ferment. The best flavored bread, I am informed by an experienced West-end baker, is made with the employment of brewer's yeast.

Instead of by fermentation, vesiculation may be effected by carbonic acid gas disengaged by incorporating carbonate of soda or ammonia with the dough, and adding muriatic, tartaric, or phosphoric acid. "Baking-powders" act in this way, and consist for the most part of tartaric acid and carbonate of soda as their basis. The employment of this process involves no loss of any portion of the flour, but it does not produce an agreeably tasted bread, and has not been therefore found to supersede the old process of fermentation.

Another plan for vesiculating bread has been recently introduced, and is known as Dr. Dauglish's process, the product being called "aërated bread." The flour is introduced into a strong, air-tight iron receiver, and afterward mixed by mechanical means with water impregnated with carbonic acid gas under a high pressure. Through an opening below, which can be enclosed when the operation of mixing is complete, the dough is forced out by the pressure existing within, and with a suitable contrivance may be received and conveyed, under the form of loaves, to the oven, without being touched by the hands. Vesiculation is produced by the expansion of the carbonic acid gas with which the dough is throughout intimately incorporated—such expansion occurring with the removal of the pressure; and, still further, from exposure to the heat of the oven. This process, it will be seen, involves the employment only of the three essential ingredients of bread—flour, water, and carbonic acid gas; but, as with other kinds of bread, some salt is also added. Nothing occurs to produce a change of any portion of the flour, except such as is induced by the action of the heat in baking. The product represents the purest form of bread, if simplicity of composition is to be taken as a criterion. As regards taste, however, it possesses, without there being anything objectionable, a distinct character of its own, and there is an absence of the agreeable flavor belonging to good bread of the fermented kind. It may be remarked that it keeps sweet and good much longer than fermented bread.

In the manufacture of bread a certain amount of salt is generally added. It improves the flavor, and gives greater whiteness and firmness to the article.

Alum, also, if it is not now, owing to the stringency of a recent Act of Parliament, was formerly frequently employed; but this constitutes an imposition, for the object of its use is to cause bread made from bad or deteriorated flour to resemble that made from good. It affords no advantage in the case of good flour, but enables bread to be made from flour that could not otherwise be used. It checks, it is said, an excess of fermentation, to which there is a tendency with bad flour; augments the whiteness of the product; and, by strengthening—that is, giving increased consistence or tenacity to—the gluten, favors the production of a light and firm loaf. Such are described as the effects of alum on bread; but the question may be asked: Is such bread to be considered as wholesome? In the first place, alum, or whatever it may be changed into or whatever the combination formed with the flour under the agency of the heat employed in baking, is not a natural article for ingestion. Its properties are not such as to be likely to occasion any immediate or strong effect, and it cannot be said that a deleterious action is to be brought home to it in a precise or definite manner; but it is believed to be capable of producing dyspepsia and constipation. "Whatever doubts," says Pereira,* "may be entertained regarding the ill effects of alum on the healthy stomach, none can exist as to its injurious influence in cases of dyspepsia." It is possible, where ill effects have been assigned to alum, that they may have been sometimes due to the bad quality of the flour, which the alum has been used to disguise.

---

* Treatise on Food and Diet, p. 311. 1843.

Lime-water, it is asserted, substituted for a portion of the water used in making the dough, may be employed with advantage, instead of alum, for improving the product from an inferior quality of flour.

The amount of bread produced from a given quantity of flour varies with the amount of water present. "Bread," says Dr. Letheby,* "should not contain more than 36 to 38 per cent. of water, and the other constituents, excepting salt, should be the same as of good flour.

"In practice, 100 pounds of flour will make from 133 to 137 pounds of bread, a good average being 136; so that a sack of flour of 280 pounds should yield ninety-five four-pound [quartern] loaves. The art of the baker, however, is to increase this quantity, and he does it by hardening the gluten through the agency of a little alum, or by means of a gummy mixture of boiled rice, three or four pounds of which will, when boiled for two or three hours in as many gallons of water, make a sack of flour yield 100 four-pound loaves. But the bread is dropsical, and gets soft and sodden at the base, where it stands."

An evaporation of water occurs, and causes bread to lose weight on keeping. The loss proceeds most actively whilst hot from the oven, and the baker sometimes endeavors to check it by throwing sacks, or something of the kind, over the loaves; but the crust thereby suffers in crispness.

Composition of Bread (Letheby's table).

Nitrogenous matter, ...	8.1
Carbohydrates, ...	51.0
Fat matter, ...	1.6
Mineral matter, ...	2.3
Water, ...	37.0
	100.0

New bread is selected by many in preference to stale. It is, however, much less digestible, and where weakness of stomach exists, is apt to excite derangement. It is its lightness or porosity which gives to bread its property of easy digestibility, and with stale bread its firmness and friability allow this porosity to be maintained during reduction by mastication. The softness of new bread, on the other hand, renders it difficult of mastication, and at the same time favors its clogging together into a heavy and close mass, which, on arrival in the stomach, will be far less easily penetrated and acted upon by the digestive juice. By heating for a short time in an oven, stale bread may be again brought into the soft condition of new, and will remain in this state for some hours. After being thus rebaked, however, it soon undergoes change and becomes unpalatable.

Besides its physical condition, which renders bread a digestible article of food, the effect of the heat which has been employed in baking is to increase the digestibility of the constituents of the flour. The state of the nitrogenous compounds becomes altered, the starch-granules ruptured, and some of the starch transformed into dextrine and sugar.

The difference in the nutritive value of brown bread as compared with white has been already referred to (vide p. 149). From the presence of the indigestible particles of bran, brown bread acts to some extent as an

---

* Lectures on Food, p. 13. 1870.

irritant, and thereby stimulates the secreting structures and the muscular walls of the alimentary canal. Hence, the service which it renders to persons, particularly those of sedentary habits, suffering from constipation. In irritable states of the alimentary canal it should be avoided; and, in the case of those who work hard or take much exercise, it may prove the source of diarrhœa.

Toast.—It is a frequent practice to cut bread into slices, and subject it to toasting, and the digestibility is thereby increased. Water is driven off, a little scorching of the surface occurs, and greater firmness is acquired. The toasting should be conducted so that crispness is imparted throughout the whole thickness of the slice. If the slice be thick, and a mere scorching of the surface be induced, the action of the heat will give increased softness to the centre (just as rebaking renders stale bread like new) and make it less digestible than the bread from which it was prepared. Buttered toast, like any article saturated with fatty matter, offers considerable resistance to digestion, and is exceedingly apt to disagree where delicacy of stomach exists.

Rusks.—These consist of tea-cakes, which are made from flour, butter, milk, and sugar, cut into slices, and the slices placed on tins and introduced for a few minutes into a sharp oven. They are turned so as to produce a little scorching of both surfaces, and afterward put into a dry-ing oven for three or four hours in order to drive off all the moisture.

Pulled bread.—For making pulled bread the crumb of a new loaf—the crust being sacrificed for the purpose—is torn or drawn out with the hands, and treated exactly in the same way as rusks. It constitutes a very digestible form of bread, and is well adapted for the dyspeptic.

Tops and bottoms.—Tops and bottoms are pretty largely used as food for infants. They are made in the same way as rusks; the form, indeed, constitutes the only essential difference between the two. Small, square-shaped cakes are, in the first place, made like the tea-cake, from flour, butter, milk, and sugar, but usually with rather less of the last ingredient. These are then cut in half—hence the name, tops and bottoms—and baked and dried.

Muffins.—Flour, water, and yeast are mixed into a liquid paste or batter. This is poured into a hoop resting on a hot tin and baked. For eating they are cut in half, toasted, and buttered.

Crumpets.—The only difference between muffins and crumpets is, that the latter are half the thickness of the former. They are toasted and buttered whole for the table. Both are very trying articles to the stomach.

Cracknels.—The process for making cracknels is somewhat peculiar. A dough is formed, composed of flour, butter, eggs, and sugar, and rolled into sheets. They are then cut into the appropriate shape, and put into boiling water. They sink, and become hardened by the coagulation of the albumen that occurs. In the course of a little time they expand, and, becoming lighter, rise to the surface, and are skimmed off. They are then immersed in cold water, and afterward placed in tins, and baked in a sharp oven.

Ginger-bread.—The ingredients of ginger-bread are flour, treacle, butter, alum, and common potashes. Its porosity or lightness is due to the liberation of carbonic acid from the last-named substance by the glucic and melassic acids of the treacle. By some makers, ground ginger or sliced candied orange-peel is introduced. Additional lightness is also sometimes given by the employment of some form of baking-powder.

Biscuits.—Biscuits are a useful wheaten product, on account of their property of keeping, which is owing to their being dried as well as baked. Some biscuits are made from flour and water only, or flour, water, and a very little butter to diminish the hard and flinty character which they otherwise possess. Such is the composition of sailors' biscuits, and nothing is employed to give them lightness. Other biscuits are made with the addition of milk, and some with the addition of sugar also; and lightness may be given either by a baking-powder or the carbonate of ammonia, which, being a volatile salt, is dissipated with the heat of the oven, and in escaping raises the dough. There are also various fancy biscuits, each kind containing, in addition to the ordinary ingredients, some special article. Plain biscuits constitute an easily digestible form of food. Biscuit-powder is often advantageously used in combination with milk where solid food cannot be borne. It also furnishes an excellent and nourishing form of food for infants.

Passover cakes belong to the biscuit class. They may be looked upon, in reality, as a very thin kind of biscuit, and are composed only of flour and water.

Stale biscuits, on being moistened and rebaked, are restored, like stale bread, to the condition of new.

Composition of Biscuit (Letheby's table).

Nitrogenous matter, ...	15.6
Carbohydrates, ...	73.4
Fatty matter, ...	1.3
Mineral matter, ...	1.7
Water, ...	8.0
	100.0

Semolina.—This substance forms a granular preparation of the heart of the wheat-grain. It is made from the hard wheats, which are rich in gluten. The grinding is performed with the mill-stones sufficiently apart to leave the product in a granular form, instead of reducing it to the state of flour. It forms a digestible and nourishing article of food, and is useful for adding to broths, soups, milk, etc. It likewise may be made into a light and nutritious pudding.

Soujee and *Manna-croup* are also names by which this granular preparation of wheat is known. The *Semoule* of the French is likewise of the same nature. It constitutes the coarse, hard granules which are a product of the grinding of the hard wheats, and are retained in the bolting machine after the fine flour has passed through. On account of the resistance which the hard wheats offer to reduction, these granules have escaped being crushed between the mill-stones. As the product fetches a higher price than flour, the skilful miller so adjusts his mill-stones as to obtain as large an amount as possible.

The *Kous-kous, Couscous,* or *Couscousou,* of the Arabs, which forms a national food in Algeria, further constitutes a granular preparation of wheat. It is cooked and eaten in a variety of ways.

Macaroni, Vermicelli, and *Italian* or *Cagliari paste.*—Italian wheat and some other kinds which are rich in gluten are employed for making the above-named preparations, which are consumed very largely in Italy. The flour is made into a stiff paste with hot water, and then pressed through holes or moulds in a metal plate, or else stamped so as to give the desired form, and afterwards dried. They are all highly nutritious, but from their closeness, where much thickness of substance exists, as, for example, with pipe macaroni, are not so easy of digestion as many other of the wheaten preparations.

Such are the alimentary products of wheat in ordinary use amongst us. Wholesome and most useful articles under ordinary circumstances, they sometimes acquire properties which render them obnoxious, upon which point a few remarks will now be offered.

Wheat is liable to be attacked by the *weevil*, a little insect which consumes the farinaceous centre of the grain. The *Acarus farinæ*, or flour mite, a microscopic animalcule, may also be encountered. Beyond deteriorating the wheat for alimentary purposes, however, it cannot be said that any harm is produced by these animals.

Certain low forms of parasitic vegetable growth also become developed upon wheat. There is the *rust*, or *smut*, with which the wheat of our own country is frequently liable to be attacked. This gives unpleasant characters to the flour and bread, but has not been ascertained to produce any specific deleterious effects upon the animal system. In some localities abroad, the cereal grains, and amongst them occasionally wheat, but most particularly rye, become infested with a species of *fungus*, which grows in such a way as to present the appearance of a spur. What is alluded to here is the *ergotized* or *spurred-corn*, which is well known to exert a poisonous action upon animal beings, the symptoms produced being of a two-fold nature, viz., those of deranged nervous action, terminating fatally, it may be, in convulsions, on the one hand; and of defective nutrition, attended with dry gangrene of the extremities, on the other.

In connection with this subject, it may be mentioned that wheat and other corn may be rendered poisonous by the accidental presence of the seeds of the *Lolium temulentum*, or Darnel grass, which has been allowed by the slovenly farmer to overrun his fields. Christison * says the *Lolium temulentum* is the only poisonous species of the natural order of the grasses. The seeds appear to be powerfully narcotic, and at the same time to possess acrid properties. " Headache, giddiness, somnolency, delirium, convulsions, paralysis, and even death," are effects that have been observed to arise from their habitual consumption as an accidental ingredient of bread. Vomiting and purging are also symptoms that have been sometimes produced.

It has been suggested that wheat and other grain may possess deleterious properties attributable to being gathered in an unripe state. Local outbreaks of illness have been ascribed to this cause in France. Dr. Christison considers that the subject requires further inquiry, and remarks that, although grain is often cut down in an unripe state in various districts of our own country, he has never heard that any disease has been produced by its consumption.

Wheat, flour, and bread may pass into an unwholesome state as a result of being kept. Under the presence of moisture, they are prone to undergo change, and to acquire a more or less strongly marked acid character. Bread made from old and bad flour may be quite sour to the taste; and, although some persons may become accustomed to such bread, and may eat it without any ill consequences arising, yet with others, who

---

* On Poisons, 4th edition, p. 944. 1845.

are unused to it, it may give rise to severe irritation of the alimentary canal, manifested by gastric derangement, griping, and diarrhœa. Good bread is only slightly acid at first, but if kept and allowed to remain moist, it becomes decidedly so in the course of a little time.

Bread also becomes the seat of development of certain species of fungi (*Penicillium oïdium*, etc.)—in other words, becomes mouldy—on keeping, and the more quickly so in proportion as it contains water. The same likewise happens with wheat and flour under the presence of moisture. The existence of this low form of vegetable growth renders the articles pervaded dangerous for use. They are liable to produce injurious and even fatal consequences. Dr. Christison states that on the Continent repeated instances have occured of severe and even dangerous poisoning by spoiled or mouldy rye-bread, barley-bread, and wheat-bread; and that several instances have been observed of horses having been killed in a short space of time with symptoms of irritant poisoning by eating such bread with their ordinary food. It has further been noticed that the consumption of mouldy oats has been followed by fatal consequences. Dr. Parkes,* quoting from Professor Varnell, states that "six horses died in three days from eating mouldy oats; there was a large amount of matted mycelium, and this, when given to other horses for experiment, killed them in thirty-six hours."

In cities and towns mouldy bread is rarely, if ever, encountered. The daily supply of fresh bread that is provided removes any necessity for keeping the article sufficiently long for a state of mouldiness to be acquired. In outlying rural districts, however, where a batch of bread is baked only at somewhat distant periods within the household, time may be given before the batch is exhausted for the last of it to become vinny or mouldy, a more or less green color being developed, and a ropy character produced.

Biscuits and rusks, on account of their dryness, are not prone, like bread, to become unwholesome from mouldiness.

OATS.—The common oat is derived from *Avena sativa*. A considerable number of varieties of the plant are cultivated, yielding oats, which may be arranged under the two heads of white oats, and red, dun, or black oats. Other species of *Avena* are also cultivated on the Continent. Scotland is specially famed for the quality of the oats it produces, and here more than half of the cultivated land is devoted to their growth.

As met with in commerce, oats consist of the seeds enclosed in their paleæ or husk. When deprived of its integument, the grain goes by the name of *groats* or *grits*, and these, when crushed, constitute *Embden groats*. They are used for making gruel.

The husk amounts to from 22 to 28 per cent. The remaining 72 to 78 per cent. comprises the kernel of the seed.

Oatmeal constitutes the product of grinding the kiln-dried seeds, deprived of their husk, or outer skin. It is not so white as wheaten-flour, and its taste is peculiar, being at first sweet and then rough and somewhat bitter. It forms the article used for making *porridge*. The Scotch oatmeal is ground coarser than the English, and is the more esteemed of the two.

In Germany and Switzerland coarsely bruised oatmeal is baked in

---

* Practical Hygiene, 3d edition, p. 223.

an oven until it becomes of a brown color, and is then used to thicken broths and soups.

Sowans, Seeds, or *Flummery,* which constitutes a very popular article of diet in Scotland and South Wales, is made from the husks of the grain. The husks, with the starchy particles adhering to them, are separated from the other parts of the grain and steeped in water for one or two days, until the mass ferments and becomes sourish. It is then skimmed, and the liquid boiled down to the consistence of gruel. In Wales this food is called *sucan.*

Budrum is prepared in the same manner, except that the liquid is boiled down to a sufficient consistency to form, when cold, a firm jelly. This resembles blanc-mange, and constitutes a light, demulcent, and nutritious article of food, which is well suited for the weak stomach.

Composition of Oatmeal (from Letheby's table).

Nitrogenous matter, ...	12.6
Carbohydrates, ...	63.8
Fatty matter, ...	5.6
Saline matter, ...	3.0
Water, ...	15.0
	100.0

Composition of Dried Oats (Payen).

Nitrogenous matter, ...	14.39
Starch, ...	60.59
Dextrine, etc., ...	9.25
Fatty matter, ...	5.50
Cellulose, ...	7.06
Mineral matter, ...	3.25
	100.00

The nitrogenous matter of the oat is formed chiefly of a principle allied to caseine, called *avenine,* which may be thus obtained : Let oatmeal be washed on a sieve, and the milky liquid which runs through be allowed to repose to deposit the suspended starch-granules. The supernatant liquid, on being heated to 200° Fahr., throws down albumen, and then, on the addition of acetic acid, a white precipitate falls, which constitutes *avenine.*

On account of the absence of gluten, oatmeal cannot be vesiculated and made into bread, like wheaten-flour. It is devoid of the tenacity or adhesiveness which is requisite to hold the vesicles of gas and give porosity or lightness to the mass. It is, however, made into thin cakes, by mixing into a paste with water, and then baking on an iron plate. Under this form it is consumed as a staple food by a large number of the inhabitants of Scotland (which is called, in consequence, " the land of cakes "), and also of the North of England.

Besides being eaten in this way, oatmeal is also consumed as porridge or stirabout, as beef- and kale-brose, and likewise as gruel.

Porridge is made by simply stirring the oatmeal into boiling water until it becomes of the consistence of hasty pudding. The water is kept boiling until the process is finished. It is usually flavored with either salt or sugar, and is frequently eaten with milk or treacle.

Brose differs from porridge in not being boiled over the fire. *Beef-brose* is made by stirring the oatmeal into the hot liquor in which meat has been boiled. *Kale-brose* is similarly made from the liquor in which cabbage, or kale, has been boiled.

Gruel is consumed in a liquid or semi-liquid form. It is prepared by first mixing groats with a little cold water, then pouring in the requisite quantity of boiling water, and afterward boiling for ten minutes and well stirring all the while.

Oats form an important and valuable article of food. With a proportion of nitrogenous matter which bears a favorable comparison with that of wheat, they stand next to maize amongst the cultivated cereals in the amount of fatty matter that is present. The percentage of saline matter is also high. "Oatmeal," says Dr. Cullen, "is especially the food of the people of Scotland; and was formerly that of the northern parts of England—counties which have always produced as healthy and as vigorous a race of men as any in Europe." Scotch oatmeal is considered preferable to English. It possesses higher nutritive value.

Oatmeal enjoys the reputation of exerting a slightly laxative action, and Dr. Christison remarks that he has in several instances found it of service in relieving habitual constipation, upon being taken at breakfast in the form of porridge. It is apt to disagree with some dyspeptics, having a tendency to produce acidity and pyrosis, and cases have been noticed amongst those who have been in the daily habit of consuming it, where dyspeptic symptoms have subsided upon temporarily abandoning its use.

Intestinal concretions, composed of phosphate of lime, agglutinated animal matter, and the small, stiff, silky hairs existing at one end of the oat, with small fragments of the husk, were formerly of not uncommon occurrence as a result of the habitual consumption of oatmeal-food. Such concretions, however, are now rarely met with, on account, it is believed, of the oats being more thoroughly deprived of their husk and better cleaned than formerly.

BARLEY.—Barley is obtained from several species of *Hordeum*, the favorite being *Hordeum distichon*, or common summer barley of England, of which several varieties are cultivated. It is met with in commerce as a grain, enclosed in the paleæ or husk. The product, when the whole grain is ground, forms barley-meal.

Scotch, milled, or *pot barley,* constitutes the grain deprived of its husk by a mill.

Pearl barley is the grain deprived of the husk, and rounded and polished by attrition.

Patent barley forms the product derived from grinding pearl barley to the state of flour.

Composition of Barley-meal (from Letheby's table).

Nitrogenous matter,	6.3
Carbohydrates,	74.3
Fatty matter,	2.4
Saline matter,	2.0
Water,	15.0
	100.0

In the composition of barley, as given by Payen, a marked discordancy with the above exists as regards the nitrogenous matter, the quantity of which, as will be seen by the following figures, is represented as rather more than double:

Composition of Dried Barley (Payen).

Nitrogenous matter, ...	12.96
Starch, ...	66.43
Dextrine, etc., ...	10.00
Fatty matter, ...	2.76
Cellulose, ...	4.75
Mineral matter, ...	3.10
	100.00

The nitrogenous matter of barley exists under the form of albumen and caseine. There is little or no gluten, and hence, like oatmeal, it cannot be made into a vesiculated bread. Barley-bread is, therefore, usually made by mixing wheaten-flour with the meal. Barley-cakes are eaten on the score of economy in some of the agricultural districts of England, Scotland, and Ireland, and in the north of Europe, but form a much less palatable food than that derived from wheaten-flour. They are also less digestible, and are regarded as possessing rather laxative properties. They certainly appear to constitute an unsuitable food in disordered conditions of the alimentary canal.

Barley-water is prepared from pearl barley, and forms a useful demulcent and slightly nutritive liquid for the sick-room.

Malt is the product yielded when barley has been allowed to germinate, and the germination has been stopped at a certain point by subjecting the grain to heat in a kiln. As a result of the process, a peculiar active nitrogenous principle, called diastase, is developed, which has the power of effecting the conversion of starch into dextrine and sugar; and, through this, malt differs from barley in a portion of the starch being represented by sugar.

Malt infused in hot water yields *Sweet-wort*, which is rich in saccharine matter. This is used for making beer. Malt is also used to some extent as food for cattle, and is thought to be more easy of assimilation than the unmalted grain, but experience has not shown that it possesses higher fattening properties.

Malt forms one of the ingredients of *Liebig's Food for Infants*, which has been introduced as a substitute for woman's milk. The article has been referred to at p. 122, under the head of milk.

RYE.—The common rye, or *Secale cereale*, is cultivated extensively on the Continent, but is little grown in England. It is of a hardy nature, and is usually sown in ground where the soil is too poor for wheat to grow.

In external appearance the rye-grain presents a closer resemblance to wheat than any of the other cereals. It is, however, darker in color and smaller in size. In the centre the grain is white and farinaceous, but toward the exterior it is brownish. As met with in commerce, it is deprived of the paleæ or husk, as in the case of wheat. It is ground, and used under the form of rye-meal.

Composition of Rye-meal (from Letheby's table).

Nitrogenous matter, ...	8.0
Carbohydrates, ...	73.2
Fatty matter, ...	2.0
Saline matter, ...	1.8
Water, ...	15.0
	100.0

Composition of Dried Rye (Payen).

Nitrogenous matter, ...	12.50
Starch, ...	64.65
Dextrine, etc., ...	14.90
Fatty matter, ...	2.25
Cellulose, ...	3.10
Mineral matter, ...	2.60
	100.00

The nitrogenous matter of rye consists of fibrine, glutine, and albumen. From the nature of its nitrogenous matter, rye approaches nearer to wheat than the other cereal grains in the aptitude of its flour for making a vesiculated bread.

Rye-bread was once a common article of food in England. It forms the dark-colored and sour-tasting bread which is still extensively used in the North of Europe. It may be spoken of as filling the place of wheaten-bread in temperate countries where poverty prevails and agriculture is the least advanced; and in some parts of Belgium, Holland, Prussia, Germany, Russia, and other countries in the north, rye-bread is found to constitute the staple food of the people.

Rye-bread falls but little short of wheaten-bread in nutritive value. Its color and acid taste, however, render it disrelishable to those who are unaccustomed to it, and it is only necessity that leads to its consumption. Moreover, it is apt to occasion diarrhœa, but custom soon overcomes this effect. On account of its laxative action, it is sometimes taken to counteract habitual constipation. Rye is imported into England for malting, and is so made use of by distillers.

Ergotized or Spurred Rye.—The cereals are subject to become the seat of growth of a parasitic fungus, which gives to the grain deleterious properties; and, of all of them, rye is the most prone to be attacked in this way. The affected grain undergoes development, so as to project considerably beyond the husk, and it may attain upward of four times its size in the ordinary state. On account of this excessive growth, it can be separated by sifting from the unaffected seed, and, unless this is done to an ergotized crop, serious consequences may arise from its consumption as food. At various times, indeed, the inhabitants of different parts of the Continent have been stricken with fatal illness from this cause. Two classes of symptoms are produced, denominated the *convulsive* and *gangrenous* forms of ergotism. In the one, the phenomena consist of weariness, giddiness, contraction of the muscles of the extremities, formication, dimness of sight, loss of sensibility, voracious appetite, yellow countenance, and convulsions, followed by death; in the other, there is also formication, that is, a feeling as if insects were creeping over the skin, and voracious appetite, and with this there occur coldness and insensibility of the extremities, followed by gangrene (Pereira).

INDIAN CORN OR MAIZE.—The common maize, or Indian corn (*Zea mays*), is a native of tropical America, and is now extensively cultivated in the United States, Africa, Asia, Southern Europe, Germany, and Ireland.

There are many varieties of the plant, as well as a distinct and smaller species, named *Zea curagua*, which forms the Chili maize or Valparaiso corn.

The grains of maize are variously colored, but those most commonly met with are yellow. The ears when nearly full-grown, and whilst in a succulent state, are a favorite delicacy in North America, where they are boiled, and the grain eaten with salt and butter, or cut off and cooked with beans, forming "succotash." The succulent grains, indeed, may be made to take the place of young peas, and are available for the table when the season for peas is over. When the ears are allowed to ripen, and the grains are afterward deprived of their hull and broken, or coarsely ground, preparations are produced known as *hominy, samp,* or *grits,* according to the size to which they are reduced. They are boiled in water, and eaten like rice.

A small variety of maize, with translucent and deeply colored grains, is specially denominated *pop-corn.* The grains possess the property, when gently roasted, of bursting, turning inside out, and swelling to many times their original size. In this condition they are sometimes sold in London, and eaten by children as a delicacy, whilst in America they are consumed at table with a little salt.

Maize or Indian corn-meal is not adapted for making bread, on account of its deficiency in gluten, without the admixture of wheaten or rye-flour. The common brown bread of New England is made from a mixture of rye- and maize-meal. Used alone, maize-meal, like oatmeal and barley-meal, is made into a cake, and this, when roasted, is called in Spanish America "*tortilla.*" In the United States it is called "*johnny-cake,*" "*hoe-cake,*" "*pone,*" or "*Indian bread.*" It is also frequently made into liquid dough and baked in thin cakes.

Maize-meal is consumed in Ireland and some other places principally in the form of porridge, which goes by the name of "*polenta*" in Italy, and "*mush*" in North America. *Polenta* is also the name applied to the maize-meal of the shops. Maize-porridge made with milk is a favorite food in British Honduras, where it forms what is called "*corn lob.*"

The flavor of maize is harsh and peculiar, and disagreeable to those who have been unaccustomed to it. Treating the meal with a weak solution of caustic soda deprives it of this unpleasantness. It also, however, removes some of the nitrogenous matter, and thus robs it of a portion of its nutritive value. Such constitutes the foundation of the process for preparing the articles so extensively sold and used under the names of *Oswego flour, Maizena,* and *Corn-flour.*

Composition of Indian Corn-meal (Letheby's table).

Nitrogenous matter,	11.1
Carbohydrates,	65.1
Fatty matter,	8.1
Saline matter,	1.7
Water,	14.0
	100.0

11

Composition of Dried Maize (Payen).

Nitrogenous matter,	12.50
Starch,	67.55
Dextrine, etc.,	4.00
Fatty matter,	8.80
Cellulose,	5.90
Mineral matter,	1.25
	100.00

Whilst containing an average amount of nitrogenous matter, maize is characterized and distinguished, as is shown by the above analyses, from the other cerealia by the large amount of fatty matter present. As regards this quality, none of the other cerealia exhibit even an approach to it. On account of the fatty matter present, maize acquires, on keeping for some time, an unpleasant rancid taste, from the usual change induced by exposure to air.

Containing, as it does, about the same percentage of nitrogenous matter as soft wheat, and upward of four times the amount of fatty matter, maize stands in a high position as regards alimentary value. It is largely used both for feeding and fattening animals; and its fattening properties, as explained by its composition, are superior to the other cereals. It is with maize that the Strasbourg geese are crammed for the production of the "*foie gras.*" Properly prepared, it furnishes a wholesome, digestible, and nutritious food for man; but with those, it is said, who have been unaccustomed to its use, it is apt to excite a tendency to diarrhœa. It is the chief food of the slaves in Brazil, as it was of those in the United States, and is largely eaten in Mexico and Peru, and by the Indians of New Spain. Since its introduction into Europe, it has in some districts superseded other grains, and it is said that twice as much maize is eaten in Piedmont as wheat-flour. In Ireland it has to a considerable extent taken the place of the potato.

RICE.—The common rice, or *Oryza sativa*, is extensively cultivated in India, China, and most other Eastern Countries, the West Indies, Central America, and the United States, and also in some of the Southern countries of Europe. It is said to supply the principal food of nearly one-third of the human race.

There is a large number of varieties of the plant cultivated, and considerably more than one hundred different kinds are grown in India and Ceylon. The best rice imported into this country is brought from Carolina and Patna. The fields in which rice is raised, called paddy fields, are periodically flooded with water, as the plant requires a constantly wet soil for its growth. Before ripening, the water is drained off, and the crop is cut with a sickle.

Paddy is the name given to the seed when enclosed in the paleæ or husk. This husk adheres very closely, and care has to be exercised to enable its removal to be effected without damaging or breaking the grain. Special machinery is employed for the purpose. After the husk has been removed, the grain is passed through a whitening machine, in order to remove the inner cuticle, or red skin. When this has been accomplished, the product forms the rice met with in the shops.

Rice is consumed as food, both in the state of grain and ground into flour.

Composition of Rice (from Letheby's table).

Nitrogenous matter, ...	6.3
Carbohydrates, ...	79.5
Fatty matter, ...	0.7
Saline matter, ...	0.5
Water, ...	13.0
	100.0

Composition of Dried Rice (Payen).

Nitrogenous matter, ...	7.55
Starch, ...	88.65
Dextrine, etc., ...	1.00
Fatty matter, ...	0.80
Cellulose, ...	1.10
Mineral matter, ...	0.90
	100.0

Rice is characterized by the large proportion of starch, and the small proportions of nitrogenous, fatty, and mineral matter it contains. In composition it must be looked upon as presenting considerable analogy to the potato.

Rice, like the potato, is largely used for the manufacture of starch. The process adopted is to treat the flour with a solution of caustic soda, which dissolves out the nitrogenous matter. The starch is then allowed to deposit itself, and is afterward washed and dried. From the alkaline solution the nitrogenous matter may be recovered, if desired, by the addition of an acid. The starch-granules of rice are remarkable for the smallness of their size. They form exceedingly minute, irregular-shaped, angular particles.

Rice is too poor in nitrogenous matter, fatty matter, and salts to yield alone what is wanted in an aliment, unless consumed in very large quantity, thereby sacrificing a considerable portion of its starch. The starch, in other words, is out of proportion to the other alimentary principles, looked at in relation to the requirements of the system. Associated with other articles, to compensate for the deficiency in the principles named, rice constitutes an exceedingly valuable food. It has the advantage of possessing an easily digestible starch-granule and hence is found a useful aliment in disordered states of the alimentary canal. In the case of persons suffering from diarrhœa or dysentery, it agrees better than any other kind of solid food. It certainly exerts no laxative action, as many of the cereals do, and is often regarded, indeed, as having an opposite effect, but probably it occupies simply a neutral position in this respect.

Rice is best cooked by thoroughly steaming. If boiled in water it loses a portion of the already small quantity of nitrogenous and saline matter it contains. It does not admit of being made into bread, but is used for mixing with wheaten-flour to furnish the very white bread which is in request in Paris.

MILLET.—The common millet (*Panicum miliaceum*) is a native of the East Indies, but is cultivated in the South of Europe and other parts of the world. *Panicum jumentorum*, or Guinea grass, is a native of Africa, but is now cultivated in the West Indies and America. There is a very large number of varieties of millet, the grain of which is mostly used as food for poultry and other domestic animals. It is sometimes made into loaves and cakes, and in some places is the principal food of the inhabitants. Its nutritive value is said to be about equal to rice.

Dhurra, *Dhoora*, or *Sorgho* grass (*Sorghum*), is sometimes called Indian millet, but it belongs to a different tribe of grasses from the true millets. It is cultivated largely in Asia and Africa, and, to some extent, in the South of Europe. The grain is round, and a little larger than a mustard-seed. In India it is ground whole and made into bread. The bread is said to be very good, and to have been issued to the English troops in the last Chinese expedition. Johnston describes the grain as quite equal in nutritive value to the average of our English wheats. Letheby speaks of it as a little more nutritious than rice, and as containing, on an average, about 9 per cent. of nitrogenous matter, with 74 of starch and sugar, 2.6 of fat, and 2.3 of mineral matter.

Manna-grass (*Glyceria*, *Festuca*, or *Poa fluitans*) constitutes one of the meadow-grasses (floating meadow-grass), and yields seeds which are sometimes consumed as human food. The plant grows plentifully in marshes and on the sides of ditches and stagnant waters in most parts of Europe, and is, also met with in Asia, North America, and Australia. It derives its name from the sweet taste which the seeds possess, a character which is particularly marked before the plant has attained its full growth. In many parts of Poland, Holland, and Germany, the seeds, which fall very readily, are collected and used in soups or consumed as gruel or puddings. They form a very palatable and nutritious product, and are sold under the name of *Polish manna*, *manna seeds*, and *manna-croup*.

BUCKWHEAT.—Buckwheat, although not a cereal, may be conveniently referred to in connection with the cereal grains.

The common buckwheat (*Fagopyrum esculentum*), belonging to the order *Polygonaceæ*, is a native of Central Asia, and is said to have been introduced into Europe either by the Moors or by the Crusaders. In France it is called *Blé Sarrasin*, or Saracen wheat, and in Norfolk and Suffolk it goes by the name of *brank*. The name buckwheat is a corruption of the German *Buckweizen* (beech-wheat), drawn from its resemblance to the seed of the beech-tree.

The plant grows very quickly, and yields abundantly, but, as it is destroyed by frost, it cannot be sown until the season for cold weather has passed. In England it is principally cultivated for feeding pheasants and other game, but in Brittany it is grown in place of wheat. No grain is eaten so eagerly by poultry, and it is sometimes given to horses instead of oats, or in combination with them. The seed is covered with a hard rind, or thin shell, which has to be removed before it is fit for being eaten by cattle.

When used for human food, it is usually consumed as hasty pudding or pottage. The flour is fine and white, but devoid of gluten, and, therefore, does not make proper bread. It is used, however, for pastry; and thin cakes, which are very good eating, are largely made from it in the United States. Crumpets made from buckwheat form a favorite dainty with the children in Holland.

Composition of Buckwheat (Payen).

Nitrogenous matter, ...	13.10
Starch, etc., ...	64.90
Fatty matter, ...	3.00
Cellulose, ...	3.50
Mineral matter, ...	2.50
Water, ...	13.00
	100.00

QUINOA.—Quinoa, like buckwheat, may also be conveniently considered in association with the cerealia.

The quinoa plant (*Chenopodium Quinoa*), belonging to the order *Chenopodiaceæ*, which includes our spinach and beet, is a native of the high table-lands of Chili and Peru, where it grows at an elevation of 13,-000 feet above the level of the sea, a height at which barley and rye fail to ripen. There are two varieties of it, viz., the sweet and the bitter. It is hardly known in this country, but forms the principal food of the inhabitants of the locality in which it grows. The leaves are used as spinach, and the grain, called "petty rice," is mixed with soup. Quinoa, judging from the subjoined analysis, forms a valuable article of food as regards the possession of nutritive ingredients. Its proportion of nitrogenous matter is very large. It is also fairly rich in fat, very rich in salts, and likewise said to be rich in iron—the richest, indeed, in this respect, of any vegetable. It thus appears to possess qualities that might render it exceedingly useful, in a therapeutic point of view. Its starch-grains are alleged to be the smallest known. The meal can only be made into cakes, not into leavened bread.

Analysis of Quinoa (Voelcker).

	Quinoa seeds dried at 212° Fahr.	Quinoa flour.
Nitrogenous matter, ...	22.86	19
Starch, ...	56.80	60
Fatty matter, ...	5.74	5
Vegetable fibre, ...	9.53	—
Ash, ...	5.05	—
Water, ...	—	16

LEGUMINOUS SEEDS, OR PULSES.

This group of farinaceous seeds, which includes beans, peas, and lentils, is characterized by the large proportion of nitrogenous matter they contain. In this respect they stand strikingly in advance of the cerealia, for the amount may be twice as much as that contained in an ordinary kind of wheat.

The form under which the nitrogenous matter is present is chiefly as a substance called *legumine*, which is a representation of vegetable cascine.

By virtue of their composition, the leguminous seeds possess a high nutritive value, and furnish a food which is more satisfying than vegetable food generally to the stomach, and more closely allied in a dietetic point of view to the alimentary products supplied by the animal kingdom. They thereby furnish an advantageous substitute for animal food for those who fast during Lent and on *maigre* days, and it is probably on this account that *haricots blanc* and lentils are so much more largely consumed in France and other Catholic countries than in England. Their large amount of nitrogenous matter adapts them for consumption in association with articles in which starch or fat is a predominating principle. With rice, therefore, they form an appropriate combination, and this admixture is found to constitute the staple food of large populations in India. Bacon and beans are also a suitable association, and form a dish which has been of repute amongst us from ancient times.

As a drawback to their high nutritive value, the leguminous seeds must be ranked as difficult of digestion. They require prolonged boiling to render them tender and digestible. They are apt, besides lying heavy on the stomach, to occasion flatulence and colic, and the flatus is charged with a considerable quantity of sulphuretted hydrogen, arising from the sulphur which the legumine contains. They are also regarded as stimulating or heating to the system, and it is on account of this property that a moderate quantity of beans proves a serviceable adjunct to the food of the horse during the winter months.

BEANS.—Beans are derived from the *Faba vulgaris*, a plant which is supposed to be a native of the East, but which has been cultivated in Britain from time immemorial. There are several varieties, one of which yields the common horse-bean, which is raised in fields; and another, the broad- or Windsor-bean, which is grown in gardens. The former is almost exclusively employed as food for cattle. It is but rarely used as food by man, and then chiefly, after grinding, as an adulterant of wheaten-flour, or to give a desired quality to the loaf made from certain kinds of flour. The latter is boiled in the young and fresh state, for use at the table as a vegetable. It is also dried and preserved, whilst still green, so as to be available all the year round. In this condition it requires to be soaked in water for some hours before being cooked.

Composition of Beans (Payen).

	Horse-bean.	Broad- or Windsor bean, dried in the green state and decorticated.
Nitrogenous matter,	30.8	29.05
Starch, etc.,	48.3	55.85
Cellulose,	3.0	1.05
Fatty matter,	1.9	2.00
Saline matter,	3.5	3.65
Water,	12.5	8.40
	100.0	100.00

Haricots or French-beans.—The common kidney-bean, or French-bean (*Phaseolus vulgaris*,) is a native of India, and was introduced into England in the sixteenth century. The scarlet-runner (*Phaseolus multiflorus*), another variety of the plant, is a native of South America, and was introduced into England in 1633. The unripe pods of both, with the young seeds in them, are cooked and eaten as a green vegetable at the table. On the Continent the pods are allowed to ripen, and the seeds form *haricots blancs*, which are consumed both in a fresh and dried state.

Composition of Haricots Blancs (Payen).

Nitrogenous matter, ... 25.5
Starch, etc., ... 55.7
Cellulose, ... 2·9
Fatty matter, ... 2.8
Mineral matter, ... 3.2
Water, ... 9.9
—————
100.0

PEAS.—There are several varieties of the pea. Some, derived from the *Pisum arvense*, are grown in fields by the farmer as food for cattle. Others, forming the garden-pea, are derived from *Pisum sativum*, a native of the South of Europe, but long known in England. The more choice kinds of the garden-pea were brought from Holland, and formed an expensive article of food in Queen Elizabeth's time. Peas are grown for the ripened and dried seeds, and also for eating as a succulent vegetable. In the latter case the pods are gathered before they have arrived at maturity, and the seeds separated and consumed in a green state. There is a kind of pea, called *sugar*-pea, the pods of which are gathered young, and cooked and eaten with the seeds in them, in the same way as French-beans.

Peas, when quite young, are tender and sweet, and far more digestible, but less nourishing, than peas in the mature state. The latter, like other leguminous seeds, require slow and prolonged cooking to render them soft and digestible. When old, no amount of boiling will soften them; indeed, the longer they are boiled the harder they become. In this condition they should be soaked in water for some time, and then crushed and stewed, or treated in the same manner as dried peas, to render them palatable and digestible.

Composition of Dried Peas (Payen).

Nitrogenous matter, ... 23.8
Starch, etc., ... 58.7
Cellulose, ... 3.5
Fatty matter, ... 2.1
Mineral matter, ... 2.1
Water, ... 8.3

The *Sea-pea* (*Pisum maritimum*) is used as an article of food in many parts of Europe, although the seeds are bitter to the taste (" Baird's Cyclo. of Natural Sciences.")

LENTILS.—Lentils form another alimentary product yielded by the leguminous tribe, and one of great antiquity. Although at present eaten in some parts of Europe and in Eastern countries, they are rarely employed as human food in England. They are derived from the *Ervum lens*, which constitutes a kind of tare.

Composition of Lentils (Payen).

Nitrogenous matter, ... 25.2
Starch, etc., ... 56.0
Cellulose, ... 2.4
Fatty matter, ... 2.6
Mineral matter, ... 2.3
Water, ... 11.5
                                        —————
                                        100.0

Revalenta and *Ervalenta*, articles which will be referred to under the head of farinaceous preparations, owe their chief composition to lentil flour.

Misos, small beans like lentils, are eaten largely by the Japanese ("Thunberg's Travels," vol. iv., p. 35).

Dolichos furnish to the poorer natives of India a pulse which they use extensively for their curries, etc. ("Baird's Cyclo. of Nat. Sci.").

The seeds of the Egyptian white *Lupine* (*Lupinus ternis*) are used by the Egyptians as an article of food, although it is difficult to rid them of their bitter taste ("Baird's Cyclo. of Nat. Sci.").

The *Lotus edulis*, a native of the South of Europe and Egypt, has the taste of peas, and is an article of food in some countries. The ancient Egyptians ate it, as do the Egyptians of the present day.

THE CHESTNUT.—The Spanish, or sweet chestnut, is an edible, farinaceous seed, which stands by itself. It is derived from a stately tree (*Castanea vesca*), which is a native of all the Southern parts of Europe, and abounds also in North America. Besides starch, the chestnut contains about 15 per cent. of sugar. No oil can be extracted from it by pressure. It is sometimes eaten in the raw state, but is more usually boiled or roasted. Even in a cooked condition it is not adapted for a weak stomach, and in the uncooked state it is decidedly indigestible. It is extensively used as an article of sustenance by the lower classes in many parts of the European Continent, as in Italy, Spain, Switzerland, and Germany, and by the Red Indians of North America (*Food Journal*, vol. i., p. 100). Sometimes it is ground into flour and made into a kind of bread, and in some districts it is specially treated to get rid of its astringent and bitter qualities. It is largely imported into England from Spain and Italy.

The seeds of some species of the genus *Cycas* are used as food, and esteemed as highly as chestnuts. The tree is found in the temperate and warm regions of Asia and America, and at the Cape of Good Hope ("Baird's Cyclo. of Nat. Sci.").

ACORNS.—*Acorns* formed a considerable part of the food of man in the early ages, and they are still used in some countries as a substitute for bread ("Baird's Cyclo. of Nat. Sci."). Bartholin says that in Norway they are used to furnish a bread. The inhabitants of Chio held out a long siege without any other food, and during a time of great scarcity in France (1709) this production was resorted to for sustenance ("Forsyth's Dict. of Diet").

OLEAGINOUS SEEDS.

There are various seeds, denominated nuts, which are devoid of starchy, but rich in oily matter. The starch of the cerealia appears to be replaced by fat. They are also rich in nitrogenous matter, which exists under the form of albumen and caseine. Thus constituted, they possess a high nutritive value, but, like all articles permeated with fatty matter, they are difficult of digestion unless reduced to a minutely divided state before being consumed. The reason of this is easily given. Digestion is effected by the agency of a watery secretion, and where a substance is permeated with oily matter, resistance is offered to the penetration of a watery liquid, and it is only by a progressive action upon the surface that it can become attacked. In a minutely divided state, however, no such obstruction is offered, and there is now only the richness belonging to an article which is largely impregnated with fatty matter. In this state, and if the stomach be not too delicate for them, they form a highly advantageous kind of food, although amongst the human race they enjoy but a limited application as an important or staple support. It must further be remarked that, on account of their fatty constituents, they are prone to become rancid in the course of time under exposure to air.

THE ALMOND.—This forms one of the most important of the oily seeds. It is derived from the *Amygdalus communis*, a small tree which belongs to Barbary and Syria, but which is now extensively cultivated in the Southern parts of Europe. It is also grown in England, but the fruit there does not arrive at perfection. The fruit, like the peach, apricot, plum, etc., belongs to the drupaceous group. The cortical part of it, however, is fibrous and juiceless, and not adapted for eating. It has been looked upon, it may be mentioned, as bearing the same relation to the peach that the sloe does to the plum, and the crab to the apple. The seed or kernel, situated within the shell, and provided with an enveloping reddish brown skin, is the only edible portion. The skin possesses a somewhat rough and bitter taste. It is easily removed after soaking for a short time in warm water, and the almond is then spoken of as *blanched*. Apart from the taste, the husk or skin is irritating to the throat and stomach, and unpleasant effects are mentioned as having been witnessed in consequence of its non-removal. Almonds, therefore, should always be blanched for the table.

Two varieties of the almond are met with, the *sweet* and the *bitter*. They both yield by pressure an odorless fixed oil, which is of a perfectly innocent nature. The bitter almond, exclusively, contains the principles for the development of poisonous products. It has been shown that these products do not exist preformed in the seed, but are generated by the reaction of two principles when water is added. It appears that the bitter almond contains a crystallizable substance, named *amygdalin*, which, by the action of the nitrogenous matter present, viz., *emulsin*, when in contact with water, is converted into a fragrant volatile oil (the essential oil of bitter almonds), hydrocyanic or prussic acid, and other products. The sweet almond contains emulsin, but no amygdalin: hence the innocent properties that belong to it.

Of the sweet almond, the Valentia, Barbary, Italian, and Jordan, form the varieties met with in commerce. The latter, imported from Malaga, are the finest. The bitter almond is chiefly brought from Mogadoce. It is extensively used for the extraction of the fixed oil, and when the residue has been mixed with water and subjected to distillation for yielding the volatile oil, it is employed for fattening pigs, etc.

Composition of Sweet Almonds (Boullay).

Emulsin, ...	24.0
Fixed oil, ...	54.0
Liquid sugar, ...	6.0
Gum, ...	3.0
Seed-coats, ...	5.0
Woody fibre, ...	4.0
Water, ...	3.5
Acetic acid and loss, ...	0.5
	100.0

Composition of Bitter Almonds (Vogel).

Volatile oil and hydrocyanic acid, .	Quantity undetermined.
Emulsin, ...	30.0
Fixed oil, ...	28.0
Liquid sugar, ...	6.5
Gum, ...	3.0
Seed coats, ...	8.5
Woody fibre, ...	5.0
Loss, ...	19.0
	100.0

The sweet almond is used dietetically in cookery and confectionery, and likewise as a dessert. For the latter purpose it is employed both in the fresh and dried state. By baking for a short time it becomes brittle and easily pulverizable, and is, doubtless, thereby rendered more digestible. On account of the demand for it as an article of food, its price is too high for the extraction of oil to be carried on from it to any extent. At my own suggestion, it has been made into biscuits for the use of the diabetic, and its composition shows that it forms a very suitable kind of food for administration in this complaint. From their richness in nitrogenous and fatty matters, the biscuits might also be advantageously employed in cases of defective nutrition, where the stomach is strong enough to bear a food of the kind.

The bitter almond is used to give flavor to puddings, sweetmeats, and liqueurs (macaroons, ratafia-cakes, and noyeau, owe their flavor to this source), but more often the essential oil, which is frequently denominated *Peach-nut oil*, is employed instead. Both, but particularly the latter, require to be cautiously dealt with, and, in proof of their dangerous properties, it may be stated that a single drop of the essential oil was observed by Sir B. Brodie to kill a cat in five minutes, and twenty seeds have sufficed, according to Orfila, to kill a dog in six hours, when measures were taken to prevent their rejection from the stomach by vomiting. Fatal results from both have been recorded as having occurred in the human subject.

THE COCOA-NUT.—The cocoa-nut is derived from the *Cocos nucifera*, a species of palm, supposed to have been originally a native of the Indian coasts and South Sea Islands, but now found in all tropical regions. The tree grows to from sixty to one hundred feet in height, and bears annually about eighty or a hundred nuts. The nut consists of a hard shell, containing a white, fleshy kernel, the central portion of which remains unsolidified, and yields the milky juice, which forms an agreeable, cooling beverage. The shell is surrounded by a thick, fibrous husk, which is turned to account for the construction of ropes, matting, etc., and in its natural state the whole fruit is about the size of a man's head. The fleshy, edible portion contains about 70 per cent. of a fixed fat, which is extracted and used under the name of cocoa-nut oil or butter. Its melting point is a little over 70° Fahr.

The cocoa-nut forms the chief food of the inhabitants of Ceylon, the South Sea Islands, the coast of Africa, and many other tropical coasts and islands. It is not only eaten as it comes from the tree, both in the ripe and unripe state, but is also prepared and served in various ways.

THE WALNUT.—This is the fruit of the *Juglans regia*, a lofty tree, with large spreading branches, a native of Persia, but long cultivated in Europe, and supposed to have been introduced into Italy in the time of the Emperor Tiberius. The ripe fruit supplies one of the finest of nuts, which in many parts of France, Spain, Germany, and Italy, forms an important article of food during the ripening season. English-grown walnuts are considered the best, but the supply from England is not equal to the demand, and large quantities are imported. In the unripe state, and before the shell has formed, it is extensively used for pickling and making ketchup. The walnut yields, by expression, a bland, fixed oil, which is consumed dietetically, and also used by painters.

The *Hickory-nut* is derived from the *Carya alba*, and the *Butter-nut* from the *Juglans cinerea*, both of which constitute species of the walnut tribe of transatlantic growth.

THE HAZEL-NUT.—The common hazel-nut is derived from the *Corylus avellana*, a native of all the temperate parts of Europe and Asia, and of North America. The plant named is the parent of many varieties obtained by cultivation. One variety, for instance, the *Corylus tubulosa*, yields the filbert, and another, *Corylus grandis*, the cob-nut. *Barcelona-nuts* are derived from another variety. Like the hazel-nut itself, the latter are largely imported into England from Spain, and other parts of Europe, having been kiln-dried before exportation.

THE BRAZIL-NUT.—The Brazil-nut is the product of the juvia tree—*Bertholletia excelsa*—large forests of which exist on the banks of the Orinoco, and in the northern parts of Brazil. The outer case of the fruit, which attains the size of a man's head, is divided into four cells, and each of these contains six or eight nuts. The kernel of the nut, which is surrounded by a hard shell, is exceedingly rich in oil and furnishes a large quantity for extraction. It is highly esteemed by the natives of the localities in which it is grown, and is largely exported from Para and French Guiana for the European market.

THE CASHEW-NUT.—The tree (*Anacardium occidentale*) which yields the *cashew-* or *acajou-nut*, is a native of the West Indies. The fruit is a kidney-shaped nut, about an inch in length, with a double shell. The outer shell is ash-colored and very smooth, and between it and the inner one there exists an acrid, black juice. The kernel is oily, agreeable to the taste, and wholesome. It is a common article of food in tropical climates, and is eaten in both the raw and cooked states.

THE PISTACHIO-NUT.—The pistachio-nut tree is a native of Persia and Syria, but is now cultivated in the south of Europe and north of Africa. The nut splits into two when ripe, and the kernel is of a bright green color. It is very oleaginous, possesses a delicate flavor, and resembles the sweet almond in its qualities. It is sometimes called the green almond. The nuts are highly esteemed in the countries where they are grown, but, as they soon become rancid, they are not much exported. ·

TUBERS AND ROOTS.

THE POTATO.—The potato may be considered as now occupying a place next in importance to the seeds of the cerealia as an article of vegetable food, although only of comparatively modern introduction amongst us.

It is derived from the *Solanum tuberosa*, a plant belonging to the order *Solanaceæ*, which, including, as it does, the belladonna, stramonium, henbane, and tobacco plants, furnishes some of the most poisonous narcotic products encountered.

It is supposed to be a native of South America, and to have extended thence to North America. It seems to have been first brought to the Continent of Europe by the Spaniards, from the neighborhood of Quito, early in the sixteenth century, and to have been then cultivated in gardens only as a curiosity. Its introduction into England and Ireland came from North America; and in "Gerarde's Herbal," published in 1597, it figures under the name of *Batata Virginiana*. John Hawkins brought it to Ireland in 1565, and Sir Francis Drake to England in 1585, but without its attracting much attention in either case. The potatoes of Shakespeare, it may be mentioned, are not the same as the potatoes under consideration; but, on the other hand, a product of the *Batatas edulis*, known by the name of *sweet potato*. The potato was a third time imported by Sir Walter Raleigh, and, as it then received notice as an article of food, the credit is usually given to him for its introduction amongst us. In 1663 the Royal Society recommended that it should be more extensively planted, but it was not grown in the open fields in England till 1684, and so little was for some time thought of it, that Bradley, in 1718, speaks of it as of "little note," and in the "Complete Gardener" of London and Wise, published in 1719, no mention at all is made of it.

The cultivation of the potato is now widely diffused over the globe, and it seems to thrive in most climates, but a considerable check to its prosperous growth has recently occurred. In 1845 a disastrous and previously unknown disease broke out amongst the crops, and has since resisted all efforts to eradicate it. The disease attacks the whole plant, beginning in the leaves and proceeding through the stem to the underground part, and in some years produces such havoc as to entail a very heavy loss. Indeed, it prevails to such an extent, and appears of such an inexterminable nature, as justly to excite serious apprehensions respecting the continuance of a supply sufficient to meet the demand for general consumption. The present aspect, it may be said, points to the possibility of the potato dying out, as an article of every-day food, amongst us.

The potato became a popular food in Ireland earlier than in England, and has ever since held its position there as one of the chief articles of sustenance. Dr. E. Smith says that an adult Irishman will consume his 10¼ pounds of potatoes daily, *i.e.*, 3½ pounds at each meal, and it has been calculated that from three-fifths to four-fifths of the entire food of the people of Ireland is derived from the potato. Since the famine, however, that arose at the commencement of the failure of the crops from the disease, Indian corn has come into greatly increased use.

The part of the plant used as food constitutes the tuber, which is connected with, or, indeed, forms an exuberant growth of, a portion of the underground stem, with which this plant, in common with some others, is provided, in addition to that which grows, as usual, above ground. The tuber develops into a thick, fleshy, mass, but retains its buds, which here go under the denomination of *eyes*, and each of these buds or eyes is capable of independent growth in a detached or isolated state. They are used, in fact, under the name of *sets* for planting and raising a crop.

The potato tuber is surrounded by a thin, grayish, epidermic covering, and beneath this is another tegumentary layer, in which coloring matter is deposited. The substance of the potato is made up of cells, penetrated and surrounded by a watery, albuminous juice, and filled with a number of starch-granules.

There are many well-known different sorts of potato met with. They are derived from corresponding varieties in the plant. In the different varieties, notable differences in size, color, and edible qualities, are observable.

Composition of the Potato (from Letheby's table).

Nitrogenous matter,	2.1
Starch, etc.,	18.8
Sugar,	3.2
Fat,	0.2
Saline matter,	0.7
Water,	75.0
	100.0

The analysis given by Payen stands as follows:

Composition of the Potato (Payen).

Nitrogenous matter,	2.50
Starch,	20.00
Cellulose,	1.04
Sugar and gummy matter,	1.09
Fatty matter,	0.11
Pectates, citrates, phosphates, and silicates of lime, magnesia, potash, and soda,	1.26
Water,	74.00
	100.00

It is thus seen that the potato contains a large percentage of starch. This, indeed, forms its characteristic feature, and renders it applicable for the extraction, that is largely carried on, of starch for domestic and other purposes. The starch obtained from it is also used for adulterating the more expensive farinaceous dietetic preparations, and likewise forms what is sold under the name of British arrow-root, tapioca, etc. Whilst less expensive, there is nothing to show that the starch of the potato differs to any sensible extent, in a nutritive point of view, from the other starchy preparations.

Potatoes require to be cooked to render them fit for eating, and this may be effected by either boiling, steaming, baking, or frying. The heat employed coagulates the albuminous juice contained within and between the cells. The starch-granules absorb the watery part of the juice, swell up, and distend the cells in which they are lodged. The cohesion of the cells becomes destroyed, and they then easily separate from each other, leading to the potato easily breaking down into a loose, farinaceous mass. When these changes are complete, the potato is spoken of as being in a floury or mealy condition. When, on the other hand, the liquid is only partially absorbed and the cells imperfectly separated, the potato remains more or less firm, and is spoken of as close, waxy, or watery.

Steaming is a better process for cooking potatoes than boiling, on account of not being attended by the loss that is occasioned by the latter. When boiling is employed, the skin should not be removed, as is so often found to be the practice; for the removal of the skin favors the extraction of the juice by the surrounding water. The waste, says Dr. Letheby, when potatoes are cooked in their skins, only amounts to 3 per cent., or half an ounce in the pound, whereas when they are peeled first it is not less than 14 per cent., or from two to three ounces in the pound. A little salt added to the water in which potatoes are boiled tends to prevent the escape of their saline constituents.

The potato constitutes a wholesome and agreeable article of food, and one of which the palate does not easily become fatigued. The amount of nitrogenous matter it contains is too small, however, to enable it to form a suitable food alone; but, with articles rich in nitrogenous matter, as meat, fish, etc., it supplies a useful and economical alimentary substance. By the peasantry in some rural districts it is employed in association with buttermilk—which, from the caseine present, furnishes the requisite nitrogenous matter—as the chief means of support; and, thus associated, a cheap, and experience shows, an efficient diet is provided.

In a floury or mealy state the potato enjoys easy digestibility; but in a close, watery, or waxy state, it is very trying to the digestive powers, and should, therefore, when in this condition, be avoided where delicacy of stomach exists. Young potatoes may be more tempting than old, but, from what has been said, will be understood to be indigestible.

The potato has a high repute for the possession of antiscorbutic properties. The concurrent testimony of numerous observers points to its forming a most efficient agent in preventing the occurrence of scurvy. It is used successfully for this purpose on board ocean-going vessels, and the inquiries of the late Dr. Baly into the diseases of prisoners showed in a conclusive manner that the addition of potatoes to the diet sufficed to arrest the prevalence of scurvy in prisons where it had before existed.

The potato is subject to various diseases, which lead to an impairment of its alimentary value. The most important, by far, is the disease that has already been alluded to and which is styled popularly "the potato disease." Ever since 1845, when it was first noticed, it has been common, some years more so than others, amongst the potato crops, not only in our own islands, but on the Continent of Europe and in America. The disease commences in the leaves of the plant, and extends thence through the stem to the tubers. Brown spots make their appearance upon the surface of the tuber, and then penetrate its substance and lead to decay. After being subjected to cooking, the affected part remains hard, whilst the healthy portion has become soft and mealy. If the diseased part be cut away, the remainder will be found good and fit for food; but considerable waste is necessarily thereby incurred, and the disease spreads as the potato is kept. Nothing has been witnessed to show that any ill effects, either in man or amongst the lower animals, have been produced by the incidental consumption of a small quantity of the diseased part; but potatoes in an advanced state of disease are prudently to be regarded as unfit food even for the lower animals.

Potatoes become deteriorated upon growing out or germinating. They cease to assume a mealy state on cooking; present a semi-translucent appearance; and possess a rather sickly, sweetish taste. It has been asserted that a poisonous principle, *solanine*, becomes developed in the buds and shoots of potatoes that are allowed to grow out on keeping. No conclusive evidence, however, has been adduced to show that the potato acquires noxious properties under such circumstances, and nothing is ever heard of any poisonous effects arising from its use, notwithstanding the universal consumption that is going on, and that it is often cooked without the aid of water, which might have the effect of dissolving out any noxious principle. If there be at any time a poison present, it must be either insignificant in amount, or be destroyed by the heat to which the potato is subjected before being sent to the table.

Exposure to frost also seriously damages the potato. The effect produced is of a mechanical nature. The watery juice contained in the cells and intercellular spaces undergoes expansion in the act of freezing, and so leads to a rupture and separation of the cells, and in this way a destruction of the organization of the tuber. Its vitality becomes thus destroyed, and, in consequence, it has no longer the power to resist, when thawed, the ordinary changes of decomposition: hence, putrefaction occurs, and, advancing, renders the article unfit for food.

THE SWEET POTATO.—The sweet potato is derived from the *Batatas edulis*, or, as it was called by the older botanists, *Convolvulus batatas*, a plant which is a native of the Malayan Archipelago, where it formerly grew wild in woods. The plant is now cultivated in most of the warm countries, and furnishes a starchy and sweet tuber, which is prized as an article of food in the East and West Indies, America, and hot climates generally. It was largely eaten in Europe before the cultivation of the potato, which has now taken its place, and also its name. The tubers were imported into England by way of Spain, and sold as a delicacy before the potato was known, and it forms the article referred to when the name is mentioned by English writers previous to the middle of the seventeenth century. It is still, to some extent, cultivated in the south of France and in Spain, and is to be obtained in Paris during the fall of the year, but is not much esteemed now, being considered too sweet to eat with meat and other articles seasoned with salt, and not sweet enough as a sweet kind of food. In North America it is a favorite article of food— more generally used than perhaps any other vegetable except the ordinary potato. When roasted or boiled, it is mealy, and may be looked upon as forming a wholesome food. It is said to possess slightly laxative properties.

There are several varieties of the Batatas cultivated. The following is the composition, according to the analysis of Payen, of a tuber of the kind grown in the south of France and America, which is characterized by richness in starchy and saccharine constituents:

Composition of the Sweet Potato.

Nitrogenous matter,	1.50
Starch,	16.05
Sugar,	10.20
Cellulose,	0.45
Fatty matter,	0.30
Other organic matter,	1.10
Mineral salts,	2.60
Water,	67.50
	99.70

THE YAM.—The yam forms a large, esculent tuber, derived from several species of the genus *Dioscorea*, a group of climbing plants belonging to tropical climates. The tuber is oblong, and sometimes grows to the length of three feet, and may weigh as much as thirty pounds. It contains a considerable amount of starch, and, when boiled or roasted, forms a mealy, palatable, and wholesome food. It is devoid of the sweetness appertaining to the sweet potato, and likewise keeps better. It is eaten by the inhabitants of New Zealand, as well as by those of the East and West Indies and the South Sea Islands, and holds as important a position as an aliment in tropical countries as the common potato does in Europe. At the period of the potato famine an attempt was made to introduce it into England, but with little success.

Of the varieties, the *Dioscorea sativa* forms the common yam of the West Indies. The *Dioscorea alata*, or winged yam, grows in the South Sea Islands and likewise the West Indies, and is met with also in a cultivated state in the East Indies. In different localities there are many other varieties. The *Dioscorea batatas* has been recently brought from China, and has been found to be susceptible of cultivation in France, yielding an abundant produce of wholesome and agreeable food, available all the year round, or readily, at least, during the greater part of the year.

The tubers of all the yams contain an acid principle, which is dissipated by boiling, but there are some species which possess poisonous properties.

THE JERUSALEM ARTICHOKE.—This vegetable product is derived from the *Helianthus tuberosus*, a plant belonging to the sunflower tribe. The word "Jerusalem," indeed, as here applied, is asserted to form a corruption of the Italian *girasole* (sunflower). The plant is said to have been brought in 1617 from Brazil, and is also believed to have been a native of Mexico. It was cultivated in European gardens before the potato was introduced. The root produces around it oval or roundish tubercles, which form the edible part, and which may amount to as many as thirty or even fifty in number. These tubercles, unlike the potato, resist the action of the frost, and thus may be allowed to remain in the ground during the winter, and collected for use as occasion may require. The herbaceous part of the plant, when dry, is also susceptible of being turned to account as fuel.

The Jerusalem artichoke is not consumed to a large extent in England. It has something of the character of the potato, but possesses a sweetish taste, is less agreeable to the palate, and does not become mealy on boiling. The absence of starch accounts for this. There are no granules, as in the potato, to swell up and absorb the moisture, and disorganize or break up the tissue into a loose, friable mass. It therefore maintains a moist or watery condition after cooking, and simply becomes softened. A body in this state must needs be of a less digestible nature than the potato. Its analysis shows that it contains a considerable percentage of sugar. The *inuline*, which is present in small amount, forms a principle isomeric with starch.

Composition of the Jerusalem Artichoke

(From the analysis of Payen, Poinsot, and Fevry).

Nitrogenous matter, ...	3.1
Sugar, ...	14.7
Inuline, ...	1.9
Pectic acid, ...	0.9
Pectine, ...	0.4
Cellulose, ...	1.5
Fatty matter, ...	0.2
Mineral matter, ...	1.3
Water, ...	76.0
	100.0

Other tuberous products are used as food. Several species of the *Oxalideæ* have tuberous roots, and are cultivated for the sake of their tubers. The *Oxalis crenata* and *Oxalis tuberosa* are natives of Peru and Bolivia. Their tubers, when cooked, become mealy, like potatoes, and are said to be much esteemed. The tubers of *Tropæolum tuberosum* are also eaten in Peru. Their taste is described as peculiar. The *Ullucus tuberosus* grows in the mountainous regions of South America; and is cultivated in Peru and Bolivia for the sake of the tubers. It was introduced into France as a substitute for potatoes. The tubers of the *Witheringia* (*Solanum*) *montana* are used as an article of food by the Peruvians. The *Phlomis tuberosa* is eaten by the Calmucs of the Caspian, after being reduced to powder. The tuberous bitter vetch, *Orobus tuberosus*, is a native of Britain, and its tubers have been used, in times of scarcity, as an article of food ("Baird's Cyclo. of Nat. Sci.").

The rhizomes or underground stems of the *Caladium seguinum*, or dumb cane, of the West Indies, are often used as a substitute for potatoes and yams. The rhizomes of the pondweed (*Potamogeton natans*) are used in Siberia as an article of food. The root of the *Arracacha esculenta*, a native of South America, is much cultivated in the neighborhood of Santa Fé de Bogota and other parts of Colombia, where it is as much eaten as potatoes or yams are elsewhere. It is boiled like a potato, and is said to have a flavor intermediate between that of the parsnep and chestnut ("Baird's Cyclo. Nat. Sci.").

THE CARROT.—The garden carrot is derived by cultivation from the *Daucus carota*, a plant which grows freely in a wild state in fields, hedgerows, and waysides in Britain. The root of the wild plant is white, slen-

12

der, and hard, and has an acrid, disagreeable taste, and strong, aromatic smell.   As the result of cultivation, the root of the garden variety is thick, fleshy, and succulent, and of a red, yellow, or pale straw color, with a pleasant odor, and a sweet, agreeable taste.   Whilst young it is very tender, but becomes hard when allowed to grow old.   It is said that the garden carrot was introduced into use in England by the Flemish refugees who settled at Sandwich in the reign of Elizabeth.

Composition of Carrots (from Letheby's table).

Nitrogenous matter, ...	1.3
Starch, etc., ...	8.4
Sugar, ...	6.1
Fat, ...	0.2
Mineral matter, ...	1.0
Water, ...	83.0
	100.0

Carrots form a wholesome and useful food, for both man and cattle. They are not adapted, however, for a weak stomach, being somewhat indigestible and apt to produce flatulence.   They are proportionately valuable as they have more of the outer, soft, red, than the central, yellow, core-like part.   On account of the sugar present, they admit of a syrup being prepared from them, and also yield, by fermentation and distillation, a spirituous liquid.   Cut into small pieces and roasted, they are sometimes used in Germany as a substitute for coffee.

THE PARSNIP.—The root of the parsnip (*Pastinaca sativa*) is of a pale yellow color, but otherwise closely resembles that of the carrot, both in general characters and alimentary properties.   The plant is a native of Britain, and is also found in many parts of Europe and the north of Asia.   In the wild state the root is white, aromatic, mucilaginous, and sweet-tasted, with some degree of acridness.   By cultivation it is rendered more fleshy and milder flavored.   It is used in the same way, but not so extensively, as the carrot, and is not so generally liked.   From custom, it forms the usual accompaniment of salt fish.

Composition of the Parsnip (from Letheby's table).

Nitrogenous matter, ...	1.1
Starch, etc., ...	9.6
Sugar, ...	5.8
Fat, ...	0.5
Salts, ...	1.0
Water, ...	82.0
	100.0

Parsnips are not only used as a vegetable, but a wine is sometimes made from them, which is spoken of as somewhat resembling malmsey. A spirit, also, is sometimes distilled from the fermented product, and in the north of Ireland, with the aid of hops, a table beer is brewed from them.

THE TURNIP.—Turnips grow wild in England, but the wild plant (*Brassica campestris*) is supposed to form the original of the Swedish turnip, or Swede, which is too coarse eating for human food, and not of the cultivated vegetable. This, the *Brassica rapa* (Lindley calls the turnip *Brassica napus*, and rape *Brassica rapa*), is said to have been first introduced as a food for cattle into this country by the celebrated agriculturist, Coke, of Holkham, afterward Earl of Leicester. It forms an agreeable and extensively used vegetable, being either cooked alone or mixed with soups and stews. From the large proportion of water it contains, its nutritive value is low.

The top shoots of such turnip plants as have stood the winter are gathered, and used as a green vegetable. Those from the Swedish turnip are the sweetest flavored.

Composition of the Turnip (Letheby's table).

Nitrogenous matter, ...	1.2
Starch, etc., ...	5.1
Sugar, ...	2.1
Salts, ...	0.6
Water, ...	91.0
	100.0

BEET-ROOT.—The common or red beet (*Beta vulgaris*) belongs to the family of saltworts, which contains the spinach, quinoa, etc., and is characterized by the large amount of alkali in combination with an organic acid existing in the plants. It is a native of the coasts of the Mediterranean, and was introduced into this country in 1548. It was at one time called beet-rave, from the French *betterave*. The root is usually of an elongated form, like that of the carrot, but in some varieties it assumes more of a turnip-shaped character. The color varies from a deepish blackish red to a light red. Beet-root is extensively grown, and employed as food both for man and cattle; and on the Continent is further used as a source of sugar. It is eaten cold, in slices, either alone or in salads, after being boiled, and is also sometimes pickled.

The mangel-wurzel (*Beta altissima*) is usually thought to constitute a large and coarse variety of the common beet, in which the red color is but little developed.

RADISHES.—The common radish (*Raphanus sativus*) is a native of China, and is mentioned by Gerard, in 1584, as then cultivated in England. The root is either long and spindle-shaped, or round and turnip-shaped. The color of the exterior varies: there being black, violet, red, and white radishes; but, in all, the central portion is white. It is usually eaten in a raw state, but is sometimes boiled and served as a vegetable. In composition the radish closely resembles the turnip.

SALSIFY.—The salsify, or purple goat's beard (*Tragopogon porrifolius*) is a hardy plant, indigenous in England. It belongs to the same tribe as the chiccory and lettuce. The root is long and tapering, and becomes by cultivation fleshy and tender, with a white, milky juice. It has a mild, sweetish taste, like the parsnip, and is boiled or stewed for the table. It is not so much eaten in England as on the Continent. In

America it is usually boiled, mashed with potatoes, and fried in small cakes; and, from the taste belonging to it when fried, it is there often called the "oyster plant."

The *Ginseng* root is highly valued by the Chinese for its supposed invigorating and aphrodisiac qualities. It is a species of *Panax;* and the *Panax quinquefolium*, which is a native of America, possesses the same qualities as the ginseng ("Barrow's Travels in China," and "Baird's Cyclo. of Nat. Sci.").

The root of the *Kalo*, or *Arum esculentum*, which is the principal food of the lower class of the Sandwich Islanders, somewhat resembles the beet, but its color is brown instead of red. It is reared with great care in small enclosures kept wet, like rice or paddy fields. A sort of paste is made from the root, which is called *poi* ("Simpson's Journey Round the World," vol. ii., p. 31).

The roots of the *Potentilla anserina*, or *goose-grass*, when roasted or boiled, taste like parsnips, and in the Western Islands of Scotland they have been known to support the inhabitants for months together in times of scarcity ("Baird's Cyclo. Nat. Sci.").

The roots of the *common fern*, or *bracken*, are largely eaten in New Zealand. They are simply washed and boiled, or beaten with a stone till they become soft and are then roasted.

HERBACEOUS ARTICLES.

These include foliaceous parts, shoots, and stems of plants. They are valuable as articles of food, not so much for the absolute amount of nutritive matter afforded—for, on account of their succulent nature, they contain but a small proportion of solid matter—as for the salts they yield and the variety they give to our diet. By cultivation they have been brought to a very different state from that in which they originally existed. To make them tender and agreeably flavored is part of the art of the gardener, and is accomplished by quick growth and, in many instances, by a partial exclusion from light. If allowed to grow slowly, the development of ligneous matter is favored, which gives them hardness, whilst full-exposure to light leads to the production, not only of green coloring matter, but of the characteristic principles of the plant, which often communicate a strong and disagreeable taste. It is found that leafy products, which have been allowed to acquire a full green color, possess more or less purgative properties. It is necessary, therefore, that the consumption of these should not be on too extensive a scale. The antiscorbutic virtue of the class of vegetables under consideration is high.

PRODUCTS OF THE CABBAGE TRIBE.—The original of the cabbage tribe is the sea-cabbage, a wild plant, named *Brassica oleracea*, which is to be found growing on many cliffs of the South Coast of England, and in some other parts. This is the true collet, or colewort (although the name is now applied to any young cabbage which has a loose and open heart), and the leaves of it are gathered by the inhabitants and consumed as a vegetable. In this state it only grows to an insignificant size in comparison with the dimensions attained as the result of cultivation. From this plant a variety of well-known and extensively consumed vegetables have been produced, including, for instance, cabbages, greens, savoys, Brussels-sprouts, cauliflower, broccoli, etc. Looked at in a gen-

eral way, these various products form a wholesome and agreeable component of the food of man. It is true, containing, as they do, about 90 per
cent. of water, their nutritive value is not high, but they are useful as
giving variety, and for the salts they supply. They also possess marked
antiscorbutic virtue. They labor under the disadvantage of being articles
of difficult digestion, which renders them unsuited where weakness of
stomach exists. Their proportion of sulphur is large, and they thus are
apt to give rise to flatulence of an unpleasant nature. To secure tenderness, they should be grown quickly, and dressed whilst young.

The common white garden cabbage is a variety of the *Brassica oleracea.* It is one of the oldest of cultivated vegetables, and has been known
in this country from time immemorial.

What is called *Sauer-kraut,* which is largely consumed in Germany,
is prepared from the leaves of cabbage. These, deprived of their stalk
and mid-rib, are cut up and placed in a tub or vat in alternate layers
with salt. They are then subjected to pressure, and allowed to remain
till acid fermentation has set in and they have become sour. The product is cooked by stewing in its own liquor.

Red cabbage.—This is another variety of the *Brassica oleracea,* which
is similar in form to the preceding. It is used chiefly for pickling, but
is sometimes stewed in a fresh state for the table.

Greens constitute all the varieties of the *Brassica oleracea* which
grow in an open way or have no hearts, and which are used as an article
of food. Some of them are called *colewort* (the name applied to the
wild plant), and others, with curled or wrinkled leaves, are known as *green
kale,* or *borecole.* They are sufficiently hardy to resist the cold of winter,
and thus yield a green vegetable when such food is scarce.

There is a variety of the cabbage-plant extensively cultivated in Jersey, which attains a height of seven or eight feet and upward. It continues to grow, and throw out leaves from the top; and these, as they
attain full size, are stripped off and used as food, both for man and cattle.
Thriving through the winter, as it does, it is a valuable plant to the inhabitants of the island. The stem is sufficiently hard and woody to be
susceptible of conversion into a walking-stick.

Savoy.—This name is applied to a variety of cabbage, which is distinguished from other close-hearted cabbages by having wrinkled leaves.
It is principally grown for winter use.

Brussels-sprouts form also a winter and early spring vegetable. They
grow with small heads, like miniature cabbages, from the axils of the
leaves of one of the many cultivated varieties of *Brassica oleracea.* The
plant is usually propagated from seed imported from Belgium, as it is
apt to degenerate by growth in England. It has been cultivated lately
to a much larger extent in the market-gardens around London than formerly.

Cauliflower.—This is one of the most delicate and highly prized articles derived from the cabbage tribe. It is entirely the product of cultivation, and constitutes the inflorescence of the plant, which by art has
been made to grow into a compact mass or head, of a white color. It was
known to the Greeks and Romans, but was not much grown in England
until the end of the seventeenth century. It was then, however, very
successfully cultivated, and even exported to Holland, from which country so many of our vegetables have been introduced.

Broccoli is distinguished from cauliflower, of which it is merely a
variety, by the color of its inflorescence and leaves, and its compara-

tively hardy constitution, which enables it to stand the winter. Its color varies greatly, through shades of buff or yellow, green, and purple. *Broccoli-sprouts* are obtained from the early purple or sprouting broccoli. The plant grows from two to three feet high, and produces sprouts of flowers from the axils of the leaves.

Kohl-rabi, Knol-kohl, or *Turnip cabbage,* constitutes a remarkable variety of cabbage-plant. The stem is enlarged just above the ground into a fleshy, turnip-like knob, of about the size of a man's fist, from which the leaf-stalks spring. The plant is of a hardy nature, and the globular enlargement is more solid and more nutritious than a turnip of the same size.

SPINACH.—The vegetable falling under this name is furnished by the leaves of the *Spinacia oleracea,* or garden spinach, a plant introduced into this country in the sixteenth century, and supposed to be a native of Western Arabia. There are several varieties of the plant, and the leaves are boiled and mashed for the table, to be eaten as a green vegetable, and are also frequently employed for introduction into soup. It is a wholesome vegetable, with slightly laxative properties.

The spinach belongs to a tribe of plants, other families of which yield leaves that are prepared and eaten in a similar way. For instance, the leaves of the *Chenopodium,* which furnishes the quinoa grain, are used as spinach by the inhabitants of Chili and Peru. The *Beet* family belongs to the same tribe, and the leaves of the *Beta maritima,* or sea-beet, a common European sea-shore plant, and of the *Beta cicla,* or white beet, are also used as spinach. The latter plant, which is supposed to be a variety of the red beet, is cultivated specially and solely for the leaves. It is a native of the sea-coasts of Spain and Portugal, and was introduced into England in 1570. What is called *mountain spinach* is derived from the *garden orache* (*Atriplex hortensis*), a member of another family belonging to the same tribe, which is a native of Tartary, and was introduced into Europe in 1548. The leaves have a slightly acid flavor, and are much esteemed as a vegetable in France.

The Romans ate the leaves of the *mallow* as a substitute for spinach, and these are still used for a similar purpose in some parts of France, Italy, and Lower Egypt. The leaves of *Mercurialis annua* are cooked and eaten as spinach in Germany (" Baird's Cyclo. of Nat. Sci.").

SORREL.—Sorrel (*Rumex acetosa*) belongs to the buckwheat order of plants. In England it is to be seen growing wild in meadows, and is now seldom used as an article of food, although in the time of Henry VIII. it was to be found in almost every garden. In France, however, it is rather extensively employed, and by cultivation is considerably improved. Sorrel possesses an acid taste of a pronounced character, which is due to the presence of the superoxalate of potash and tartaric acid.

RHUBARB.—This is also a member of the buckwheat tribe, and yields one of the most useful of garden productions. Whilst the leaves were formerly boiled and made into a sauce for meat in England, the stalks have only been of comparatively recent introduction into dietetic use amongst us. The *Rheum rhaponticum* and *Rheum hybridum* constitute the species usually grown for alimentary purposes. The *Rheum palmatum,* commonly known to gardeners as the true Turkey rhubarb, also yields an excellent edible product. The stalks of the leaves, after being peeled, are cooked and eaten precisely in the same way as gooseberries, for which they form a good substitute, if even they are not to be preferred. Rhubarb occupies, indeed, in an alimentary point of view, the position of a fruit, but it is not eatable in the raw state. It is also sometimes used for making wine. On account of oxalate of lime forming a constituent of rhubarb, it should be avoided by persons suffering from the oxalate of lime diathesis.

LAVER.—Laver is the name given to various kinds of sea-weed used as food. *Green laver*, as dressed for the table, closely resembles spinach in appearance, but has a bitterish taste. It is obtained from the *Ulva latissima*, a common sea-weed on the British shores. Amongst the other marine plants employed are the *Porphyra vulgaris* and *laciniata ;* *Chondrus crispus*, or *carrageen*, or *Irish moss ; Laminaria digitata*, or seagirdle ; *Laminaria saccharina ;* and *Alaria esculenta*, or bladderlock.

Basing his remarks upon the analyses of Dr. Davy and Dr. Apjohn, Dr. Letheby states that sea-weeds, in a moderately dry condition, contain from 18 to 26 per cent. of water, 9½ to 15 per cent. of nitrogenous matter, and, upon an average, about 60 per cent. of starchy matter and sugar, (vegetable mucilage ?)—a composition which places them amongst the most nutritious of vegetable substances. He urges the advisability of extending the use of so valuable and abundant a stock of food, which already enters largely into the diet of some of the coast inhabitants of Great Britain, Ireland, and the Continent. Before being cooked, they require to be soaked in water to remove their saline matter. They are then stewed in water or milk until they become tender and mucilaginous. Sometimes they are pickled, and eaten with pepper, vinegar, and oil, or with lemon-juice. The consumption of laver is thought to be useful in scrofulous affections and glandular tumors.

Sea-weeds are eaten by the Chinese, and a jelly is likewise made by them from the leaves of *fucus* ("Barrow's Travels in China," pp. 551-2).

It may be mentioned here that certain varieties of *Lichen* are consumed as food. Captain Franklin and his party, in their voyage to the Polar Sea, subsisted principally, during a part of the year 1821 (when suffering great privations), on lichens of the genus *Gyrophora*, which the Canadians term *tripe de roche*. Under this diet, however, the party became little more than skin and bones, and after a time the unpalatable weed became quite nauseous to all, and produced bowel complaint amongst several ("Franklin's Journey," p. 403).

CELERY.—The common celery (*Apium graveolens*) is a native of Britain, and in its wild state is known as *smallage*, which grows freely by the sides of ditches and in marshy places. In this state it has a coarse, rank taste, and a peculiar smell. By the process of cultivation which is now resorted to, and which was introduced from India about a century and a half ago, it loses its acrid nature, and becomes mild and sweet. The plan adopted is to earth it up as it grows, and thus keep it white by exclusion from light, the tops of the leaves only being allowed to appear above the ground. Several varieties of the plant are met with. Eaten raw, it must undoubtedly be looked upon as difficult of digestion. It is frequently stewed, and is employed also for introducing into soups.

SEA-KALE.—The Sea-kale (*Cramba maritima*) forms a hardy plant, which grows on the sea-shores of various parts of Britain and the Continent. It has long been eaten by the common people, but was not cultivated in gardens until the eighteenth century. It is now brought to a high state of perfection, and is one of the most esteemed of vegetables. Properly cooked, it is delicate, easy of digestion, and nutritious. Like celery, it is blanched by exclusion from light during its growth, and unless this is carefully attended to, the shoots acquire an acrid taste. The vegetable is but little known on the Continent.

ARTICHOKE.—The green artichoke constitutes the flower-head of one of the *Compositæ*, viz., the *Cynara scolymus*, which is a native of the South of Europe, and was introduced into England in 1548. The flower-head is gathered before the flowers expand. The succulent bases of the leafy scales and the central disc form the edible portion, and furnish a delicate-flavoured vegetable.

The term *chard* is applied to the leaf-stalks, which have been blanched by tying up the leaves and wrapping all of them over expect the tops. In this state the stalks are tender and white, and are sometimes thus prepared for the table.

The fleshy receptacle of the carline thistle (*Carlina caulescens*), a native of the South of Europe, exceeds that of the artichoke in size and is said to equal it in flavor.

The *cardoon* (*Cynara carduncellus*) also yields an edible article. The plant closely resembles the common artichoke. The thick, fleshy leaves are blanched, and, when cooked, taste very much like the artichoke. It is not much used in England, but is in considerable request on the Continent.

ASPARAGUS.—The *Asparagus officinalis* belongs to the lily tribe, and in its wild state is a sea-coast plant. It is a native of Europe, and is now extensively cultivated as a garden vegetable. The young shoots form the portion that is eaten, and, by cultivation, these have been greatly increased in size and altered from their original condition. They are universally esteemed as a choice and delicate vegetable. They contain a special crystallizable principle, called *asparagine*, which possesses diuretic properties, and gives a peculiar odor to the urine.

Other vegetable products are sometimes dressed and eaten in the same way as asparagus. The flower-stalks, for instance, of the *Ornithogalum pyrenaicum* are used as asparagus in some parts of Gloucestershire, and sold in Bath under the name of Prussian asparagus. The stalks of the *salsify* are likewise sometimes similarly employed, and also the leaf-stalks and mid-ribs of the great white or sweet *beet* (*Beta cicla*). The latter is denominated *beet chard*. The young shoots of one or two species of *Typha* are eaten by the Cossacks like asparagus. The young buds of hops are said to be scarcely inferior to asparagus in taste.

ONION.—The onion (*Allium cepa*), like the asparagus, although differing so much from it in its dietetic properties, belongs to the lily tribe of plants. In common with, but to a higher degree than, the other members of the allium species, which includes also the garlic, chive, shallot, and leek, it contains an acrid, volatile oil, which possesses strongly irritant and excitant properties. Grown in Spain and other warm places, the onion is milder and sweeter than when grown in colder countries.

The chief use of the onion reared in our own gardens is as a condiment or flavoring agent, whilst the large onions imported from Spain are sufficiently mild to be eaten as an ordinary vegetable, and are stewed and roasted for the table.

LETTUCE.—The garden lettuce (*Lactuca sativa*), is a hardy plant, of which a great number of varieties exist. It is supposed to be a native of the East Indies, but has been cultivated in Europe from a remote period of antiquity. Most of the lettuces grown for use form one or other of two kinds—*cos* and *cabbage*. The leaves of the former are oblong and upright, and are tied together for the purpose of being blanched; whilst those of the latter are rounder and of a more spreading character, and at the same time grow nearer to the ground.

The lettuce supplies a wholesome, digestible, cooling, and agreeable salad. It is occasionally made use of as a boiled vegetable. It contains a milky juice, especially when the plant has been allowed to run to flower, which possesses mild soporific properties, and is collected and inspissated, and used as a medicinal agent, under the name of *lactucarium* or *lettuce opium*.

ENDIVE.—The endive (*Cichorium endivia*) is a native of China or Japan, and was introduced into Europe in the year 1548. It is largely used as a winter salad, but is less tender than lettuce, and has a decidedly bitter taste. It is sometimes stewed and eaten as a cooked vegetable.

CRESS.—The common or garden cress (*Lepidium sativum*) is a native of the East, but has been cultivated in our gardens since 1548. The young leaves are used as salad, and they possess a pungent and agreeable flavor. It ranks as one of the principal of the small salads, and a variety with curled leaves is especially esteemed.

MUSTARD.—The white mustard (*Sinapis alba*) is a native of Britain, and grows in waste places. It is sown in gardens, and forced under glass for the production of a small salad, which, like cress, possesses an agreeable, pungent flavor.

RAPE.—The Rape (*Brassica napus*) is frequently grown and used as a substitute for mustard and cress. It is devoid, however, of the agreeable pungency which belongs to these latter articles.

WATER-CRESS.—The water-cress (*Nasturtium officinale*) is a creeping plant, which grows in slow-running streams, and thrives best on a bottom of sand or gravel. It is a native of almost all parts of the world, and forms a favorite and wholesome edible product, which is seldom out of season. There are two varieties, the green and brown

The young shoots of the common poke, or American grape (*Phytolacca decandra*), are eaten by the natives of America and the West Indies as a vegetable, and in Austria the plant is cultivated for the same purpose ("Baird's Cyclo. Nat. Sci.").

The leaves of the common daisy are used as a pot-herb in some countries ("Baird's Cyclo. Nat. Sci.").

The leaves of the dandelion are eaten as a salad, and are little inferior to endive ("Forsyth's Dictionary of Diet").

The large purple flowers of the *Abulilon esculentum* (called in Brazil, Bençao de Dios), are dressed and eaten with their food by the inhabitants of Rio de Janeiro ("Baird's Cyclo. Nat. Sci.").

The leaves of the *Lithospermum maritimum*, which belongs to the same tribe as the borage, and grows on the sea-coast in certain northern parts of the United Kingdom, are said to have a strong taste of oysters. It is hence sometimes called the "oyster-plant" in Scotland.

FRUITY PRODUCTS CONSUMED AS VEGETABLES.

CUCUMBER.—The common cucumber (*Cucumis sativus*) is a native of the South of Asia, but has long been cultivated in all civilized countries. It furnishes a fleshy fruit, which forms an edible product. It is grown both in the open air and under glass, the fruit varying in size, tenderness, and flavor, accordingly: that which is forced or grown quickly possessing choicer qualities than that which is grown slowly.

Cucumber, in the raw state, must be looked upon as a cold and indigestible article; and it is apt to disagree with many. Stewed, it forms a light and wholesome vegetable.

Young cucumbers are pickled in vinegar and called *gherkins*. In this state they form an agreeable relish at a meal, and serve to give zest for other food.

VEGETABLE MARROW.—Vegetable marrow constitutes the fruit of the *Cucurbita ovifera*, a plant which is supposed to be only a variety of the pumpkin. It was introduced into Europe from the East Indies at the commencement of the present century, and is now extensively cultivated in England. It is dressed in various ways, and its name is derived from the softness of its fleshy substance. It forms a delicate-flavored and easily digestible vegetable, but, on account of its highly succulent nature, its nutritive value is very low.

The pumpkin (*Cucurbita pepo*), and melon-pumpkin, or squash (*Cucurbita melopepo*), are products of an allied nature to vegetable marrow, and are sometimes used as food.

TOMATO.—The tomato, or love-apple (*Solanum lycopersicum*), is a native of South America, and was introduced into Europe in 1596. The ripe fruit is used in various ways, and has an agreeable acidulous taste. It is more, perhaps, as a relish, than for its nutritive value, that it is useful, and its popularity has rapidly increased of late. In the unripe state it is said to make an excellent pickle. In America it is very largely used, and is eaten raw as a salad, or after being stewed; and of late years an important industry has sprung up in that country, embracing their preservation by partial cooking and enclosure in hermetically sealed tins.

A variety of the *Solanum melongena*, or egg-plant, yields a fruity product, known as the *egg-apple, aubergine*, or *brinjal*. This is of an elongated form and purple color. It is somewhat largely eaten on the Continent, and to some extent also in England; but it is dry and spongy, and devoid of the agreeable qualities belonging to the tomato. In America it is a favorite vegetable, and is there usually sliced and fried.

ESCULENT FUNGI.

The fungi are low vegetable products, which are characterized chemically by the large amount of nitrogenous matter they contain. In this respect, indeed, they are closely allied to animal substances. On the Continent a considerable number of varieties are consumed, but in England, from suspicion of the possession of dangerous properties, the selection is restricted mainly to three, viz., the *mushroom*, *morel*, and *truffle*. The following is the chemical composition of these, according to the analyses of Payen:

Composition of Edible Fungi (Payen).

	Mushrooms.	Morels.	White truffles.	Black truffles.
Nitrogenous matter and traces of sulphur, ...	4.680	4.40	9.958	8.775
Fatty matter, ...	0.396	0.56	0.442	0.560
Cellulose, dextrine, saccharine matter, mannite, and other non-nitrogenous principles, ...	3.456	3.68	15.158	16.585
Salts (phosphates and chlorides of the alkalies, lime, and magnesia), silica, ...	0.458	1.36	2.102	2.070
Water, ...	91.010	90.00	72.340	72.000
	100.000	100.00	100.000	100.000

In the dried state, mushrooms contain, Payen states, 52, morels 44, white truffles 36, and black truffles 31 per cent. of nitrogenous matter.

MUSHROOMS.—Belonging to the mushroom tribe is a large number of varieties, many of which are suitable for eating, whilst other possess poisonous properties. The *Agaricus campestris* constitutes the common edible mushroom. It is found springing up spontaneously in our pastures during the months of August, September, and October, and is also cultivated in beds, and thence obtainable all the year round. It is a native of most of the temperate regions of both hemispheres. It produces a spreading filamentous or thread-like underground structure, called the mycelium or spawn. From this, little tubers spring, which rapidly enlarge, and grow into a stalk, bearing at its summit a rounded head, which, in a short time, expands into a pileus or cap. This, which forms the edible portion, constitutes the fructification, and presents upon its undersurface a number of parallel plates or gills, that bear the sporules of the fungus.

Mushrooms are employed for flavoring, and as an occasional delicacy, rather than as a common article of food. Although difficult of digestion, and, therefore, not adapted for the weak stomach, they may, nevertheless, be consumed by most healthy persons without proving hurtful. Sometimes, however, probably from idiosyncrasy on the part of the individual, they give rise to more or less serious derangement. They are eaten in the fresh state, either broiled, baked, or stewed, and are also preserved by pickling. The young or button mushrooms are used for the latter purpose. *Ketchup* (besides being made from the walnut) is prepared from their juice, flavored with salt and aromatics.

The resemblance between mushrooms and their companion non-edible growths—toadstools—is so close, that mistakes have sometimes arisen and serious consequences resulted from the wrong fungus being eaten. It is not easy to give precise rules that will serve to distinguish the wholesome from the poisonous product; but, as affording some assistance, the following particulars bearing on the point may be furnished. Mushrooms, when young, are like a small, round button, with the exterior of both the stalk and head white. As they grow larger, the head expands, assuming a flat or discoidal shape, and the gills underneath are at first of a pale flesh color, but afterward become dark brown or blackish. The skin upon the top of the cap or disc peels off easily. The flesh is white, compact, and brittle, not soft and watery. They have an agreeable odor, and grow, for the most part, in open, closely fed pastures—rarely in woods. Toadstools, on the other hand, grow freely in woods, or shady, damp places. They have, in general, an unpleasant smell, and the gills are of a brown color. A sure test, says Dr. Christison, indicative of a poisonous fungus, is an astringent, styptic taste, and perhaps, also, a disagreeable, but certainly a pungent odor. He says, also, that most fungi which have a warty cap, and more especially if fragments of membrane are seen adhering to their upper surface, are poisonous. In the absence of practical knowledge of the different varieties, the golden rule to observe is, to reject all kinds of fungi, which are disagreeable to smell and taste—or stated conversely, to select those only which possess the well-known agreeable aroma and flavor of the common edible mushroom. The effects produced by the poisonous fungi are of a narcotico-acrid nature. The usual symptoms are pain or uneasiness in the stomach, vomiting, purging, a sense of constriction in the throat, distress of breathing, giddiness, fainting, prostration, and stupor. Sometimes the brain symptoms predominate, and the sufferer is thrown into a state of coma; at other times the effects are chiefly manifested upon the alimentary canal, and symptoms allied to those of cholera are observed. Sometimes, also, the effects have come on within a few minutes after the fungi have been eaten, whilst at other times they have been delayed for several hours. Recovery has generally occurred after a longer or shorter period, but a few instances have been recorded where a fatal termination has been observed. Some persons, as already mentioned, are, through idiosyncrasy, injuriously affected by the ordinary edible mushrooms, but the effects in such cases are usually confined to vomiting, purging, and colic.

The active principle of the poisonous fungi has recently been separated from the *Agaricus muscarius* by Schmiedeberg of Strasburg, and named by him *muscarin.* From the investigations conducted by its discoverer, it appears to have the power of checking in a very striking manner the action of the heart. Dr. Lauder Brunton * has also found that it causes marked contraction of the pulmonary vessels, and thereby diminishes the flow of blood through the lungs to such an extent that the general arteries are brought to a nearly empty condition. A further discovery, which promises to prove of practical importance, is that these effects of muscarin are in a very complete manner counteracted by the active principle of belladonna. The merest trace of muscarin, it is stated, will almost instantaneously arrest the pulsations of the frog's heart, and the

---

* British Medical Journal, p. 617, November 14, 1874.

effect will be permanent unless a little atropine be afterward employed, when the pulsations will be resumed. It remains to be seen whether the administration of belladonna, or the subcutaneous injection of atropine will prove effectual as an antidote in cases of mushroom-poisoning.

Although fungi constitute an important article of diet of large numbers of people in France, Germany, Russia, and Italy, the prejudice from mistrust in England is such that nearly all except the common mushroom (*Agaricus campestris*) are neglected. Rocques has called them "the manna of the poor," and so large is the consumption of fungi in Rome, that the appointment of an official inspector was made in 1837. In Terra del Fuego, the inhabitants almost live upon a species of mushroom (*Cyttaria Darwinii*) which grows on the bark of the beech of that country; and in Australia, many species of Boletus are eaten by the natives, one of them (*Mylittus Australis*) is commonly known as Australian bread ("Baird's Cyclo. of Nat. Sci.").

Dr. Badham, in his work on "The Esculent Funguses of England," writes: "No country is perhaps richer in esculent funguses than our own; we have upward of thirty species abounding in our woods. No markets might therefore be better supplied than the English, and yet, England is the only country in Europe where this important and savory food is, from ignorance or prejudice, left to perish ungathered." Dr. Badham's work (1847) contains descriptions of twenty-nine species of Agaricus, three of Boletus, three of Polyporus, and many others.

Attempts have been made of late years to break through the popular prejudice against many species of edible fungi, and the Rev. M. J. Berkeley, the most distinguished mycologist in England, attended the Food Committee of the Society of Arts (*Vide Journ. of the Soc. of Arts*, p. 467, May 15, 1868), to give information on the subject.

The members of the Woolhope Naturalists' Field Club have paid special attention to the discovery of edible fungi, and on October 9, 1868, a meeting was arranged at Hereford for the purpose of making a "Foray among the Funguses." A large number were collected, which were eaten at the dinner that was given after the excursion. Among these were the *Fistulina hepatica*, the liver fungus or vegetable beef-steak, one specimen of which was nearly two feet in diameter and weighed about 10 or 12 lbs., and the *Agaricus prunulus* or *Orcella*, called vegetable sweet-bread.

THE MOREL.—The common morel (*Morchella esculenta*), though a native of this country, is usually imported for use from the Continent. It is kept in a dried state, and sold at Italian warehouses, and by the herbalists at Covent Garden. In the fresh state it consists of a hollow stem and rounded head continuous with each other. It enters as a flavoring ingredient into some made dishes, and is sometimes also stewed and eaten separately, like the mushroom.

TRUFFLES.—The truffle forms a subterraneous fungus, which never appears above the surface. It grows in light, dry soils, and is found in several parts of England: more especially on the Downs of Wiltshire, Hampshire, and Kent. It is more plentiful in France, and there acquires a larger size and choicer flavor. The most esteemed, on account of the richness of their aroma, are those which are obtained from the oak forests of Perigord. There are three varieties: the black, white, and red or violet. The latter is rare, and of the two former the black is held in by far the higher repute. The white, indeed, is considered of comparatively little value. To be in perfection, truffles should be quite fresh, much of their aroma being lost by keeping. The black truffle is nodulated on the surface, and, as met with in the market, varies in size from that of a filbert or plum to that of the fist. Internally, it is marbled with white, filamentous streaks, which have been regarded as constituting a sort of mycelium.

As they do not appear above the surface, there is nothing to indicate the locality of their growth, but their odor leads to their being scented out by animals employed for the purpose. In England, dogs are trained for this work. They scratch and bark over the spot where the truffles grow, and then men dig them out. In France, pigs are used in the same way. This animal appears to be very fond of them, and on discovering their situation turns up the ground with its snout in search of them.

Truffles are considered, particularly on the Continent, an article of the greatest delicacy. Their firm and toughish consistence renders them indigestible, but they are esteemed for the sake of their peculiar aroma. Whilst being seldom eaten alone, they are often used as a stuffing, and form also a frequent ingredient of made dishes, besides being employed to flavor gravies and sauces.

FRUITS.

The term fruit, in botanical language, signifies the seed, with its surrounding structures, in progress to or arrived at maturity. In a popular and dietetic sense it has a more limited signification, and refers in a general way only to such product when used in the manner of a dessert. Botanically, wheat, peas, beans, etc., constitute fruits, but popularly the term is restricted to articles like apples, pears, plums, grapes, etc.

Fruits consist of two parts—the *seed*, and what is technically called the *pericarp*. The latter comprises that which surrounds the seed, and is composed of the *epicarp*, the external integument or skin; the *endocarp* or *putamen*, the inner coat or shell; and the *sarcocarp* or *mesocarp*, the intermediate part, which generally possesses a more or less fleshy consistence. It is the sarcocarp which forms the edible succulent portion of the fruit.

The flower, and thence the fruit, is formed from modifications of the leaf, and in an early stage the fruit is *green*, and exhibits much the same chemical composition and general comportment as the leaf. It is only as maturity advances that its special characteristics become developed. At first, like other green parts of the plant, it absorbs and decomposes the carbonic acid of the atmosphere under the influence of light, liberating oxygen and assimilating the carbon. During its progress, it increases more or less rapidly in bulk and weight; and, as it approaches maturity, it loses its green color, becomes brown, yellow, or red, and no longer acts on the air like the leaves, but, on the contrary, absorbs oxygen and gives out carbonic acid. As this process advances, some of the proximate principles contained in the unripe fruit, particularly the vegetable acids and tannin, in part disappear, apparently by oxidation, and, thus, it becomes less sour and astringent. At the same time the starch undergoes transformation into sugar, and the insoluble pectose into pectin and other soluble substances of allied composition and having more or less of a gelatinous character. The fruit in this way arrives at a state of perfection for eating. Oxidation, however, still advances, and now the sugar and remaining acid become destroyed, giving rise to the loss of flavor which occurs after the full ripened state has been attained and deterioration has set in. Finally if the changes are allowed to pursue their ordinary course, the pericarp undergoes decay and the seed is set free.

The agreeable taste of fruits partly depends on the aroma, and partly on the existence of a due relation between the acid, sugar, gum, pectin, etc., and likewise the amount of water and the soluble and insoluble constituents. Luscious fruits like the peach, greengage, and mulberry, which seem to melt in the mouth, contain a very large proportion of soluble substances. A due proportion of gum, pectin, and other gelatinous substances, serves to mask the taste of the free acid, if present in a somewhat large proportion as compared with the sugar. Such is the case with the peach, apricot, and greengage, which contain but a small amount of sugar as compared with the free acid, but a large proportion of gum and pectous substances. The sour taste of certain berry fruits, as the currant and gooseberry, arises from the presence of a considerable quantity of free acid, with only a small amount of gum and pectin to disguise it. By cultivation, the proportion of sugar may be increased in fruits, as is instanced by the difference existing between the wild and cultivated strawberry and raspberry ("Watts' Dictionary of Chemistry," Art. Fruit).

Fruit forms an agreeable and refreshing kind of food, and, eaten in moderate quantity, exerts a favorable influence as an article of diet. Its proportion of nitrogenous matter is too low, and of water too high, to allow it to possess much nutritive value. It is chiefly of service, looking at the actual material afforded, for the carbohydrates, vegetable acids, and salts it contains. It enjoys in a high degree the power of counteracting the unhealthy state found to be induced by too close restriction to dried and salted provisions. The preserved juice acts in this way equally as well as the fresh fruit, and the juice of certain fruits—the lemon and lime, for instance—as is well-known, is specially and largely used for its antiscorbutic efficacy.

Whilst advantageous when consumed in moderate quantity, fruit, on the other hand, proves injurious if eaten in excess. Of a highly succulent nature, and containing free acids and principles prone to undergo change, it is apt, when ingested out of due proportion to other food, to act as a disturbing element, and excite derangement of the alimentary canal. This is particularly likely to occur if eaten either in the unripe or over-ripe state: in the former case, from the quantity of acid present; in the latter, from its strong tendency to ferment and decompose within the digestive tract. The prevalence of stomach and bowel disorders, noticeable during the height of the fruit season, affords proof of the inconveniences that the too free use of fruit may give rise to.

The effect of fruit is to diminish the acidity of the urine. The alkaline vegetable salts which it contains become decomposed in the system, and converted into the carbonate of the alkali, which passes off with the urine. By virtue of this result, the employment of fruit is calculated to prove advantageous in gout and other cases where the urine shows a tendency to throw down a deposit of lithic acid.

In the following description of fruits no strict classification will be attempted. There are some fruits, however, that admit of being conveniently grouped together, and these will be made to follow each other. The *pomaceous* group, for instance, forms a natural assemblage, and includes the apple, pear, quince, etc. The *orange* or *citron* group includes, besides the orange and citron, the lemon, lime, shaddock, and pomelo. *Drupaceous* fruits are those provided with a hard stone, surrounded by a fleshy pulp, such as the plum, peach, cherry, olive, date, etc. Fruits of the *baccate* or *berry* kind comprise the grape, gooseberry, currant, cranberry, barberry, and others. Strawberries, raspberries, blackberries, and mulberries, although in name compounded of the word berry, constitute a fruit of quite a different nature.

THE APPLE.—The apple (*Pyrus malus*), of which there are now very numerous varieties, is derived by cultivation from the wild crab, a native of Britain and other parts of Europe. The smallest apples grow in Siberia, and the largest in America, where many new varieties have originated, and the fruit has attained its highest perfection. Their Newtown pippin is considered by the Americans to stand at the head of all apples, native or foreign.

The apple forms one of the most useful and plentiful of British fruits. It is introduced into tarts and puddings, besides being employed at the dessert-table and made into sauce, preserve, and jelly. It also furnishes the fermented beverage called cider. Verjuice is the fermented juice of the crab-apple.

In a raw state the apple must not be looked upon as easy of digestion. In a cooked state, however, it is light and digestible. Roasted apples exert a slightly laxative action, and are often employed as an agreeable means of overcoming habitual constipation.

Large quantities of apples are dried and flattened in America and Normandy, producing what are known as "biffins" and "Normandy pippins." These are prepared for use by stewing.

Composition of Apples (Fresenius).

	White dessert.
SOLUBLE MATTER—	
Sugar,	7.58
Free acid (reduced to equivalent in malic acid),	1.04
Albuminous substances,	0.22
Pectous substances, etc.,	2.72
Ash,	0.44
INSOLUBLE MATTER—	
Seeds,	0.38
Skins, etc.,	1.42
Pectose,	1.16
[*Ash from insoluble matter included in weights given*],	[0.03]
WATER,	85.04
	100.00

THE PEAR.—The pear (*Pyrus communis*), like the apple, is indigenous to this country, but the wild pear is a very insignificant fruit. It flourishes in a warm, moist atmosphere, and Jersey is considered to be the most favorable situation for its growth in all Europe. There is a larger number of the varieties of the pear than of the apple. The jargonelle, bergamot, and Beurré form three of the most highly esteemed varieties. The fruit is chiefly used for dessert, but is also stewed and made into compote and marmalade. Perry is obtained from the fermented juice. The best varieties of pear form a very choice and delicate fruit, and when in proper condition for eating, it is soft and more digestible than the apple. Hard pears to be rendered wholesome, require to be subjected to cooking.

Composition of Pears (Fresenius).

	Sweet	Red.
SOLUBLE MATTER—		
Sugar, ...	7.000	7.940
Free acid (reduced to equivalent in malic acid), .	0.074	trace.
Albuminous substances, ...	0.260	0.237
Pectous substances, etc., ...	3.281	4.409
Ash, ...	0.285	0.284
INSOLUBLE MATTER—		
Seeds, ...	0.390 ⎫	
Skins, etc., ...	3.420 ⎬	3.518
Pectose, ...	1.340	0.605
[Ash from insoluble matter included in weights given],	[0.050]	[0.049]
WATER, ...	83.950	83.007
	100.000	100.000

THE QUINCE.—The quince (*Pyrus cydonia* or *Cydonia vulgaris*) was cultivated by the ancient Greeks and Romans, and is now grown throughout temperate climates. The fruit, which, like the apple and pear, belongs to the pomaceous group, is in some varieties globose, in others pear-shaped, and has a rich yellow or orange color, with an agreeable odor taken singly, but a strong, disagreeable smell when stowed away together in quantity. In Persia it ripens so as to be eatable in a raw state, but in Europe it never ripens sufficiently to allow of its being eaten previous to being cooked. It is stewed with sugar, and frequently added to apple-tarts, the flavor of which it greatly improves. It also furnishes an excellent marmalade—a preserve which takes its name from the Portugese word for quince, *marmelo*. The seeds are employed for the mucilage they yield.

THE MEDLAR.—The medlar (*Mespilus germanica*) is a native of various parts of Europe, and grows wild in Great Britain. The fruit, which is only eaten when its tough pulp has become soft by incipient decay, has a very peculiar flavor.

THE SERVICE.—The service (*Pyrus domestica* or *Sorbus domestica*) is a native of Italy, Germany, and France, and has been found wild in England. The fruit has a peculiar acid flavor. It requires, like the medlar, to be kept until it is over-ripe. It is not much eaten in England, as it is considered inferior to the medlar.

THE ORANGE.—The common or sweet orange (*Citrus aurantium*) is supposed to be a native of the Eastern and Central parts of Asia. It does not appear to have been known to the Greeks and Romans, and was probably introduced into Italy in the fourteenth century, above a thousand years after the citron.

The orange is one of the most useful and agreeable of common fruits.

13

It is exceedingly grateful and refreshing to the palate, and in the ripe state is so little likely to occasion disorder as to be admissible under almost every condition both of sickness and of health.

Several varieties of orange exist. The following are the chief encountered in ordinary use. The Portugal or Lisbon orange, which is characterized by the thickness of its rind, is the most common of all. The China orange, which is said to have been brought by the Portuguese from China, has given rise to the St. Michael's as a sub-variety, and this is one of the most highly esteemed on account of its sweet and abundant juice. Its rind is smooth and thin. The Maltese or blood-orange is remarkable for the blood-red color of its pulp. The Tangerine orange is small and flat, and valued chiefly for the aroma belonging to it. The peel, particularly, is charged with a large quantity of volatile oil lodged in round or vesicular receptacles, easily discernible beneath the outer surface. The egg orange is known by its oval shape. The Majorca orange is seedless. The sweet orange is pretty largely used by the cook and confectioner, as well as being consumed as a fresh fruit.

The *Seville* or *bitter orange* (*Citrus vulgaris*) is characterized by its taste and the amount of aromatic volatile oil contained in its rind. It is too bitter to be agreeable for eating in the raw state, but forms the best kind of orange for making wine and marmalade, and, for these purposes it is extensively employed. The rind is used for its aromatic bitterness as a stomachic and tonic, and also simply as a flavoring agent. The flavor of Curaçoa is derived from it. The best orange-flower water is distilled from the flowers of this variety of the orange tree.

THE LEMON.—The lemon (*Citrus limonium*) is a native of the North of India. The fruit is oblong, wrinkled or furrowed, and of a pale yellow color. In the common variety the pulp is very acid, but in the variety called the sweet lemon the juice is sweet.

Lemons are extensively used to give flavor to many articles of food. The juice possesses valuable anti-scorbutic properties, and made into lemonade constitutes one of the most popular of refreshing beverages. The rind contains a volatile oil and bitter principle which renders it useful as an aromatic and stomachic. In a candied state it is employed as a dessert and in confectionery. The fruit is occasionally made into wine in the same way as the orange.

THE CITRON.—The fruit of the citron tree (*Citrus medica*) is larger and less succulent than the lemon, and of a strongly acid taste. The peel is very thick and the surface warty and furrowed. The citron is not suitable for eating in the natural state. Its juice mixed with water and sweetened forms an excellent refrigerant and antiscorbutic drink. Its peel is candied in the same way as that of the orange and lemon.

THE LIME.—The common lime (*Citrus acida*) is a native of India and China, but has long been cultivated in the West Indies and the South of Europe. The fruit is similar to the lemon, but smaller in size. It has a thin rind and an extremely acid juice, which is largely used for its antiscorbutic virtue. The sweet lime (*Citrus limetta*) is a variety cultivated in the South of Europe, which has a pulp of a less acid nature.

THE SHADDOCK.—The fruit of the shaddock (*Citrus decumana*) is large, and from the thickness of its skin will keep longer on sea voyages than any of the other species of citrus. The pulp is of a mixed red and white color and has a moderately acid taste. It forms a pleasant re-freshing fruit and is frequently made into a preserve.

THE POMELO.—The pomelo or pompelmoose (*Citrus pompelmoos*) closely resembles the shaddock, of which it is sometimes regarded as a va-riety. Its flavor is pleasant and approaches that of the orange. It is this fruit which is sometimes sold in the London shops as the "forbidden fruit."

THE POMEGRANATE.—The pomegranate (*Punica granata*) has been cultivated in Asia from ancient times, and has long been naturalized in the South of Europe. The fruit is of about the size of a large orange, and possesses a thick leathery rind of a fine golden yellow color with a rosy tinge on one side. The central part is composed of cells filled with numerous seeds, each of which is surrounded with pulp and separately enclosed in a thin membrane. The pulp has a sweetish, styptic, and slightly bitter taste. The rind is much more strongly astringent, and is sometimes used in medicine on account of this property. The fruit is also sometimes employed for its refrigerant and mildly astringent qualities.

THE PLUM.—The common plum (*Prunus domestica*) is supposed to be a native of Asia Minor, but it has long been naturalized in England. The wild sloe (*Prunus spinosa*) which is found growing in hedges, forms the parent of the plum. From this is first derived the bullace (*Prunus insititia*), and from the bullace, afterward the plum. The varieties of the plum are numerous. They range in quality from a delicious dessert fruit to one fit only for tarts and preserves.

The *Damson* or Damascene plum is so called from being derived originally from Damascus. The *Greengage*, which is known in France as the *Reine Claude*, may be looked upon for sweetness and richness of flavor as the choicest kind of plum. The purple gage is a new variety lately introduced by the French under the name of *Reine Claude violette*.

Composition of Plums (Fresenius).

	Mirabelle, common yellow.	Dark black-red.	Common Mussel.	Greengage, large green, very sweet.
SOLUBLE MATTER—				
Sugar, ...	3.584	2.252	5.793	3.405
Free acid (reduced to equivalent in malic acid), . .	0.582	1.331	0.952	0.870
Albuminous substances, . .	0.197	0.426	0.785	0.401
Pectous substances, etc., . .	5.772	5.851	3.646	11.074
Ash, ...	0.570	0.553	0.734	0.398
INSOLUBLE MATTER—				
Seeds, ...	5.780	3.329	3.540	2.852
Skins, etc., ...	0.179 }	1.020	{ 1.990	1.035
Pectose, ...	1.080 }		{ 0.630	0.245
[*Ash from insoluble matter in-cluded in weights given*], .	[0.082]	[0.063]	[0.094]	[0.037]
WATER, ...	82.256	85.238	81.930	79.720
	100.000	100.000	100.000	100.000

Large quantities of plums are imported and consumed as a dried fruit. The commoner kind are known by the name of *Prunes*, the choicer kinds by that of *French plums*.

Plums are more apt than most other fruits to produce disorder of the bowels, attended with griping and diarrhœa, and should, therefore, only be eaten in moderate quantity. In both the unripe and over-ripe state they must be regarded as decidedly unwholesome. Cooking renders them less objectionable. Some kinds possess so marked an astringency as scarcely to be eatable in a raw state. Prunes are often used for their laxative effect by persons suffering from habitual constipation.

THE CHERRY.—The common cherry (*Ceracas duracina*) is supposed to have been a native of Syria and other parts of Western Asia. The varieties differ greatly in color. The pale, sweet, firm-fleshed *Bigarreau* forms the cherry most esteemed for dessert. The dark-skinned *morello* constitutes the favorite for making preserves and for cherry brandy.

Cherries, like plums, require to be eaten in moderation, on account of their tendency to disorder the bowels. In the unripe and unsound state they are particularly apt to do so.

Kirchwasser is the name of a liqueur obtained from cherries. *Maraschino*, a sweeter and more agreeable liqueur, is also prepared from a delicately flavored variety of cherry grown in Dalmatia, and called marasca or marasquin.

In speaking of cherries, it may be mentioned that serious results have sometimes arisen from the stones having been swallowed. These, like the stones of other fruits, are liable, if swallowed, to become impacted in the alimentary canal, and thence to occasion inflammation and its consequences.

Composition of Cherries (Fresenius).

	Sweet, light red-heart.	Very light heart, rather sour.	Sweet black.	Sour.
SOLUBLE MATTER—				
Sugar, ...	13.110	8.568	10.700	8.772
Free acid (reduced to equivalent in malic acid), . .	0.351	0.961	0.560	1.277
Albuminous substances, . .	0.903 }	3.529	{ 1.010	0.825
Pectous substances, etc., . .	2.286 }		} 0.670	1.831
Ash, ...	0.600	0.835	0.600	0.565
INSOLUBLE MATTER—				
Seeds, ...	5.480	3.244	5.730	5.182
Skins, etc., ...	0.450	0.464	0.366	0.808
Pectose, ...	1.450	0.401	0.664	0.246
[*Ash from insoluble matter included in weights given*], . .	[0.090]	[0.070]	[0.078]	[0.067]
WATER, ...	75.370	81.998	79.700	80.494
	100.000	100.000	100.000	100.000

THE PEACH.—The peach (*Amygdalus persica*) is a native of Persia and the North of India, and is now cultivated in all temperate climates. It thrives very freely and produces most plentifully in the United States.

The peach forms one of the choicest and most luscious of fruits. The skin is downy or velvety, and its color varies from a dark reddish violet through many shades of crimson, green, or yellow, to the beautiful clear white of the American snow peach. The composition shows that the peach is notable for the small quantity of saccharine matter it contains in comparison with the other kinds of edible fruits.

Composition of Peaches (Fresenius).

	Large Dutch.	Similar variety.
SOLUBLE MATTER—		
Sugar, ...	1.580	1.565
Free acid (reduced to equivalent in malic acid),	0.612	0.734
Albuminous substances, ... 0.463		11.058
Pectous substances, etc., ... 6.313		
Ash, ...	0.422	0.913
INSOLUBLE MATTER		
Seeds, ...	4.629	6.764
Skins, etc., ... 0.991		2.420
Pectose, ...		
[Ash from insoluble matter included in weights given],	[0.042]	[0.163]
WATER, ...	84.990	76.546
	100.000	100.000

THE NECTARINE.—The nectarine constitutes merely a variety of the peach, probably produced by cultivation. It has been sometimes found growing on peach trees, and the Boston nectarine, which forms the finest kind known, was produced originally from a peach-stone. It differs from the peach in having a smooth and wax-like skin, and being of smaller size.

THE OLIVE.—The olive-tree (Olea Europœa) is supposed to be originally a native of Greece, but it has long been naturalized in France, Italy, and Spain. The fruit in the ripe state is black, and its fleshy part abounds in oil, which is expressed and used with us as salad oil and largely on the Continent for cooking. The ripe fruit is also sometimes eaten abroad, but it has a strong and, most persons would consider, a disagreeable taste.

The olives imported into this country have been gathered green and soaked, first in strong lye and then in fresh water, to remove their rough and bitter taste before being preserved in a solution of salt. French, Spanish, and Italian olives are imported. The Spanish are much larger, and more bitter, rich, and oily than the others. Olives enter into the constitution of various dishes, are sometimes used to stimulate the appetite at the commencement of dinner, and also eaten at dessert as a relish and to cleanse the palate for the enjoyment of wine.

THE DATE.—The date is derived from the Phœnix dactylifera, the date palm or palm tree of Scripture, a native of Africa and parts of Asia, and now brought into cultivation in the South of Europe. The tree bears its fruit in bunches which weigh from twenty to twenty-five pounds.

Dates, both fresh and dried, form the chief food of the Arabs. Cakes of dates, pounded and kneaded together into a solid mass, constitute also the store of food, called the "bread of the desert," provided for African caravans on their journey through the Sahara. The fruit is of a drupaceous nature, and the fleshy part contains, according to the analysis of Reinsch, 58 per cent. of sugar, accompanied by pectin, gum, etc.

THE APRICOT.—The apricot (*Prunus armeniaca*) is a native of Armenia, and was introduced into England in the time of Henry the Eighth. A good apricot, when perfectly ripe, is an excellent fruit, but when of inferior quality it eats dry and insipid. Unless quite ripe it is apt to prove laxative, and should not be eaten by delicate persons. In the cooked state it is more easy of digestion, and green apricots are often used for tarts. It makes one of the most highly esteemed of preserves. The kernels of some are sweet, of others bitter. From the bitter kind, *Eau de Noyaux* is distilled in France.

Composition of Apricots (Fresenius).

	Fine, rather large.	Large, fine flavored.	Small.
SOLUBLE MATTER—			
Sugar, ...	1.140	1.531	2.736
Free acid (reduced to equivalent in malic acid), ...	0.898	0.766	1.603
Albuminous substances, ...	0.832	0.389	0.411
Pectous substances, etc., ...	5.929	9.283	5.562
Ash, ...	0.820	0.754	0.723
INSOLUBLE MATTER—			
Seeds, ...	4.300	3.216	3.415
Skins, etc., ...	0.967	0.944	1.248
Pectose, ...	0.148	1.002	0.750
[Ash from insoluble matter included in weights given], ...	[0.071]	[0.104]	[0.060]
WATER, ...	84.966	82.115	83.552
	100.000	100.000	100.000

THE GRAPE.—The grape-vine (*Vitis vinifera*) is indigenous in the East, but was introduced into the South of Europe at a very early period. It produces fruit in the form of a globular or oval berry with a smooth skin. The color of the fruit is very various, from white, yellow, amber, green, and red, to black. More than 1,500 varieties are described in works on the culture of the plant.

In England the summer is not long and warm enough to thoroughly ripen the fruit in the open air, but some of the finest grapes produced are grown in the hot-houses of Great Britain.

The grape is one of the most useful and highly esteemed of fruits. The skin and seeds are indigestible and should be rejected, but the juicy pulp possesses wholesome, nutritious, and refrigerant properties, and may usually be safely taken by the invalid. If eaten freely, the fruit exerts a diuretic and laxative action. Besides being useful as a fresh fruit, it is dried and imported under the form of raisins and currants, and, as is well known, furnishes the choicest of wines and spirits.

The juice of ripe grapes, according to the analyses of Proust and

Bérard, contains a considerable quantity of grape-sugar, small quantities of a glutinous substance and of extractive matter, bitartrate of potash, tartrate of lime, a little malic acid, and other ingredients suspended or dissolved in water.

Composition of Grapes (Fresenius).

	White Austrian (quite ripe).	Klienberger (quite ripe).
SOLUBLE MATTER—		
Sugar, ...	13.780	10.590
Free acid (reduced to equivalent in malic acid),	1.020	0.820
Albuminous substances, ...	0.832	0.622
Pectous substances, etc., ...	0.498	0.220
Ash, ...	0.360	0.377
INSOLUBLE MATTER—		
Seeds, ... }	2.592	1.770
Skins, ... }		
Pectose, ...	0.941	0.750
[*Ash from insoluble matter included in weights given*], .	[0.117]	[0.077]
WATER, ...	79.997	84.870
	100.000	100.000

The amount of sugar varies considerably in different kinds of grape. In Fresenius' analysis of very ripe Oppenheim grapes it amounted to 13.52 per cent.; over-ripe Oppenheim, 15.14 per cent.; red, very ripe Asmannshäuser, 17.28 per cent.; and Johannisberg, 19.24 per cent.

Raisins constitute grapes in a dried state. The process of drying is effected either by exposure to the sun or by the heat of an oven. The sun-dried grapes are the sweeter and better of the two. Sometimes the stalks of the ripened bunches of grapes are partially cut through, and the fruit allowed to dry spontaneously upon the vine. The *muscatels*, which form the finest sort, and are eaten at the dessert table, are prepared in this way. The *Lexias* are so called on account of being dipped into a lixivium of wood-ashes and olive oil before being dried. This disposes them to shrink and wrinkle, the alkaline solution serving to remove the waxy coat which impedes the drying of the berry. *Sultanas* are characterized by an absence of stones, whereby they save a great amount of trouble in the kitchen, but they are not sufficiently rich in flavor and sweetness to be advantageous for employment alone in puddings. Raisins abound more in sugar and less in acid than the fresh fruit. They are, therefore, more nutritious but less refrigerant. They are apt to derange the digestive organs if eaten freely.

The so-called *currants* which are used in cakes and puddings, constitute the dried fruit of a vine which grows in the Ionian Islands (especially Zante and Cephalonia) and yields a very small berry. The word currant, as here employed, is a corruption of Corinth, where the fruit was formerly produced. After being gathered and dried by exposure to the sun and air, the currants are heaped together and stored in magazines, where they become so firmly caked as to require digging out for packing into casks for exportation. Currants are of so indigestible a nature that they frequently pass through the alimentary canal without betraying any decided evidence of being acted upon.

THE GOOSEBERRY.—The common gooseberry, or feaberry as it was in former times called (*Ribes grossularia*), grows wild in thickets and rocky situations, and is a native of many parts of Europe and the North of Asia. This fruit is comparatively neglected on the Continent, but has been brought to a high state of perfection in size and flavor in England by the attention which has been paid to its cultivation, more especially since the middle of the eighteenth century.

The gooseberry forms a wholesome and useful fruit. Malic and citric acids blended with sugar give it its chief characteristics. It is made into tarts and puddings and eaten at the dessert table, besides furnishing a good preserve and a very passable wine.

Composition of Gooseberries (Fresenius).

	Large red.	Small red.	Middle-sized yellow.	Large smooth red.
SOLUBLE MATTER—				
Sugar,	8.063	6.030	6.383	6.483
Free acid (reduced to equivalent in malic acid),	1.358	1.573	1.078	1.664
Albuminous substances,	0.441	0.445	0.578	0.306
Pectous substances, etc.,	0.969	0.513	2.112	0.843
Ash,	0.317	0.452	0.200	0.553
INSOLUBLE MATTER—				
Seeds,	2.481 }	2.442	3.380 }	2.803
Skins, etc.,	0.512 }		0.442 }	
Pectose,	0.294	0.515	0.308	0.390
[*Ash from insoluble matter included in weights given*],	[0.146]	[0.069]	[0.100]	[0.133]
WATER,	85.565	88.030	85.519	86.958
	100.000	100.000	100.000	100.000

THE CRANBERRY.—The common cranberry (*Oxycoccus palustris*, formerly *Vaccinium oxycoccus*) is a native of the colder regions of the Northern Hemisphere. The fruit is too acid to be eaten raw, but is in much request for tarts.

Wine is made from it in Siberia.

The American cranberry (*Oxycoccus macrocarpus*) furnishes a larger fruit, but is not so highly esteemed.

Another species, brought from Nova Scotia in 1760, is called *snowberry*, from the fruit being white.

THE BARBERRY.—The common barberry (*Berberis vulgaris*) grows widely distributed through the North of Europe, Asia, and America. It is found in woods, coppices, and hedges in England, especially on a chalky soil. The old English name for the plant is Pipperidge, or Piprage bush. The berries are of an elongated oval form, and, when ripe, generally of a bright red color, more rarely whitish, yellow, or almost black. They are too acid to be eaten in the fresh state, but make excellent preserves and jelly, and are also used to garnish dishes. Malic acid is prepared from them in France.

THE CURRANT.—There are two varieties of the currant, viz., the red (*Ribes rubrum*) and the black (*Ribes nigrum*). Both are natives of Europe and some parts of Asia and North America. Cultivation has produced the white currant from the red, and in Russia there are varieties of the black currant with yellow berries. The name currant is derived from the resemblance of the fruit to the Corinth raisins, or small grapes of Zante, commonly called Corinths or currants.

Currants are employed in the same way as gooseberries, with which they pretty closely agree in their alimentary properties. A wine is made from the red currant and a liquor from the black.

Composition of Currants (Fresenius).

	Middle-sized red.	Very large red.	Middle-sized white.
SOLUBLE MATTER—			
Sugar, ...	4.78	6.44	5.647	7.12
Free acid (reduced to equivalent in malic acid), . .	2.31	1.84	1.695	2.53
Albuminous substances, . . .	0.45	0.49	0.356	0.68
Pectous substances, etc., . .	0.28	0.19	0.007	0.19
Ash, ...	0.54	0.57	0.620	0.70
INSOLUBLE MATTER—			
Seeds, ...	4.45 }	4.48	3.940	4.85
Skins, etc., ...	0.66 }			
Pectose, ...	0.69	0.72	2.380	0.51
[*Ash from insoluble matter included in weights given*], . }	[0.11]	[0.23]	[0.185]	[0.14]
WATER, ...	85.84	85.27	85.355	83.42
	100.00	100.00	100.000	100.00

THE ELDERBERRY.—Elderberries are derived from the *Sambucus nigra* (the bourtree of the Scotch), which forms a native of Europe, and the North of Asia and of Africa. The berries are black in color (sometimes, however, white), and have a faintly acid with an after-sweetish and unpleasant taste. They are rarely used except for making *elder wine.* The purple juice obtained by expression is called *elder rob.* It possesses mildly aperient, diuretic, and sudorific properties.

THE BILBERRY.—The whortle-, hurtle-, bil- or blae-berry (*Vaccinium myrtillus*) is a native of Great Britain, and grows in woods and on heaths or waste places in the North of Europe and of America. It furnishes a small round purple or almost black fruit, covered with a delicate azure bloom. This is sweet and agreeable to the taste, and is either eaten uncooked with cream or made into tarts. The bog whortleberry or great bilberry (*Vaccinium uliginosum*) has a larger fruit, but its flavor is inferior.

The red whortleberry (*Vaccinium vitis idæa*) is often called cranberry, from the similarity of its acid fruit to the true cranberry. It is much esteemed for preserves.

Composition of Bilberries (Fresenius).

SOLUBLE MATTER—

Sugar, ...	5.780
Free acid (reduced to equivalent in malic acid),	1.341
Albuminous substances, etc., ...	0.794
Pectous substances, etc., ...	0.555
Ash, ...	0.858

INSOLUBLE MATTER—

Seeds, ...	
Skins, etc., ...	} 12.864
Pectose, ...	0.256
[*Ash from insoluble matter included in weights given*],	[0.550]
WATER, ...	77.552

100.000

THE STRAWBERRY.—The common wood strawberry (*Fragaria vesca*) is indigenous in almost all temperate climates. The products which have been obtained by cultivation from this plant rank among the choicest and most tempting of summer fruits, and afford an example of one of the greatest triumphs of the gardener's art. The Alpine strawberry (*Fragaria collina*) is a native of Switzerland and Germany. The fruit is small, but produced in great abundance.

Composition of Strawberries (Fresenius).

	Wild.		Light red pine (quite ripe).
SOLUBLE MATTER—			
Sugar, ...	3.247	4.550	7.575
Free acid (reduced to equivalent in malic } acid), ... }	1.650	1.332	1.133
Albuminous substances, ...	0.619	0.567	0.359
Pectous substances, etc., ...	0.145	0.049	0.119
Ash, ...	0.737	0.603	0.480
INSOLUBLE MATTER—			
Seeds, ... }			
Skins, etc., ... }	6.032	5.580	1.960
Pectose, ...	0.299	0.300	0.900
[*Ash from insoluble matter included in* } *weights given*], ... }	[0.315]	[0.345]	[0.154]
WATER, ...	87.271	87.019	87.474
	100.000	100.000	100.000

THE RASPBERRY.—The raspberry (*Rubus idæus*) is a native of Great Britain and most parts of the world, but it has only been cultivated in gardens during the last one or two centuries. The fruit is wholesome and agreeable, but is not so much eaten at dessert in England as on the Continent. It is, however, largely used for tarts and puddings under the form of a preserve, and for making raspberry vinegar. A wine is sometimes prepared from the fermented juice.

Rubus arcticus, a smaller variety, takes the place of the common raspberry in the colder regions of Northern Europe.

Composition of Raspberries (Fresenius).

	Wild red.	Cultivated.	
		Red.	White.
SOLUBLE MATTER—			
Sugar, ...	3.597	4.708	3.703
Free acid (reduced to equivalent in malic acid), ...	1.980	1.356	1.115
Albuminous substances, ...	0.546	0.544	0.665
Pectous substances, etc., ...	1.107	1.746	1.397
Ash, ...	0.270	0.481	0.380
INSOLUBLE MATTER—			
Seeds, ...	8.460	4.106	4.520
Skins, etc., ...			
Pectose, ...	0.180	0.502	0.040
[*Ash from insoluble matter included in weights given*], ...	[0.134]	[0.296]	[0.081]
WATER, ...	83.860	86.557	88.180
	100.000	100.000	100.000

THE BLACKBERRY.—The blackberry (*Rubus fruticosus*) is indigenous in Great Britain and the greater part of Europe, and grows wild as a shrubby bramble in hedges. The fruit is gathered by children for eating, and also for making into puddings. Jelly and jam are sometimes prepared from it as well as a wine.

Composition of Blackberries (Fresenius).

SOLUBLE MATTER—   Very ripe.

Sugar, ...	4.444
Free acid (reduced to equivalent in malic acid), .	1.188
Albuminous substances, ...	0.510
Pectous substances, etc., ...	1.444
Ash, ...	0.414

INSOLUBLE MATTER-

Seeds, ...	5.210
Skins, etc., ...	
Pectose, ...	0.384
[*Ash from insoluble matter included in weights given*], .	[0.074]
WATER, ...	86.406
	100.000

THE DEWBERRY.—The dewberry or gray bramble (*Rubus cæsius*) is a native of Britain and many parts of Europe and Asia; it is closely allied to the blackberry, but grows on the ground and not in hedges. The fruit is very sweet and agreeable, and makes an excellent wine. The dewberry of North America (*Rubus procumbens*) bears a more acidulous and superior fruit to that of Britain.

THE MULBERRY.—The black or common mulberry (*Morus nigra*) is a native of Persia, but is supposed to have been brought to Europe by the Romans. The fruit is of a purplish black color, with dark red juice, fine aromatic flavor, and acidulous and sweet taste. It possesses wholesome, refrigerant, and slightly laxative properties, and is highly esteemed for dessert. An excellent preserve and an agreeable wine are made from it.

Composition of Mulberries (Fresenius).

SOLUBLE MATTER—	Black.
Sugar, ...	9.192
Free acid (reduced to equivalent in malic acid), .	1.860
Albuminous substances, ...	0.394
Pectous substances, etc., ...	2.031
Ash, ...	0.566
INSOLUBLE MATTER—	
Seeds, ...	} 0.905
Skins, ...	
Pectose, ...	0.345
[*Ash from insoluble matter included in weights given*],	[0.089]
WATER, ...	84.707
	100.000

THE MELON.—The melon (*Cucumis melo*) belongs to the gourd tribe. The fruit varies greatly in size, color, and the character of the rind. In some the rind is smooth and thin, in others thick and warty, and cracked in a net-like manner. The color of the flesh is green, red, and yellow. It is eaten with sugar at dessert, or with pepper and salt at dinner. When in perfection it forms a rich and delicious fruit, but, like its congeners, the cucumber, etc., it is sometimes apt to disagree.

The *watermelon* (*Cucumis citrullus*) is highly prized for its flavor and juiciness. This fruit is round, with a dark green spotted rind, and pink or white flesh. It is only eaten at dessert.

THE PINEAPPLE.—The pineapple (*Ananassa sativa*) is a native of South America, whence it has been introduced into Africa and Asia. It was first cultivated in hot-houses in Holland and England at the end of the seventeenth century. It may be looked upon as furnishing the finest of dessert fruits. Besides being eaten in the fresh state, it is made into a preserve with sugar, and otherwise employed by the confectioner. It is also used to flavor rum.

THE FIG.—The common fig (*Ficus carica*) is a native of Asia and Barbary, and has been naturalized in Greece, Italy, Spain, and the South of France, where the fruit forms an important part of the people's food. The fig-tree also grows in the open air in some of the milder parts of England, but its fruit fails to acquire the perfection in flavor belonging to that produced in a warmer climate. The varieties cultivated are numerous, and the color of the fruit of some is bluish black, of others, red, purple, green, yellow, or white. The fruit is pear-shaped, and consists of a pulpy mass, containing many seed-like bodies. The amount of sugar present is exceedingly large. The figs grown in England have but little taste, and that of a somewhat sickly nature. Grown in warm countries, however, they form a rich and luscious fruit. Figs are largely imported in a dried and compressed state. The best are brought from Smyrna, and are known as Turkey figs. If freely eaten, they are apt to irritate and disorder the stomach and bowels.

THE PRICKLY PEAR.—The prickly pear, or Indian fig (*Opuntia vulgaris*), is a native of America, but is now naturalized in many parts of the South of Europe and North of Africa. It grows freely on the barest rocks, and spreads over expanses of volcanic sand and ashes too arid for almost any other plant to live. The fruit is somewhat like a fig, of a deep rose color, and rather larger than a hen's egg. The pulp is juicy, and its flavor, which to most palates will be considered of a sickly nature, combines sweetness with acidity. It is not much known in England, but is largely eaten in some localities abroad.

THE TAMARIND.—There are two varieties of the tamarind—the East Indian (*Tamarindus Indica*), and the West Indian (*Tamarindus occidentalis*). The fruit consists of a brown, many-seeded pod, filled with a sweet and acidulous, reddish black pulp. The pod of the East Indian is much longer than that of the West Indian variety. According to the analysis of Vauquelin, tamarinds contain 9.40 per cent. of citric acid; 1.55 per cent. of tartaric acid; 0.45 per cent. of malic acid; 3.25 per cent. of bitartrate of potash; and 12.5 per cent. of sugar, besides gum, vegetable jelly, parenchyma, and water. They are preserved by placing alternate layers of the fruit and sugar into a cask, and pouring over them boiling syrup.

THE PLANTAIN AND BANANA.—The plantain (*Musa paradisiaca*) is a native of the East Indies, but is now diffused all over the tropical and sub-tropical regions of the globe. It is so called on account of having been supposed to have furnished the fruit which tempted Eve in Paradise. The banana (*Musa sapientum*) appears to be only a variety of the plantain, bearing smaller, softer, and more delicately flavored fruit. Its name is due to its having formed the chief food of the Brahmins or wise caste of India. They both constitute exceedingly productive plants, and it is asserted that an extent of ground which would only grow wheat enough for the support of two persons, would maintain fifty if cultivated with the plantain. Plantains and bananas furnish important and valuable articles of food to the inhabitants of many tropical regions. They even afford in some localities the chief alimentary support of the people. The fruit occurs in large bunches or clusters, which may weigh as much as fifty pounds. On stripping off the tegumentary part, a softish core is met with, which is chiefly farinaceous in the unripe, and saccharine in the ripe state; the starch becoming converted, it is stated, during maturation, first into a mucilaginous substance, and then into sugar. Plantain-meal is prepared by powdering and sifting the dried core of the plantain whilst in the green or unripe state. It has a fragrant odor, and a bland taste, like that of common wheat-flour. It is said to be easy of digestion, and to be extensively employed in British Guiana as the food of infants, children, and invalids. The larger proportion of it consists of starch, but it also contains a certain percentage of nitrogenous matter, and is, therefore, of higher alimentary value than the starchy preparations, as sago, arrow-root, etc.

Composition of the Pulp of Ripe Bananas (Corenwinder).

Nitrogenous matter, ...	4.820
Sugar, pectose, organic acid, with traces of starch, .	19.657
Fatty matter, ...	0.632
Cellulose, ...	0.200
Saline matter, ...	0.791
Water, ...	73.900
	100.000

THE GUAVA.—The common or white guava (*Psidium pyriferum*) is said to be a native of both the East and West Indies, where it is now much cultivated. It has also been grown as a stove plant in England. The fruit is roundish or oblong in shape, and rather larger than a hen's egg in size. It has a smooth and yellow rind and a flesh-colored firm pulp full of hard seeds. It possesses a sweet aromatic taste, and is eaten raw and made into a preserve and jelly. The red guava (*Psidium pomiferum*), which is also common in both the East and West Indies, has a beautiful fruit crowned like a pomegranate; but it is strongly acid and not so agreeable to eat as that of the white. The China guava (*Psidium Cattleyanum*) is a native of the country its name bears, but it has been brought over to and grown in Europe, and is found to flourish in the open air in the South of France. The fruit is round and of a fine claret color. It has an agreeable acidulous taste and makes an excellent preserve. A dwarf species of guava called Marongaba (*Psidium pygmæum*) grows on some of the mountains of Brazil. The fruit is about the size of a gooseberry, and is much esteemed on account of its delicious flavor, which bears some resemblance to that of the strawberry.

THE MANGO.—The common Mango (*Mangifera Indica*) grows into a large spreading tree, and is a native of India, but was introduced into Jamaica toward the end of the eighteenth century, and is now extensively cultivated in warm countries. The fruit, which contains a large flattened stone covered with fibrous filaments, is smooth and kidney-shaped, and varies in color and size, sometimes being as large as a man's fist. From its luscious character, and sweet and yet slightly acidulous taste, it is highly prized for dessert. The green or unripe fruit is made into tarts and also into pickles. In times of scarcity the kernels have been cooked and used as food.

THE BREAD FRUIT.—This is derived from the *Artocarpus incisa*, a native of the islands of the Pacific and the Moluccas. The fruit is of a round or oval shape, and attains a size as large as that of a small loaf of bread. In an alimentary point of view, it occupies the same position amongst the inhabitants of Polynesia that is held by corn in other parts of the world. The *Artocarpus integrifolia* is cultivated throughout Southern India and all the warmer parts of Asia. Its fruit, called *jak fruit*, is considerably employed as an article of food in Ceylon.

The fruit of the *Carob tree*, or St. John's bread (*Ceratonia siliqua*), is eaten in time of scarcity by the country people of the districts where it grows, and, as implied by its name, it has been supposed to have been the food of John the Baptist. It is a native of the countries skirting the Mediterranean, and is almost the only tree that grows in Malta (" Baird's Cyclo. of Nat. Sci.").

The *Date plum* of China, or key fig of Japan (*Diospyros kaki*), is a native of China and Japan, and is frequently sent to Europe in a dried state (" Baird's Cyclo. of Nat. Sci.").

The fruit of the *Persimmon tree* (*Diospyros virginiana*), a native of the United States, when fully ripe, is sweet and palatable. The fleshy part is separated from the seeds, and made into cakes, which are dried and preserved (" Baird's Cyclo. of Nat. Sci.").

The fruit of the *Chilian pine* (*Araucaria imbricata*) is the chief food of the inhabitants of Chili and Patagonia. It is asserted that the produce of one large tree will maintain eighteen persons for a year (" Johnston's Chemistry of Common Life," vol. i., p. 108).

BARK.

The bark of trees is to some extent eaten in certain localities. The Jakuts of Northern Siberia grate the inner bark of the larch, and sometimes of the fir, and mix it with fish, a little meal and milk, or by preference with fat, and make it into a sort of broth (" Wrangell's Polar Sea," p. 23). The inhabitants of New Caledonia eat the bark of a tree after they have roasted it (" Cook's Second Voyage," vol. ii., p. 123); and the Laplanders and Fins make a kind of bread with the triturated internal layers of the bark of the pine (" Baird's Cyclo. of Nat. Sci.").

SAW-DUST AND WOODY FIBRE.

In Sweden and Norway saw-dust is sometimes converted into bread, for which purpose beech, or some wood that does not contain turpentine, is repeatedly macerated and boiled in water to remove soluble matters, and then reduced to powder, heated several times in an oven, and ground. In this state it is said to have the smell and taste of corn-flour (" Tomlinson's Cyclo. of Useful Arts," vol. ii., p. 926).

Bread has been made in times of famine of a variety of substances; thus, in the years 1629, 1630, and 1693, very good, wholesome, white bread was made in England from boiled turnips. The moisture was pressed out of the turnips, and they were then kneaded with an equal quantity of wheaten-flour (" Beckman's History of Inventions," vol. i., p. 349, 1846).

During the late siege of Paris, the bread served out constituted a very coarse and mixed article. In Sheppard's " Shut up in Paris," p. 309, it is stated to have been found by analysis to be comprised of one-eighth wheat; four-eighths potatoes, beans, peas, oats and rye; two-eighths water; and the remaining one-eighth straw, hulls of grain, and the skins of vegetable products.

VEGETABLE BUTTER.

A vegetable butter is obtained from several species of *Bassia*, a genus of plants indigenous to tropical India and Africa. The seeds of the *Bassia butyracea*, or Indian butter-tree, contain a substance which in the fresh state resembles butter, but which hardens by degrees and becomes like suet ("Baird's Cyclo. of Nat. Sci.").

The Shea or African butter-tree (*Bassia Parkii*) is named after Mungo Park, who describes in his "Travels in the Interior Districts of Africa" the mode adopted by the natives to obtain the butter. "These trees," he says (vol. i, pp. 198–9, 1816), "grow in great abundance all over this part of Bambarra. They are not planted by the natives, but are found growing naturally in the woods; and in clearing woodland for cultivation, every tree is cut down but the shea. The tree itself very much resembles the American oak; and the fruit, from the kernel of which, being first dried in the sun, the butter is prepared, by boiling the kernel in water, has somewhat the appearance of a Spanish olive. The kernel is enveloped in a sweet pulp, under a thin green rind, and the butter produced from it, besides the advantage of its keeping the whole year without salt, is whiter, firmer, and to my palate of a richer flavor than the best butter I ever tasted made from cow's milk. The growth and preparation of this commodity seem to be among the first objects of African industry in this and neighboring states; and it constitutes a main article of their inland commerce."

SACCHARINE PREPARATIONS.

Sugar forms an important alimentary principle, and is met with widely, and in certain cases largely, amongst vegetable products, from some of which it is extracted for use. It also constitutes, under the name of *lactine*, one of the ingredients of the animal food provided by nature for the support of the young mammal—viz., milk.

Sugar was known to the ancient Greeks and Romans, and its manufacture is said by Humboldt to be of the greatest antiquity in China.

Sugar evidently contributes toward force-production in the body, and, likewise, as is shown by ample evidence, toward the formation and accumulation of fat. Being of a soluble and diffusible nature, it needs no preliminary digestion for absorption, and, therefore, sits lightly on the stomach. It is, however, apt in some dyspeptics to undergo acid fermentation, and give rise to preternatural acidity of stomach and likewise flatulence. A popular notion prevails that it has a tendency to injure the teeth, but no trustworthy evidence that such is the case exists.

The consumption of sugar in Great Britain in 1700 amounted to 10,000 tons. In the year 1863–64 it had risen to 536,226 tons of unrefined, 14,879 tons of refined, and 40,165 tons of cane-juice, syrup, and molasses. In relation to population, the amount stood at 30 pounds per head. In 1866, the quantity consumed in England was at the rate of 38 pounds per head.

Besides employment as a daily article of food, sugar constitutes the base of a variety of products of the confectioner's art. On account of its antiseptic virtue, it is also extensively used as a preservative of other substances. Vegetable products, as fruits, etc., are those which are chiefly subjected to the influence it exerts in this direction, but animal substances can be equally well preserved by it.

There are two main varieties of sugar. The one is familiar to us as the produce of the sugar-cane, and the other as contained in grapes and other kinds of fruit. The former variety is characterized by the facility with which it crystallizes, and by its strong sweetness of taste. It not only exists in the sugar-cane, but also in beet-root, in the sap of certain species of maple, in the stems of maize, and in some other vegetable products. It is distinguished by the appellation *crystalline* or *cane-sugar*. The latter is imperfectly crystallizable, and of much inferior sweetness. It abounds in grapes and many other fruits and vegetable articles, and may also be obtained by the action of acids and ferments on cane-sugar, starch, gum, and licorice. It is known by the name of *glucose* or *grape-sugar*. These two varieties differ further in their chemical relations, and in the amount of the elements of water they contain. The various saccharine products in common use consist in one or other of these varieties.

Cane-sugar.—This, looked at as a specific product, is derived from the sugar-cane, or *Saccharum*, a plant which appears to have come originally from the interior of Asia, whence it was transplanted to Cyprus. It was introduced into the West Indies, where it is now extensively cultivated, early in the sixteenth century. There are several varieties of *Saccharum* grown for the extraction of sugar, but the Creole cane, or *Saccharum officinarum*, is that which was first introduced into the New World.

The sugar is contained in the juice of the cane, and the first step in its manufacture is to obtain the juice by means of pressure, which is usually applied by iron rollers. The cane, when ripe, is cut close to the ground, stripped of its leaves, and then twice passed between the iron rollers. The expressed juice is next clarified and evaporated. This is effected by the combined use of heat and the addition of lime. Passing through a series of evaporating vessels, the scum and deposit are removed, and the liquor brought to the proper consistence. It is now transferred into coolers, for the crystals to form and separate from the uncrystallizable portion, which is allowed to drain off. The solidified product constitutes *muscovado*, or *raw sugar*, and is packed in hogsheads and distributed to the consumer. The uncrystallizable portion, containing changed products resulting from the action of the heat, is called *molasses*. The juice of the sugar-cane contains about 18 to 22 per cent. of sugar, and six to eight pounds of it are required to yield one pound of the crystallized article.

A large portion of the raw sugar is refined or transformed from brown or moist into white or loaf sugar before being used, and the process of refining is extensively carried on in this country. The object is to clarify and decolorise, and this is usually effected by boiling the dissolved sugar with bullock's blood, filtering, and allowing the liquor to percolate through coarsely grained animal charcoal. The nearly colorless liquid thence obtained is concentrated to the requisite degree in a vacuum pan heated with steam, and then transferred to conical moulds, where solidification occurs. The unsolidified portion, which constitutes treacle, is afterward permitted to drain off, and loaf sugar is left. The article is still to some extent colored, and, as a finishing process, a saturated solution of sugar is allowed to percolate through the loaf. This washes out the remaining coloring matter, and leaves the product in the white and porous condition observed to belong to the fully refined article.

Sugar is also extracted from the root of the *beet* (*Beta vulgaris*), which contains nearly one-tenth part of its weight of the principle. The cultivation of the beet was recommended for the purpose as early as 1747, at Berlin, but nothing was practically carried out until Napoleon the First encouraged the proposal, and now the manufacture is successfully and extensively pursued in France, Belgium, and Russia. In England a beet-sugar factory has been established at Lavenham, in Suffolk. The juice of the root is obtained and submitted to the same kind of treatment

14

as that of the sugar-cane, and in the refined state the two sugars resemble each other.

A considerable portion of the sugar used in the northern parts of North America is obtained from a variety of *maple*, the *Acer saccharinum*. Incisions are made into the tree, to allow the sap to escape. This is collected and concentrated to crystallizing point. It yields then a coarse sugar, which, however, admits of being purified and brought into the same state as the refined sugar of the cane and beet.

The green stalks of *maize*, or *Indian corn*, are largely impregnated with sugar, and are sometimes employed for its extraction. Sugar was obtained from this source by the ancient Mexicans. The *Sorghum saccharatum*, or sugar-grass, is also gradually growing into importance as a source of sugar, both in North America and the south of Europe. In India a large amount of sugar, called *jaggary*, is obtained from the juice of various trees of the palm tribe. The date-palm (*Phœnix dactylifera*), the wild date-palm (*Phœnix silvestris*), and the gomuto-palm (*Saguerus saccharifer*), are all turned to account for this purpose, and the sugar is to some extent imported into England and used for mixing, but it is said not to be of sufficient "strength" to pay for refining.

Barley-sugar.—When a concentrated solution of sugar is rapidly boiled down, its tendency to crystallize is diminished, and, it may be, even destroyed. On being allowed to cool, it solidifies into a transparent, amorphous mass, of a vitreous nature. It is in this way that barleysugar is prepared, and the same principle also determines the production of acidulated drops, hardbake, toffee, etc. Sometimes a little cream of tartar is introduced to favor the action of the heat, and in the case of acidulated drops, tartaric acid is added whilst the liquid is boiling.

Sugar-candy.—This is crystallized sugar, and is prepared by allowing a concentrated syrup to slowly deposit crystals on the surface of the vessel in which it is contained, and on threads stretched across it. Crushed sugar-candy forms the coarse crystalline article which is often sold for sweetening coffee.

Molasses constitutes the dark-colored, viscid liquid which drains off during the preparation of raw sugar. The molasses which separates from beet-root sugar has a disagreeable taste, and is thereby unfit for employment in the same way as that which is derivable from the sugar of the cane.

Treacle.—As molasses constitutes the uncrystallized liquid which drains from raw sugar, so treacle forms that which escapes from the moulds in which refined sugar concretes. Both liquids contain uncrystallizable sugar, crystallizable sugar, gum, extractive matter, free acid, various salts, and water. They are used as a cheap substitute for sugar. If consumed to any great extent, they exert a laxative action.

Golden syrup is produced by reboiling the liquid which drains from refined sugar, and filtering through animal charcoal. It therefore constitutes a purified form of treacle.

Caramel.—When crystallized sugar is heated to about 400° Fahr., it suffers decomposition, gives off the elements of water, loses its power of crystallizing, becomes dark-colored, and acquires a bitter taste in the place of a sweet one. The article thus produced is called *caramel*, and is used by the cook and confectioner as a flavoring and coloring agent.

Glucose, or grape-sugar.—It has been already stated that it is to this modification of sugar that grapes and many other fruits owe their sweet taste, and that it may be produced artificially from cane-sugar, starch, and some other substances. Its separation from the juice of grapes, and likewise its manufacture from potato-starch and sago, have been to some extent carried out, and the product has formed an article of commerce, but its chief employment has been as an adulterant of cane-sugar. It is not used dietically upon its own merits in the same way as the latter. Its taste is less agreeably sweet, and its sweetening power is so far inferior, that five parts of grape-sugar are said to be required to raise a given volume of water to the same degree of sweetness as is effected by two parts of cane-sugar. It is also much less soluble in water, and less disposed to assume a crystalline form, on which account it is not susceptible of the same facility of purification.

HONEY.—Honey may be most conveniently referred to here, although not a preparation standing in precisely the same position as the other products included in the group.

It is an article collected by the bee for its own use, which man takes possession of and consumes instead. It is an exudation from the nectariferous glands of flowers, which the bee sucks up and passes into the dilatation of the œsophagus forming the crop or honey-bag. From this it is afterward disgorged, probably somewhat altered in its properties by the secretion of the crop, and deposited in the cell of the honey-comb. In Europe, it is principally through the *Apis mellifica* that honey is obtained, and it is by the neuter or working member of the hive that the office is performed. The honey of Surinam and Cayenne, furnished by the *Apis amalthea*, is red, and that supplied by the *Apis unicolor* of Madagascar is of a greenish color.

Honey is a concentrated solution of sugar, mixed with odorous, coloring, gummy, and waxy matters. It usually resolves itself into a fluid and a solid crystalline portion, which are separable from each other by pressure in a linen bag. Chemically, the saccharine matter is of two kinds: the one resembles that from the grape (glucose), whilst the other is uncrystallizable, and analogous to the uncrystallizable sugar which exists along with common sugar in cane-juice. Mannite, a non-fermenting kind of sugar, has also been met with.

Honey varies in flavor and odor, according to the age of the bees and the flowers from which it has been collected.

Virgin honey, or that procured from young bees which have never swarmed, is held in higher estimation than that collected from a hive that has swarmed; but the term virgin honey is also applied to that which flows spontaneously from the comb, on account of its being better than that obtained by the aid of pressure, and especially heat and pressure, this being contaminated with foreign matter derived from the comb. The honey, again, of certain countries and districts is well known to possess special qualities dependent on the flora of the locality. Hence the fragrant odor and choice taste belonging to the honey of Mount Ida in Crete; the neighborhood of Narbonne, where the labiate flowers abound; the valley of Chamounix; and of the high moorlands of Great Britain when the heather is in bloom. Hence, also, the deleterious qualities which the honey of Trebizonde, upon the Black Sea, has long been known to possess, and which are due to its collection from a species of rhododendron, the *Azalea pontica*, which grows upon the neighboring mountains. The effects produced consist of headache, vomiting, and a kind of intoxication; and, if eaten in large quantities, a loss of all sense and power for some hours may occur. It is said to have been probably this kind of honey which poisoned the soldiers of Xenophon, as described by him in the " Retreat of the Ten Thousand." Many other instances of honey exerting poisonous effects have been recorded.

Honey formed an alimentary article of great importance to the ancients, who were almost unacquainted with sugar; and certain localities, as Hybla in Sicily, and Hymettus near Athens, were specially celebrated for its production. It is still pretty largely consumed dietetically in some districts, and possesses the same alimentary value as sugar. It exerts a slightly laxative action, and is frequently employed therapeutically as an emollient and demulcent.

MANNA.—Manna is a sweet substance, which solidifies from the juice of certain species of ash, especially *Fraxinus ornus* and *rotundifolia*. Incisions are made into the stem of the tree, and the juice allowed to escape and dry into solid masses. It contains a peculiar kind of sugar— *mannite*—which forms about four-fifths of the best manna. Mannite, which also exists to some extent in the beet-root and some other vegetable products, constitutes a white, crystallizable, odorless, and sweet principle, which differs from ordinary sugar in not being susceptible of undergoing alcoholic fermentation in contact with yeast.

The chief use to which manna is applied is as a mild and safe laxative. It possesses some nutritive value. Different sorts of manna are eaten by the natives of Australia (" Eyre's Central Australia," vol. ii., p. 250). The peasants of Mount Libanus in Syria it is said, eat manna ordinarily as others do honey; and in Mexico they have a manna which is eaten as we eat cheese (" Forsyth's Dict. of Diet ").

FARINACEOUS PREPARATIONS.

Farinaceous or starchy matter is a product which is yielded by the vegetable kingdom only. Here, however, it is widely and often very largely met with. It occurs under the form of little granular bodies (starch-granules) lodged in the vegetable tissues, but readily susceptible, under appropriate treatment, of isolation. These granules possess a distinctly organized construction, and are made up of a series of superposed layers, the outermost of which is the thickest and hardest. Thus are produced the concentric lines which are visible when the granule is submitted to microscopic examination, and which are arranged around a spot which is called the *hilum*. The granules from different sources present distinctive features as regards size, form, and appearance, which may be recognized with the aid of the microscope.

Starch forms an important alimentary article. Being devoid of nitrogen, it can contribute only toward force and fat-production. The hardness of the external envelope renders the granule in its original state difficult of digestion—and digestion, which involves transformation into sugar, must occur before absorption and utilization can ensue. On this account, when starch is consumed in the raw state, more or less of it passes off with the undigested residue from the alimentary canal. By boiling, or otherwise exposing to heat, the granules rupture and become far more easily attacked by the digestive juices. Starchy matter, therefore, should be subjected to cooking before being consumed.

There are various starchy preparations in common use, an account of which will now be furnished.

SAGO.—Sago is obtained from the central or medullary part, commonly called pith, of the stems of several species of palm. When the tree is sufficiently mature, it is cut down near the root and split perpendicularly. The medullary matter is extracted, reduced to powder, mixed with water, and strained through a sieve. From the strained liquid the starch is deposited, and, after washing with water and drying, forms the *sago-flour*, or *meal*, of commerce. A single tree is said to yield from five to six hundred pounds of sago. What is called *sago-bread* is made in the Moluccas by throwing the dry meal into heated earthenware moulds, which leads, in the course of a few minutes, to its incorporation or caking together into a hard mass.

Granulated sago is prepared from sago-flour by mixing it with water into a paste, and then granulating. It consists of *pearl sago*, which occurs in small spherical grains, and constitutes the kind now commonly employed for dietetic purposes; and *brown* or *common sago*, which occurs in larger grains, and was the only kind used in England prior to the introduction of the first. Both sorts are met with variously tinted, but the tint is not uniform throughout, the surface of the grain being deep on one side and pale on the other. It may be rendered white by bleaching.

Sago constitutes an important article of food in some parts of the East. It is used in household economy in England for introduction into soup, and under the form of pudding. It serves as a light and digestible alimentary material for the invalid and dyspeptic. It absorbs the liquid in which it is cooked, and becomes transparent and soft, but retains its original granular form. In 1863–64 the amount of sago imported into Great Britain was 7,300 tons.

CASSAVA AND TAPIOCA.—These starchy preparations are obtained from the large, thick, fleshy, tuberous roots of the *Manihot utilissima*, formerly known as the *Jatropha manihot*, a native of tropical America, but now cultivated in Africa, India, and other hot countries. The plant in question constitutes what is popularly called the *bitter cassava*, but there is another variety from which cassava and tapioca are also obtained, called the *sweet cassava*. Both plants, like others of the order *Euphorbiaceæ*, to which they belong, have a milky juice. This, in the case of the bitter variety, contains, amongst other deleterious principles, hydrocyanic acid, and gives to the root highly acrid and poisonous properties. In the case of the sweet variety, the juice is devoid of poisonous properties, and the root by boiling or roasting becomes soft, and is used as an edible article. . In the bitter variety it is only the juice that is poisonous, and when this has been expressed or otherwise removed, the residue is of a harmless nature.

To procure the farinaceous preparations, the root, after being washed and scraped, is reduced to a pulp by being rasped or grated. The pulp is then subjected to pressure, to express the juice. From the compressed residue cassava-meal and bread are obtained; and from the juice, cassava-starch and tapioca.

The residue, for instance, dried over a brisk fire, and afterward pounded, forms *cassava-meal*. If baked on a hot plate, it yields *cassava-bread*. Both these products form important and valuable articles of food to the inhabitants of tropical America. They contain starch, vegetable fibre, and nitrogenous matter. The expressed juice, in the next place, contains suspended starch, which is allowed to subside. This, after being washed and dried in the air without the aid of heat, constitutes *cassava-*

starch, or what is known in commerce as *tapioca-meal* or *Brazilian arrow-root*. *Tapioca* is made by heating the cassava-starch, before being dried, on hot plates, and stirring it with an iron rod. By these means the mass agglomerates into small, irregular, transparent granules, forming the article imported into England under the name in question from Bahia and Rio Janeiro.

Tapioca forms an agreeable, light, and easily digestible farinaceous article of food. It is useful both for the sick and healthy, and is employed under the form of pudding and for introduction into soup and broth. Consisting, as it does, of starchy matter only, it possesses a less nutritive value than cassava-meal and bread. In consequence of the heat to which it has been subjected, many of the starch-granules are in a ruptured state, which leads to its being partially soluble in cold water.

ARROW-ROOT.—Genuine arrow-root, or, as it is called, West Indian arrow-root, in contradistinction to spurious representatives of the article, constitutes a pure form of starch from the tuberous root of the *Maranta arundinacea*, It owes its name to the belief of the Indians of South America, that the root of the plant was an antidote to the poison of their enemies' arrows. The plant grows in tropical climates, and was originally cultivated in the West Indies, but has been transferred to the East Indies, Ceylon, and Africa.

The following is the process by which the product is obtained. The roots are dug up when they are about ten or twelve months old, washed, and reduced to a state of pulp. This is mixed with water, cleared of fibres by means of a coarse sieve, and the starch allowed to settle. Successive washings are employed for further purification, and the arrow-root is then either dried on sheets in the sun, or in drying-houses, care being exercised to exclude dust and insects.

Arrow-root is imported into England from the West Indian Islands, Calcutta, and Sierra Leone, and is usually distinguished by the name of the island or place producing it. That derived from Bermuda is held in the highest estimation. It forms a white, odorless, and tasteless substance, and is met with either in the state of powder or of small pulverulent masses. When rubbed between the fingers it feels firm, and produces a slight crackling noise. It consists of starch-granules, which are readily distinguished by their microscopic characters from those derived from other sources.

Consisting, as arrow-root does, of pure starch, it has no alimentary value beyond that belonging to this principle. It is chiefly used as a bland article of food for invalids, but, of course, requires to be conjoined with other alimentary matter, as alone it possesses only a limited sustaining power. As an ordinary dietetic agent, it is employed under the form of pudding and blanc-mange, and, with other materials, is made into a biscuit.

The spurious arrow-root consists of starch derived from other sources, and substituted on the score of greater cheapness. For example, *Tahitan* arrow-root, or *Tacca* starch, also sometimes called *Otaheite salep*, is obtained from the root of the *Tacca oceanica*, a native of the South Sea Islands (the *Tacca pinnatifida* of the tropical parts of Asia also yields a large quantity of beautifully white starch, which constitutes an important article of food to the natives); *Portland* arrow-root (so called from being manufactured in the island of that name) from that of the *Arum maculatum; Brazilian* arrow-root, from that of the plant which yields tapioca; *East Indian* arrow-root, from that of the *Curcuma angustifolia,* a species of turmeric plant; and *English* arrow-root, from the potato.

Tous-les-mois.—This name is given to the starch obtained from the tuberous *root* of the *Canna edulis,* a native of the West Indies. It is extracted in the same way as arrow-root, viz., by reducing the tuber to a pulp, straining, washing, decanting the supernatant liquid, and drying the starchy deposit. It is imported from St. Kitts, and was only introduced into England as recently as about the year 1836. Its granules are characterized by exceeding in size those of all other starches. It is very soluble in boiling water, and appears to be readily susceptible of digestion. It is used for invalids in the same way as arrow-root, and in alimentary value resembles the other farinaceous preparations.

Salep.—Salep constitutes the prepared tubercles of several orchideous plants. It is imported from India, Persia, and Turkey, and is met with under the form of small ovoid tubercles, which have been subjected to boiling for a few minutes in water, rubbing with a coarse linen cloth to remove the skin, and drying in an oven. When required for use, they are ground to a fine powder, and mixed with boiling water. Salep consists of, besides other ingredients, mucilaginous matter and starch. It, therefore, possesses demulcent as well as nutritive properties.

Revalenta Arabica.—*Revalenta* and *Ervalenta* form preparations the chief portion of which consists of the flour of the lentil, or *Ervum lens* (hence *ervalenta*), a plant belonging, like peas and beans, to the leguminous tribe.

Du Barry's Revalenta Arabica is thus composed, according to the analysis of Dr. Hassall. Three samples, he says, were examined, and one consisted of a mixture of the *red* or *Arabian lentil* and *barley-flour;* another of the same ingredients mixed with *sugar;* and the third of the *Arabian lentil* and *barley-flour,* with saline matter, chiefly *salt,* and a flavoring principle tasting as though consisting of *celery seed.* Such, according to Dr. Hassall, was found to be the composition of samples of an article which is vaunted in the advertising columns of the daily press as a specific for almost all the aliments that the human frame is heir to, and sold at an enormous price, looked at in relation to the cost of its ingredients.

A sample of *Wharton's Ervalenta,* examined by Dr. Hassall, consisted of the *French* or *German lentil,* mixed with a substance resembling *maize* or *Indian corn.*

The object of the admixture of barley- and other flours with the lentil powder is not, remarks Dr. Hassall, that of gain, for the cost of the latter is less than that of the former, but to diminish the strong flavor which lentils possess, and which is so distasteful to many.

Regarded dietetically, a preparation which owes its chief composition to lentil-flour is rich, like leguminous seeds in general, in nitrogenous matter, but in that form of it which is of a more indigestible nature than the nitrogenous matter belonging to the *Cerealia.*

BEVERAGES.

A supply of water under some shape or other is one of the essential conditions of life. It is just as needful as solid matter. It not only enters largely into the constitution of the different parts of the organism, but is required for various purposes in the performance of the operations of life. Without it, for instance, there could be no circulation nor molecular mobility of any kind. It forms the liquid element of the secretions, and thereby the medium for dissolving and enabling the digested food to pass into the system and the effete products to pass out. A constant ingress and egress are occurring, and the former requires to stand in proper adjustment to the latter. Under ordinary conditions of exercise and temperature, it may be estimated that about five pints of fluid pass off through the kidneys, skin, lungs and alimentary canal from an average-sized adult in the course of the twenty-four hours, and this has to be replenished by supply from without. But it is not necessary that this amount should be drunk. A large proportion of our solid food, in many cases as much as 70, 80, or 90 per cent., consists of water, and the quantity required in an ordinary way to be taken daily in the form of drink may be roughly assumed to amount to from two and a half or three to three and a half or four pints or more. The loss going on, however, represents such a fluctuating product dependent on exercise or work and the temperature to which the body is exposed, that great variation must ensue in the amount of fluid required. The effect of muscular exertion in leading to increased cutaneous transpiration is familiar to all. Exposure to heat also is well known to act in the same way, and where a particularly elevated temperature has to be endured, the loss of fluid by the skin is very great—indeed, it is by this loss and the evaporation which follows, that the cooling influence is exerted whereby the temperature of the body is kept down within natural limits. In the case of men, as particularly the stokers of large steam-vessels, who remain for some time in a highly heated atmosphere, the loss of fluid occurring entails the consumption of an enormous quantity (some quarts in the course of a few hours) of liquid, and it is the practice with such persons to drink from a store of water into which a little oatmeal has been thrown. Now, according to the amount required, so is the supply provided for by the sensation of thirst—a sensation which creates an irresistible desire to drink when the want of fluid in the system exists.

If a plain and wholesome liquid be drunk, the error is not likely to be committed of taking too much. After compensating for the loss by the skin and with the breath, the surplus passes off through the urinary channel, and it is desirable that this surplus should amply suffice to carry off the effete products forming the solid matter of the urine in a thoroughly dissolved state. The notion has been started that it is advisable to restrict the amount of liquid taken with the meals with the view of avoiding the dilution of the gastric juice. Whether as the result of the influence of this notion upon the public mind or not, mischief, I believe, is frequently occasioned, especially amongst the higher ranks of society, by a too limited consumption of fluid. Instead of taking a draught of some innocent and simple beverage, it is at many tables the fashion to sip fluid —and this a more or less strongly alcoholic one—only from the wine-glass. It is a mistaken notion to think that when we drink with a meal we are diluting the gastric juice. The act of secretion is excited by the arrival of the meal in the stomach, and the gastric juice is not there at the time of ingestion. It happens, indeed, that the absorption of fluid takes place with great activity, and the liquid which is drunk during a meal becoming absorbed, may be looked upon as proving advantageous by afterward contributing to yield the gastric juice which is required.

Water constitutes the essential basis of all our drinks, taken purely as such. The liquids consumed are of various kinds, but water is the element physiologically and indispensably required. Many of the beverages in use, however, are far from simply fulfilling the office of supplying water for the purposes of life. The accessory ingredients they contain give them special properties, for the sake of which their employment is often mainly, if not solely, dictated. It may be said, however, that a large quantity of fluid is required to be consumed to compensate for the loss occurring under violent exercise * or exposure to a high temperature, and that nothing is equal to a simple aqueous liquid, and the softer and purer the water the better. As already mentioned, those who work in unusually hot situations are in the habit of consuming, and wisely so, plain water, the rawness of which is removed by the addition of a little oatmeal.

Before treating of the beverages having special properties, as tea, coffee, etc., and the various liquids of the alcoholic class, all of which are products of artificial resources, something will be said regarding water, which forms the drink that has been placed at our disposal by nature.

---

* In Appendix II. to Dr. Parkes' publication, On the Issue of a Spirit Ration During the Ashanti Campaign of 1874, an account is given setting forth the good effect produced by the employment of oatmeal drink during the heavy work recently accomplished in the conversion of the broad into narrow-gauge on the Great Western Railway.

One portion of the undertaking consisted of narrowing the gauge on the South Wales section of the railway for a length of about 400 miles of single line. The number of men employed was 1,500, and the work lasted from seventeen to eighteen hours a day for several successive days. According to the report of the superintending engineer, the men worked in gangs of about thirty each, and were housed in lodges built along the line about six miles apart. They were directed to bring with them the food they would want for about two weeks, and, as a rule, they provided cocoa, coffee, sugar, bacon, bread, and cheese. At early dawn, water was heated at the lodges and breakfast made. That over, the day's work was commenced. Two men went in advance provided with a large iron pot, and oatmeal in 28 lb. packages. Water being found, a fireplace of stones was constructed and the pot boiled. Oatmeal was then sprinkled into it and added until their gruel was made. As soon as the shout for drink was heard, buckets were filled and carried round, small tins being used to drink it from. The men soon got to like it exceedingly, and used it very largely to supplement their solid food. It was the only drink taken during the day.

The engineer superintending the portion of the work which was carried out in the month of June, 1874, on the Wilts, Somerset, and Weymouth branch of the line, reported that the men worked from daylight to dark. Each man was allowed one pound of oatmeal and one-half pound of sugar per diem, and a man was appointed to cook and serve it out to each gang of twenty-one men. The men very much appreciated this drink, and had nothing else, no beer or spirits being allowed on the work. The work from beginning to end of the conversion lasted nearly a fortnight. The oatmeal supplied the place of water, beer, tea, and coffee. For meals the men had bread and cheese, or meat, and in some cases they had beer at night after their work was over, but never in the work. It is further stated that there was a strong feeling on the part of the engineers that the good conduct of the men and the hard work done by them was due to the liberal supply of oatmeal which they had ; as it not only quenched their thirst, but sustained them, and enabled them upon one occasion to keep on continually working very hard from four o'clock on Friday morning till nine o'clock on Saturday evening, with very little intermission.

WATER.—Water is derivable from various sources, and is denominated accordingly.

Rain-water constitutes the aqueous vapor which has existed in the atmosphere and, becoming condensed, has descended in a liquid form. It holds an analogous position to distilled water, and differs from it only in being impregnated with volatile products which have been abstracted from the air. It is found to be highly aërated, and to contain traces of ammonia, nitric acid, etc., and also a little organic matter. It is likely to be contaminated by the surfaces upon which it has fallen, and, unless special care has been taken in its collection, is not well adapted for potable purposes, although from its freedom from the earthy salts it is particulary eligible for domestic use. Its purity, indeed, as far as freedom from the earthy salts is concerned, renders it specially prone to acquire dangerous properties from lead contamination should it chance to be brought into contact with this metal.

Spring-water is rain-water which has percolated through the earth, and made its escape through some opening at a lower point admitting of its flow. It is charged with gaseous and saline principles, dependent in nature upon the character of the soil it has permeated. Many spring-waters furnish one of the best kinds of water for drinking. Some are charged with special ingredients—the mineral waters are alluded to—which render them unfit for ordinary use, but may give them a high value in a therapeutic point of view.

Well- or *pump-water* is of the same nature as spring-water. Deep well-water, unless there should be any defect in the construction of the well, allowing a leakage into it from above, mostly yields a safe and wholesome drink. The water of surface or superficial wells, however, cannot be spoken of in a similar way. Derived as it is from soakage from the surrounding surface, through a comparatively shallow stratum only, and this often consisting of a loose porous soil, it is liable to be contaminated with organic impurities that may cause it to give rise to the most serious consequences. Superficial well-water should always be regarded with suspicion. It may be clear, bright, sparkling, cool, and agreeable, and yet possess dangerous properties.

River-water consists partly of spring-water and partly of rain-water that has run off from the surrounding surface of land. A large portion of the water consumed is drawn from rivers, and whilst varying considerably in character, according to local circumstances, some river-waters possess qualities that render them highly suited for our use. The main drawback to their employment as a source of supply is their liability to pollution by the refuse of cities and towns being allowed to reach them. Rivers, however, possess a purifying power of their own. The effect of a running stream, and the influence of vegetation, are to oxidize and destroy impurities; and thus if the pollution be only of a limited extent, the water may be maintained fit for use.

Distilled water is now extensively used at sea. Most large vessels are furnished with the necessary appliance for subjecting sea-water to distillation to afford the water required, instead of, as formerly, shipping it from shore. Thus, a plentiful supply of pure water, in a strict sense, is at command. From the absence of air it has a flat taste, and, therefore, drinks less agreeably than that obtained from other sources. There are means, however, of submitting it to aëration, and overcoming this objection. On account of its purity it readily takes up lead, and many instances have occurred of injurious effects having been produced by contamination through the medium of the pipes or their joints belonging to the condensing apparatus.

Speaking now of water generally, it is almost needless to say that to be suitable for drinking purposes it should be bright and clear, and devoid of taste and smell. As a natural product, impregnation with a certain amount of gaseous and solid matter may be looked for. The gaseous matter, when consisting, as it only properly should do, of air and carbonic acid, gives an agreeable briskness, and may be considered a desirable accompaniment. The solid matter, unless of a specially noxious character from the presence of organic impurities, or unless existing in considerable amount, cannot be regarded as detracting from the fitness of the water for consumption, although it must be said that the less the extent of impregnation with solid matter—in other words, the purer the water—the better it is suited for our use.

Unwholesome water.—The chief sources of unwholesomeness of water are: 1st, An excess of saline matter; 2d, the presence of organic impurities; and 3d, contamination with lead.

First.—The presence of a moderate amount of saline matter does not render a water objectionable for drinking, although the less the amount the more wholesome it may be considered to be. A large amount of saline matter may prejudicially influence (increasing or diminishing according to its nature) the action of the secreting organs of the alimentary canal and so occasion constipation or diarrhœa; may aggravate the deranged condition existing in cases of dyspepsia; and possibly prove, in some instances, the source of calculous disorders, or, at least, if not the source, may favor the formation of urinary gravel or calculi when a tendency exists that way.

Second.—There is conclusive evidence to show that the most serious consequences have arisen from the consumption of water polluted with organic matter. This, in fact, is the impurity that is most to be dreaded. Outbreaks of diarrhœa have been very distinctly traced to the use of contaminated water of this kind. It is acknowledged to be one of the most common causes of dysentery, and has been alleged, when derived from a marshy district, to be capable of inducing malarious fever and its concomitant enlargement of the spleen.

From the facts that have been recently made known, there can be no doubt that typhoid or enteric fever has been frequently communicated through the medium of water. Some well-established instances have lately been brought to light where milk adulterated with polluted water has been the cause of serious outbreaks of fever. Whether water simply charged with general organic impurity will suffice to produce the disease has not been settled, but certain it is that if it be contaminated with the intestinal excreta of a fever patient, either by the discharge of sewage into a river, percolation from a drain or cesspool into a superficial well, or in any other way, it will do so. Probably the presence of sewage impurity in a particular state, apart from the specific poison, will occasion the disease, and it appears that it may be induced by impregnation with sewer-gases allowed, through a defective service arrangement, to become absorbed during storage in a cistern. Cholera is another disease which may be considered as having been traced to contaminated water, and probably this forms the chief mode of its spread through a community. As with typhoid fever, the discharges from a cholera patient, in any way reaching water that is subsequently consumed, may suffice to be the cause of a widely spread outbreak of the disease.

Third.—Water may possess unwholesome properties from contamination with lead, acquired by transit through leaden-pipes or storage in leaden-cisterns. A portion of the metal becoming dissolved, the prolonged use of the water gives rise to the ordinary phenomena of lead-poisoning. It is only certain kinds of water that are liable to become contaminated in this way. Water charged with a moderate quantity of the earthy salts may be preserved in contact with lead with impunity. Protection is afforded by the formation of an insoluble compound upon the surface of the metal. With a purer water, on the other hand, a solvent action is allowed to come into play. Distilled water very readily becomes impregnated with lead, and if a cistern be provided with a leaden-cover, the water which has evaporated and condensed in drops upon the surface, in falling back may lead to a contamination which, from the character of the water, would not otherwise occur.

Purification of Water.—It follows from what has been stated, that water has much to answer for in the causation of disease, and that care should be taken to secure a pure supply for drinking purposes. It is wise to be cautious in drinking water that has been derived from a superficial source, unless it has been subjected to a preparatory purification. In the case of spring-water issuing from a depth, and of deep well-water, there is but little chance of any serious harm arising. The extent of soil through which it has percolated is sufficient to ensure an absence, certainly, of noxious organic impurity. The danger especially lies with river-water and the water of shallow wells, and these should always be regarded with suspicion.

A considerable number of processes have been proposed for the purification of water. Only those in common use in this country need be referred to.

Water from certain sources is treated on a large scale by what is known as *Clark's process*, which consists of the addition of a definite amount of lime-water. The object of the process is to diminish the hardness by reducing the amount of earthy matter, and it is usefully applied to water derived from chalk districts. By combining with the carbonic acid, which is holding in solution carbonate of lime, the lime leads to a precipitation of newly formed carbonate, and at the same time of almost the whole of the carbonate previously present. The hardness produced by sulphates and chlorides still remains, but suspended, and perhaps some dissolved, organic matter is thrown down.

Boiling, by driving off the carbonic acid, has the effect of diminishing the hardness due to the earthy carbonates. It also acts upon organic matter. If it does not remove organic matter it may be spoken of as having the power of destroying the activity of that which possesses specifically poisonous properties. Where fear is entertained respecting the transmission of cholera or typhoid fever, the water should be subjected to thorough boiling, and it may then be considered safe for use. *Toast and water*, which is made by pouring boiling water on toasted and partially charred bread or biscuit and allowing it to cool, forms, on this account, a safer drink for water-drinkers than plain and fresh water, unless dependence can be placed upon the purity of the source.

Filtration is very extensively practised, and contributes in a most important manner toward the purification of water. Before being distributed to the metropolis the supply of the London Water Companies is submitted to filtration through sand and gravel. Suspended matters, both mineral and organic, are thereby removed, and dissolved mineral matter may be to some extent diminished, but dissolved organic matter fails to undergo any material alteration, and such filtration must not be viewed as rendering water safe for use when contaminated with noxious excreta. Animal charcoal, however, possesses a purifying power which is not enjoyed by other agents, and percolation through a good filter composed of this material effects a removal not only of suspended matters, but of a large proportion of the dissolved organic matter that may be contained in water. It is alleged that animal charcoal, in arresting, exerts at the same time a chemical alteration of the organic matter. The best domestic filters owe their action to this agent, and it is probable that they have the power of completely depriving water of any noxious property of an organic source that it may have possessed. There is always the possibility, however, that through defective action some active matter may pass through, and where room for suspicion exists that water may be dangerously contaminated, it is prudent to subject it to boiling instead of relying solely on filtration. The purifying power of animal charcoal is not unlimited. When water is charged with much organic matter it soon ceases to be effective. With the ordinary drinking-waters, however, where the organic impurity is small in amount, a filter will continue to act satisfactorily for many months, or even longer, provided, as is always necessary, the passage of the water is not too quick. After ceasing to act properly, the animal charcoal may be cleansed and again fitted for use, and to secure a constant state of efficiency a filter should from time to time be subjected to this process.

NON-ALCOHOLIC EXHILARATING AND RESTORATIVE BEVERAGES.

The group of dietetic articles of which tea, coffee, and cocoa form the chief representatives, are only of comparatively modern introduction into Europe, although now so extensively consumed amongst us. They must be regarded as exerting a great influence on the social condition of mankind, possessing the innocent properties they do, and consumed as largely as they are in the place of articles belonging to the alcoholic class, from which, when used in excess, such baneful physical and moral results take their source.

It is certainly a remarkable circumstance that the articles of this group should have independently come into use in different parts of the globe purely upon their own merits; that they should also be derived from plants widely separated in their botanical affinities, and from different structures of the plant, and yet that they should be found to possess the same physiological properties and dietetic virtue, and, moreover, should be discovered, long subsequently to their introduction, to contain the same active chemical principle. In 1820, *caffeine* was discovered in coffee by Runge, and in 1827 *theine* in tea by Oudry; and in 1838 these two principles were found by Jobst and Mulder to be identical. In 1840, the same substance was recognized by Martius in Guarana—an article used in some parts of South America in the same way as we use tea and coffee; and in 1843 it was found by Stenhouse also to exist in Paraguay tea—a kind of tea obtained from the leaves of quite a different plant from that which yields the Chinese tea. *Theobromine*, the peculiar principle belonging to cocoa, is certainly not strictly identical with, but, on the other hand, is very closely allied to caffeine and theine. *Cocaine*, the active principle of the leaves of the *Erythroxylon coca* which are used in South America in the same way as tea, coffee, etc., and possess the same dietetic properties, has been further found to bear a close chemical relation to the other principles, and to agree with them in physiological action. Now that caffeine and theine, and what were originally called guaranine and paraguaine, have been shown to be identical, it would prove a source of convenience if some suitable generic name were invented and employed by chemists to represent them. The action of these various principles has been made the subject of inquiry by the Committee of the British Medical Association appointed to investigate the antagonism of medicines; and the results showing the resemblance they bear to each other, and the antagonistic position they hold in relation to morphia, are to be found in the second volume of the *British Medical Journal* for 1874.

TEA.—Tea constitutes the dried leaves of a plant belonging to the genus *Thea* of Linnæus, which, according to the more recent authority of Bentham and Hooker, forms a section only of the genus *Camellia*, a tribe of plants with which all are familiar in England. The tea-plant is indigenous in China, Cochin China, Japan, and the northern parts of the eastern peninsula of India, and has been introduced into British India on the southern declivities of the Himalayas, Java, the Kong Mountains in Western Africa, Brazil, Madeira, and other warm and temperate countries. It is capable of flourishing in all latitudes between 0° and 40°.

The two chief varieties of the plant are *Thea bohea* and *Thea viridis*, but besides these *Thea sasangua* is grown and used for some of the choicest sorts of tea.

It was formerly supposed that *Thea bohea* yielded black tea only, and *Thea viridis* green; but Mr. Fortune ascertained, and it has since been fully corroborated by others, that black and green are both obtained from each variety of the plant, it being upon the mode of preparation adopted that the difference in the nature of the article depends. *Thea viridis* abounds in the northern districts of China, where it is cultivated on the fertile slopes of the hills. *Thea bohea* is cultivated in the southern parts of China, especially about Canton.

The first gathering of tea is conducted in April, and consists of young leaf-buds, the removal of which to some extent injures the plant. The tea thus obtained, called *yutien*, is insignificant in amount, and not an article of commerce, but only intended for choice gifts to friends. It is used on occasions of ceremony, and although very strong in taste, scarcely colors the water in which it is infused. The showers of spring bring on fresh leaves, and the second gathering, which is the most important of the season, takes place in May. A third and last gathering supplies only inferior teas.

Green tea is prepared from the *young* leaves, which within an hour or two after being gathered are roasted in pans over a brisk wood fire. After four or five minutes' roasting they are rolled by hand, and again thrown into the drying pans, where they are kept in rapid motion for about an hour and a half. The process is simple, and speedily accomplished. Prussian blue, turmeric-root, gypsum, and sometimes indigo and copper, are used to give an attractive bloom, but this artifice is only resorted to for the foreign market. The Chinese, it is said, never dye the teas for their own consumption.

For *black tea*, the leaves are allowed to lie in heaps for ten or twelve hours after they have been gathered, during which time they undergo a sort of fermentation. They are then tossed about till they become soft and flaccid, and, after being rolled, are alternately heated and rolled three or four times. The leaves are afterward dried slowly over charcoal fires. Various sorts of both black and green tea are manufactured. Of green, Singlo or Twankay is the lowest in quality. The chief of the others, in upward order of excellence, are Hyson-skin, Hyson, Imperial, Gunpowder, and the choicest Young Hyson. The chief varieties of black tea, arranged in a similar order, are Bohea, Oolong, Congou, Campoi, Souchong, Souchy or Caper, and Pekoe.

Certain teas possess a characteristic aroma, dependent on the district in which they are grown; but the Chinese also adopt the plan of scenting some kinds of tea with various flowers, such as roses, jasmine, and orange-blossoms. The dry tea and the freshly gathered flowers are mixed and allowed to remain together for twenty-four hours. The flowers are then sifted out.

Lie tea is the name applied to an article produced from the dust and sweepings of tea-warehouses, cemented with rice-water, and rolled into grains. It is made either of a black color, to imitate Caper; or green, to resemble Gunpowder. It is manufactured for the purpose of adulterating the better kinds of tea.

Brick tea is made from the refuse, siftings, sweepings, and the broken leaves and twigs of tea moulded into forms. The Tartars use this tea. They reduce it to powder, and boil it with the alkaline water of the step-pes, to which salt and fat have been added; and this decoction, mixed with milk, butter, and a little roasted meal, they consume as an article of subsistence. It is also used in the same manner as other tea.

Tea appears to have been used from time immemorial in China, and is known to have been common at the beginning of the sixth century. It is said to have been introduced into Japan about the beginning of the ninth century. The Dutch East India Company introduced it into Europe early in the seventeenth century. The first reference to tea made by an Englishman was in the year 1615, and is found in the records of the English East India Company. In 1657 a rather large consignment fell into the hands of Mr. Thomas Garraway, the person who established Garraway's Coffee House. The consumption of tea in the United Kingdom in 1853 amounted, according to Johnston, to 58,000,000 pounds (25,000 tons), or about one forty-fifth part of the estimated produce of China.

In 1866 the amount entered for home consumption had risen to 98,-000,000 pounds. In 1871, according to the published Custom House Returns, the quantity consumed was 3 lbs. 15 oz. for each member of the community.

The most important constituents of tea are:

First.—An astringent matter of the nature of tannic acid, which constitutes the source of the bitter styptic taste it possesses. In the analyses furnished below, the amounts of this astringent matter stand in round figures at 13 and 18 per cent.

Second.—A volatile oil, to which it owes its peculiar aroma, and which only amounts to about ½ or ¾ per cent.

Third.—A crystallizable body, of an alkaline nature, and rich in nitrogen, called *theine*. This, according to the subjoined analyses, only amounts to about ½ per cent., but Stenhouse has found from 1 to 1.27 per cent., and Peligot's results give more than double this, viz., from 2.34 to 3 per cent.

There is, therefore, considerable diversity in the results that have been obtained by different chemists upon this point. *

Composition of Tea (Mulder).

	Black tea.	Green tea.
Essential oil,	0.60	0.79
Chlorophyll,.	1.84	2.22
Wax, .	0.00	0.28
Resin, .	3.64	2.22
Gum, .	7.28	8.56
Tannin,	12.88	17.80
Theine,	0.46	0.43
Extractive matter,	21.36	22.80
Coloring substance,	19.19	23.60
Albumen,	2.80	3.00
Fibre, .	28.32	17.08
Ash (mineral substances), .	5.24	5.56

Tea is consumed under the form of infusion, made by pouring *boiling* water upon it and allowing it to stand for a short time. If boiled, a loss of its characteristic flavor would occur through the dissipation of its aromatic principle, which is very volatile.

The water used should be neither particularly hard nor soft, as the former impedes the extraction of the soluble principles, and the latter favors the absorption of too much of the general extractive matter, at the sacrifice of delicacy of flavor. River-water is the best, and this is employed by the Chinese. The water should not be allowed to remain long on the leaves, as by standing, or stewing, the infusion loses its aroma and takes up an excess of extractive matter which gives a rough and bitter taste. Thus, the liquid quickly poured off contains more aroma and less coloring and astringent matters, and thereby possesses a choicer flavor than that which has been allowed to stand. In China, tea is sometimes infused in a teapot and sometimes in the cup, from which it is drunk off the leaves. In Japan, the tea-leaves are ground to powder and, after infusion in a teacup, the mixture is beaten up till it becomes frothy, and then the whole is drunk.

Dr. Letheby says that it is experimentally proved that an infusion of tea is strong enough when it contains 0.6 per cent. of extracted matter, and that a moderate-sized cup, holding five ounces, would thus contain about thirteen grains of the extract of tea.

Tea is usually measured by the spoon for use, but the weight of a spoonful varies much with the different sorts of tea, and as green tea is rolled much closer and weighs heavier than black, a spoonful of the former, apart from any difference in composition, will make a stronger infusion than that of the latter. Dr. E. Smith has instituted a comparison in reference to this point, and the following is the table given by him showing the weight in grains of an evenly taken moderate-sized caddy-spoonful of tea, and the number of such spoonfuls required to make a pound.

---

* In the Food Journal, vol. i., p. 162, it is stated that Stenhouse's observations show a range in the amount of theine in various teas from 0.70 to 2.13 per cent.; and that Peligot's results vary, but that in his last and most complete experiment he obtained 6.21 per cent.

Kind of tea.		Weight of a spoon-ful in grains.	Number of spoon-fuls in a pound.
BLACK—			
Oolong, ...		39	179
Congou, inferior quality, . . .		52	138
Flowery Pekoe, ...		62	113
Souchong, ...		70	100
Congou, fine, ...		87	80
GREEN—			
Hyson skin, { Not now imported } .		58	120
Twankay, { into England } .		70	100
Hyson, ...		66	106
Fine Imperial, ...		90	77
Scented Caper, an artificial preparation, .		103	68
Fine Gunpowder, ...		123	57

With regard to these results, something may be due to the condition as to form of the tea, some teas holding together in the spoon more than others, otherwise a pound packet of the first on the list ought to be three times the size of that of the last.

The Chinese drink their tea in a pure state. The Russians frequently squeeze the juice of lemon into it, and this is said to form an agreeable addition. The Germans often flavor it with rum, cinnamon, or vanilla. In England it may be said to be customary to add milk or cream, and sugar; the one having the effect of diminishing the astringent taste, and the other being employed to please the palate.

Tea is not to be looked upon as constituting an article of nutrition. The quantity of material furnished to the system in the manner it is used is too small to be of any significance per se in contributing to the chemical changes which form the source of vital action. If not occupying the position of an article of nutrition, however, its extensive and widely spread employment may be taken as indicating that some kind of benefit is derivable from its use, and it is probably through the nervous system that this is mainly, if not entirely, produced.

Much discordancy exists in the statements that have been made regarding the effects of tea upon the system, and an unfortunate want of uniformity prevails amongst medical practitioners in the recommendations given to the public upon the subject of its employment. The diametrically opposite advice that is frequently found to be given to patients, one member of the profession recommending, and another immediately afterward prohibiting, the use of tea, exhibits an arbitrary course of procedure which testifies to the want of some definite guiding principle of action. An attempt will be made to furnish a concise representation of what is known, and from this may be drawn a basis for greater uniformity of procedure.

Tea forms a light beverage, which is neither heating to the system nor oppressive to the stomach, in which respects it differs from coffee. Taken in moderate quantity, it may be spoken of as exerting an exhilarating and restorative action without stimulating or inebriating like alcohol. By such action it exerts a reviving influence when the body is fatigued, but perhaps some of the effect is also attributable to the warmth belonging to the liquid consumed. It disposes to mental cheerfulness and activity, clears the brain, arouses the energies, and diminishes the tendency to sleep —to such an extent, it may be, in some sensitive persons, as to occasion a painful state of vigilance or watchfulness, and sleeplessness.

15

The phenomena produced when tea is consumed in a strong state, and to a hurtful extent, show that it is capable of acting in a powerful manner upon the nervous system. Nervous agitation, muscular tremors, a sense of prostration, and palpitation, constitute effects that have been witnessed. It appears to act in a sedative manner on the vascular system. It also possesses direct irritant properties, which lead to the production of abdominal pains and nausea. It promotes the action of the skin, and, by the astringent matter it contains, diminishes the action of the bowels. Green tea, as is well known, possesses far more active properties than black, although, as previously stated, the two are obtained from the same plant. The difference between them is dependent on the mode of treatment to which the leaf is subjected and the period of gathering it.

Tea, like coffee, appeases the sensation arising from the want of food, and enables hunger to be better borne. Lehmann was of opinion that it lessened the waste of the body, but Dr. E. Smith asserts that it increases slightly the amount of carbonic acid exhaled, and he thereby speaks of it as promoting rather than checking chemico-vital action. More conclusive evidence, it may be considered, is required in reference to this matter to show that any decided action either way is exerted.

To express in a few words the advantages derivable from the use of tea, it may be said that it forms an agreeable, refreshing, and wholesome beverage, and thereby constitutes a useful medium for the introduction of a portion of the fluid we require into the system. It secures that the water consumed is rendered safe for drinking by the boiling which is necessitated as a preliminary operation in making tea. It cools the body when hot, probably by promoting the action of the skin; and warms it when cold, by virtue, it would seem, of the warm liquid consumed. In a negative way it may prove beneficial to health by taking the place of a less wholesome liquid. Through the milk and sugar usually consumed with it in England, it affords the means of supplying a certain amount—and not by any means an insignificant amount, viewed in its entirety—of alimentary matter to the system. Experience shows that it often affords comfort and relief to persons suffering from nervous headache. It also tends to allay the excitement from and counteract the state induced by the use of alcoholic stimulants; and, further, on account of its antisoporific properties, like coffee, it is useful as an antidote in poisoning by opium.

Its use, particularly green tea, is objectionable, in a strong state, in the case of persons who are rendered watchful by it, and in all irritable conditions of the stomach. The astringent matter it contains will cause it to impede digestion, if taken strong and in any large quantity during or shortly after a meal.

REPRESENTATIVES OF TEA.—Before concluding this section on tea, reference may be made to the leaves of certain plants, which are prepared and extensively used in some localities in the same manner as those of the Chinese tea-plant.

Maté, or Paraguay Tea.—This is derived from the dried leaves of the *Ilex Paraguayensis*, or Brazilian holly, a plant belonging to the same tribe as the holly of our own country. It is a native of South America, where it grows in a wild state; and in some parts of that portion of the world the leaves are extensively employed dietetically as tea and coffee are in Asia and Europe. The leaves, after being dried, are reduced to a coarse kind of powder before being used for yielding the infusion. It is not correct to look upon Paraguay tea as a spurious substitute for Chinese tea. It is consumed upon its own merits, and it forms a curious and interesting fact that it contains an active principle which was at first called *paraguaine*, but which has since been found to be identical with *theine* and *caffeine*.

The chief constituents of Paraguay tea are:

First.—An astringent principle analogous to tannic acid, which is present in sufficient proportion to render the fresh leaves an article of use to dyers in the Brazils.

Second.—A volatile oil.

Third.—Theine, amounting in quantity to about 1.20 per cent.

Paraguay tea is spoken of as being more exciting than Chinese tea; and, when used in excessive quantity, is said to produce a kind of *delirium tremens*.

Additional varieties of Paraguay tea are made from the leaves of the *Ilex gongonha* (called Brazilian tea), *Ilex theœzans*, *Psoralea glandulosa* (called Mexican tea), and *Capraria biflora*.

Coffee-leaves.—In the islands of the Eastern Archipelago, the leaves of the coffee-plant, which somewhat resemble in outside character those of the common laurel, are dried and used in the manner of tea. They yield an infusion which even more approximates to that of Chinese tea than does the infusion of maté, or Paraguay tea. It contains the same kind of constituents, and the *theine* amounts to about 1.26 per cent. It forms the favorite tea of the dark-skinned population of Sumatra. In taste and odor it resembles a mixture of tea and coffee.

Labrador tea is made from the dried leaves of the *Ledum palustre* and *Ledum latifolium*. It is very strong in astringent and narcotic properties.

Abyssinian tea, called *chaat,* consists of the dried leaves of the *Catha edulis,* a small tree allied to the *Sageretia theœzans.* It is cultivated and used extensively in Northern Africa.

In "Johnston's Chemistry of Common Life" a list of several other plants is given, the leaves of which are used for infusing and consuming in the same manner as Chinese tea.

COFFEE.—Coffee-beans constitute the seeds found within the fruit of the *Coffea Arabica,* a small tree belonging to the tribe *Coffeaceæ,* of the family *Rubiaceæ,* which is indigenous in Southern Abyssinia.

The tree is said to have been transplated into Arabia at the beginning of the fifteenth century, and the cultivation has since been extended to Egypt, the West Indies, Peru, Brazil, Java, Ceylon, and other warm countries. When the climate is dry, abundant irrigation is required while the tree is growing, but as the fruit begins to ripen the water is cut off.

The fruit forms a succulent berry, similar in appearance and color to a small cherry. Each berry contains usually two seeds, forming the coffee-bean of commerce, surrounded by a parchment-like envelope and the fleshy pulp.

To extract the seeds, the fresh, ripe berries are sometimes bruised between rollers, and the thick, juicy pulp is then separated by passing through sieves, upon which the beans are retained. They are afterward washed with water, and dried. The parchment-like envelope is next detached by a heavy wooden wheel, and the chaff removed by winnowing. Sometimes the berries are dried in the sun, by which the pulp and membranous envelope become friable, and are removed by lightly crushing and winnowing.

The coffee-bean is usually imported in the above-mentioned decorticated state. It then constitutes a horny body, rounded on one side and flat, with a longitudinal furrow, on the other, and of a yellowish, bluish, or greenish color. Sometimes, however, it is met with surrounded by its membranous envelope, and is then called in commerce " *coffee in the husk.*"

The coffee produced by different countries presents variations in quality and the physical characters of the bean. The smallest bean is considered the best. *Mocha* or *Arabian* coffee is the most highly esteemed. The bean is small and round, and of a dark yellow color, with a tinge of green. This variety develops a more agreeable aroma than the others. *West Indian* coffee is usually of a greenish gray tint, with the ends of the beans rounded. A slight difference exists in the production of the various islands. *Jamaica* coffee, for instance, does not exactly resemble that from *Martinique*, and the coffee from *St. Domingo* is less esteemed than either, and is pointed at the two extremities. *Java* and *East Indian* coffee is large, and of a pale yellow color. *Ceylon* coffee is the least prized of all.

Coffee is said to have been in use in Abyssinia from time immemorial, and in Persia from A.D. 875. It was used in Constantinople about the middle of the sixteenth century, in spite of the violent opposition of the priests; and in 1554 two coffee-houses were opened in that city. It was introduced into Europe in the seventeenth century, but the precise date is variously stated by different authorities. It was drunk in Venice soon after 1615, and brought to England and France about forty years subsequently.

To show the progress in the consumption of coffee, it may be mentioned that in 1699 one hundred tons of coffee were consumed in the United Kingdom, seventy of which were used in England (Tomlinson). In 1858 the consumption in the United Kingdom is stated to have been sixteen thousand tons (" Chambers's Encyclopædia "). About the same time the total European consumption was something like seventy-five thousand tons (Johnston), and the entire weight of coffee raised over the world was guessed to be about six hundred millions of pounds (Johnston). Nearly as much coffee is consumed in the United Kingdom as in France; and, proportionately to its size, Belgium, Payen says, consumes five times as much as France.

The coffee of commerce is formed of the raw bean, and subjection to the process of roasting is required to place it in a suitable condition for the consumer. This is performed in an iron cylinder, made to revolve over a fire. It leads to the development of the aroma and other qualities for which the article is esteemed. From the volatile nature of the aroma the roasted coffee greatly deteriorates by keeping; hence the process of roasting should not be performed long before the coffee is made use of.

Under the process of roasting, the coffee-bean loses in weight and gains in bulk by expansion. It at the same time changes in color, assuming a reddish brown, chestnut-brown, or dark brown, according to the extent to which the roasting has been carried. The quality of the coffee a great deal depends upon the manner in which the roasting has been performed. If the seeds are roasted too little, the desired aroma and empyreumatic products are not sufficiently developed, whilst if roasted too much they are partially dissipated, and an unpleasant flavor substituted. If a full-flavored coffee be desired, the darker shade of color should be chosen. In England, the operation of roasting is conducted in large establishments devoted to the purpose, but on the Continent it is not uncommon for it to be performed from time to time on a small scale by a member of the household. Before being used, coffee requires to be ground, and the remark that has been made about the roasted bean losing its aroma by keeping, applies with still greater force to the article when ground. To grind it as it is required forms the best plan, but when this is not adopted it should be preserved in a well closed bottle or tin.

The chief constituents of coffee are of the same nature as those mentioned for tea. They are as follows:

First.—A volatile oil, which gives to coffee the aroma it possesses, and is developed by the process of roasting. The amount of it is less than that existing in tea.

Second.—Astringent matter constituting a modification of tannin, and called caffeo-tannic and caffeic acids. It is present in much smaller quantity than tannic acid in tea, and amounts to about 5 per cent. in *raw* coffee.

Third.—Caffeine. This principle, as already mentioned, is identical with theine. The amount of it, as estimated by different observers, in coffee varies considerably. Stenhouse gives it as about 0.75 to 1 per cent., others at 3 to 4 per cent.

Composition of Unroasted Coffee (" Chambers' Encyclopædia ").

Caffeine,	0.8
Legumine (vegetable caseine),	13.0
Gum and sugar,	15.5
Caffeo-tannic and caffeic acids,	5.0
Fat and volatile oil,	13.0
Woody fibre,	34.0
Ash,	6.7
Water,	12.0
	100.0

An elaborate analysis is given by Payen,* from his own results, with which the above is in close accord. It is as follows:

Composition of Coffee (Payen).

Cellulose,	34.
Water,	12.
Fatty matter,	from 10 to 13.
Glucose, dextrine, undetermined vegetable acid,	15.5
Legumine, caseine, etc.,	10.
Chloroginate [caffeo-tannate] of potash and of caffeine, from 3.5 to	5.
Nitrogenized structure,	3.
Caffeine,	0.8
Essential oil,	0.001
Aromatic essence,	0.002
Mineral substances,	6.697
	100.000

* Substances Alimentaires, p. 414. Paris, 1865.

Coffee is prepared for drinking both in the form of infusion and de-coction. In Arabia and the East a decoction of the unroasted article is usually drunk, and the custom prevails of consuming the grounds, which are looked upon as nutritious, with the liquid. In Europe, however, cof-fee is always roasted before it is used. The old practice in England was to place the coffee-pot over the fire for the coffee to boil. In this way a larger amount of material is extracted, but at the sacrifice, it must be said, of flavor, for the aroma of coffee is of a volatile nature, and becomes dis-sipated during the process of boiling. To preserve the aroma, an infusion only should be made, and the appliances that have been devised for mak-ing coffee in this way are exceedingly numerous. The most general plan adopted is to allow the boiling water to percolate through the coffee, dis-posed in such a manner as to prevent the grounds passing with the liquid.

As boiling leads to a loss of aroma, so infusing only involves a waste of some of the extractive matter, which escapes being taken up. If econo-my is no object this need not be considered, a large amount of coffee be-ing taken for use. If it be desired, however, to turn the coffee to the utmost account, both a decoction and an infusion should be made; and this may be accomplished by boiling the grounds from which an infusion has been made with water, and pouring the boiling decoction over a fresh portion of recently ground coffee. The boiling water has fully extracted what the grounds would yield, and on being poured over the fresh coffee, carries with it the aroma and the principles contained in an ordinary infu-sion. The grounds last left, in their turn, will serve to boil with more water, and yield a decoction for pouring over another fresh portion of coffee. In this way all the goodness is obtained without any sacrifice of aroma.

As is the case with tea, soft water extracts more from coffee than hard, and the addition of an alkali, as carbonate of soda, augments the extract-ing capacity.

The extent to which the coffee has been roasted influences the amount of matter susceptible of extraction. Payen says that one litre (about 1¾ pint in English measure) of boiling water allowed to filter through 100 grammes (about 3½ oz.) of recently ground coffee—and this he gives as about the proper proportion for making coffee—when the roasting has been carried only to the production of a reddish brown color, extracts 25 per cent. of its substance, and only 19 per cent. when the roasting has been carried to a chestnut-brown.

According to Dr. Letheby, an infusion of coffee is strong enough when it holds in solution 3 per cent. of extracted matter. Charged to this ex-tent, a moderate-sized cup (5 ounces), he adds, should contain 66 grains of extract of coffee, and such proportion will be obtained when 2 ounces of freshly roasted coffee are infused in a pint of boiling water.

Coffee forms a favorite and useful beverage. The properties it pos-sesses fully justify the estimation in which it is held. Like tea, it pro-duces an invigorating and restorative effect on the system, without being followed by any depression. It, however, exerts a more heating and stimulating action than tea, and increases in a decided manner the force and frequency of the pulse. It also differs in being heavier and more op-pressive to the stomach. It arouses the mental faculties and the energies generally, and so disposes to wakefulness, but in this latter respect its influence is not so powerful as that of tea. Taken in immoderate quantity it may induce feverishness, and various manifestations of disordered ner-vous action, as tremor, palpitation, anxiety, and deranged vision.

One of the most valuable properties of coffee is its power of relieving the sensation of hunger and fatigue. It exerts a marked sustaining influence under fatigue and privation, and thus enables arduous exertion to be better borne under the existence of abstinence or a deficiency of food. To the soldier on active service it forms a most useful article on this account. The experiments of Lehmann led him to conclude that coffee diminishes the waste of the tissues, and causes food to go further, but whether this is true is doubtful. Gasparin, however, from his observations, also says that coffee has the property of rendering the elements of the body more stable; and thus, if not affording much nourishment itself, that it economizes other nourishment by diminishing the waste going on. On the other hand, Mr. Squarey * could not find that the elimination of urea and chlorides was diminished, as might be looked for if the above view were correct, under the use of large doses of coffee, and some later researches of E. Roux † furnish evidence of a corroborative nature.

"In some constitutions," says Pereira, "coffee acts on the bowels as a mild laxative." "I have known," he adds, "several persons in whom it has this effect; yet it is usually described as producing constipation."

Whilst heating and stimulating to the system in hot weather, coffee is most serviceable in giving warmth to the body under exposure to cold. Something, it must be admitted, is due to the warm liquid consumed, but an action beyond this is exerted.

Consumed, as coffee usually is, with milk and sugar, it further forms a medium for supplying direct nourishment, and this of no inconsiderable amount, to the system. Payen remarks that a litre (about a pint and three quarters) of *café au lait*, such as is usually taken with the morning meal, contains between 5 and 6 ounces of solid matter, of which about 1¾ ounce consists of nitrogenous matter.

In addition to its dietetic value, considerable benefit is often derived from the employment of coffee as a therapeutic agent. By virtue of its antisoporific properties it is advantageously administered as an antidote in cases of opium-poisoning. It is also of service in subduing the effects produced by the immoderate use of alcoholic stimulants. It frequently affords relief in some forms of nervous headache, and is well known to constitute one of the most valuable agents we possess for controlling the paroxysms of spasmodic asthma.

Fictitious coffee.—A number of articles, consisting of various beans, seeds, berries, and roots, have been used as substitutes for coffee, but in none of them does there exist the characteristic and active principle— caffeine, and none therefore are endowed with the virtue of coffee. The roasted acorn is much used on the Continent under the name of *acorn coffee*, and has been imported into England. The best substitute for coffee yet discovered is said to be that which is known by the name of *Swedish coffee*, and is prepared from the *Astralagus Bæticus.*

CHICCORY.—Chiccory is prepared from the root of the wild succory or endive (*Cichorium Intybus*), the type of a great division of the order *Compositæ*, known by their milky juice, and to which also belong the dandelion and lettuce. It was formerly used medicinally from possessing properties resembling those of the dandelion; and for about 100 years has been employed as a substitute for and admixture with coffee. The plant

---

* Medico-Chirurgical Transactions, vol. xlix., pp. 1–19, 1866.
† Comptes Rendus, vol. lxxvii., p. 365-7, 1873.

is cultivated in England, Belgium, Holland, Germany, and France, and the foreign is considered much superior to the English growth. The roots after being washed are cut into small pieces and dried on a kiln. They are then roasted in iron cylinders, which are kept revolving, just as is done in the case of coffee.

Roasted chiccory contains, like coffee, an empyreumatic volatile oil, which forms the source of its aroma, and a bitter principle, but no caffeine. According to the analysis of John, 25 per cent. consists of watery, bitter extractive matter.

Chiccory yields a drink closely allied in flavor and color to coffee. It is very largely consumed on the Continent, not merely as an adulterant of coffee, but as an independent beverage. In Belgium, as much as 5 pounds a head are used in the year, counting the whole population; and in some parts of Germany, women, it is said, are regular chiccory-topers.

It gives increased color and flavor to coffee, and, used as an admixture to a moderate extent, is considered by most persons to furnish an improvement upon coffee alone. The preference shown is quite independent of any consideration of economy. It is employed upon its own merits, and, when there is no concealment, its addition to coffee cannot be looked upon in the light of an adulteration.

The root of the *dandelion* is sometimes roasted and used in the same way as chiccory.

GUARANA.—Brazilian cocoa, or guarana, is obtained from the seeds of the *Paullinia sorbilis*, a tree belonging to the order *Sapindaceæ*, or soapworts, which, according to most botanists, includes the common horse-chestnut. The tree grows abundantly in the province of Amazonas, along the banks of the Tapajos, Rio Negro, etc., as well as in Guiana and Venezuela. It is used extensively in Brazil, Guatemala, Costa Rica, and other parts of South America as a nervous stimulant and restorative, and also as a refreshing beverage. According to late reports, 16,000 pounds are annually exported from the city of Santarem.

The fruit, which is about the size of a small walnut, contains five or six seeds. These seeds are roasted, and, after being pounded, are made into a thick paste with water and formed into round or oblong cakes, which are dried in an oven or by the heat of the sun, and called guaranabread. The cakes are scraped or grated when required for use, and the powder produced possesses a light brown color, an odor faintly resembling roasted coffee, and a bitter, astringent taste.

It contains, in addition to empyreumatic oil (developed by the process of roasting), and tannic acid, a substance called *guaranine* by Theodore von Martius, but shown by Dr. Stenhouse to be identical with theine. This alkaloid is stated by Dr. Stenhouse to be present to the extent of 5.07 per cent., or, according to the results of the same observer, to the extent of twice the amount contained in good black tea, and five times that contained in coffee: the actual figures given for tea being 2.13 per cent., and for coffee 0.8 to 1.0 per cent. For Paraguay tea the amount mentioned is 1.25 per cent.

The large amount of tannic acid that enters into the composition of guarana gives it marked astringent properties, whilst, owing to the guaranine it contains, it exerts the same kind of effect on the nervous system as tea and coffee.

Guarana is used in South America to some extent dietetically, but chiefly therapeutically, as a stomachic and febrifuge, and as an astringent in catarrhal diarrhœa and dysentery. It is either eaten with cassava or chocolate, or taken as a drink in sweetened water. In the United States it is employed as a nervous stimulant and restorative, and attention was directed to it some years ago in France by Dr. Gavrelle, who had held the post of physician to Don Pedro of Brazil.

Alcohol, it is stated, forms the only agent which completely extracts its active principles. Ether and water only do so imperfectly. A watery infusion, therefore, will fail to possess the virtue belonging to guarana.

Guarana appears for some time to have enjoyed a high repute in France as a remedy for *migraine,* or sick headache, and attention has been recently directed to its employment for this purpose, in England, by my colleague, Dr. Wilks. Articles upon the subject may be seen in the *British Medical Journal* for 1872, and another article, by Mr. M. C. Cooke, is to be found in vol. i., third series, of the *Pharmaceutical Journal,* p. 221. As far as experience goes, it seems that in some cases of sick or nervous headache it is capable of affording the most marked relief, whilst in others it utterly fails to produce any good effect. Its virtue is, in all probability, due to the *guaranine* (theine or caffeine) it contains, which, as already remarked, is, according to the analysis of Stenhouse, present in much larger proportion than in either tea or coffee. Employed for the medicinal purpose above referred to, the quantity generally used is about 15 grains of the powder administered in coffee, water, or some other suitable vehicle.

Cocoa.—Cocoa constitutes a product derived from the seeds of the *Theobroma cacao,* a tree indigenous in South America, Mexico, and the West Indies, and cultivated also in the Mauritius, the Isle of Bourbon, and some parts of Asia and Africa. The term cocoa, as applied to this product, must not be looked upon as signifying that it has any relation to the well-known cocoanut. It is employed as a corruption of cacao, which through want of euphony has been excluded from popular use. The generic name *Theobroma* (food for gods—θεος βρώμα) was given by Linnæus to the tribe of plants, which includes several species, to mark the estimation in which he held the product under consideration.

From the cacao tree small flowers grow on stalks, springing directly from the stem. The flower is succeeded by an elongated thick fruit somewhat resembling in form the vegetable marrow. The fruit consists of a number of seeds (from twenty to fifty) arranged in regular rows, with partitions between them, and surrounded by an acid and slightly saccharine pulp. When the fruit is ripe, it is gathered and collected in earthen vessels or into heaps on the ground, where it is allowed to remain a few days, during which time it ferments, heats, and softens. It is then opened, and the seeds, which are about the size of or rather thicker than a plump almond, are separated, cleansed, and dried in the sun. The fruit is sometimes covered instead with earth until the pulp has become rotten and soft, and the cocoa yielded is said to be sweeter and better.

The use of cocoa is of great antiquity in Mexico and Guatemala, and chocolate was introduced into Europe in 1520 by the Spaniards, who long kept its preparation a secret. Cocoa was sold in the London coffee-houses soon after their establishment, about the year 1652, and in 1660 its use spread over Europe, and as far as Turkey and Persia. The present total annual consumption is said to amount to about 100,000,000 pounds. A large quantity is used in France, Germany, Italy, and Spain. In England the consumption is on a smaller scale.

Cocoa is imported in the state of dried and cleansed seeds, consisting of a crisp, dark-colored central portion or kernel, surrounded by a somewhat brittle husk. The first step in preparing it for use is to subject it to the process of roasting, which is performed in an iron cylinder like a coffee-roaster, and has for its object the development of aroma. From the roasted seeds, chocolate and the various forms of cocoa supplied for use are prepared.

Cocoa nibs constitute the kernels of the roasted seeds deprived of husk, and roughly crushed in a machine called a "kibbling mill." Nibs are used for furnishing a decoction. They are gently boiled in water for about a couple of hours, and the dark-brown decoction is then simply poured off the undissolved part of the nib. Used in this way, only a portion of the kernel is extracted and consumed, and the beverage presents a closer analogy to tea and coffee than that derived from the other cocoa products, which, from being prepared in such a way as to lead to the whole substance of the kernel being drunk, furnish liquids possessing in addition to the common properties of the class, a high nutritive value.

In the other preparations of cocoa, the kernel is ground to a paste and usually incorporated with some diluting material of a starchy or saccharine nature to diminish its oily consistence. Numerous kinds of cocoa are sold, some of them being named from the form given, the nature of the admixture, or after the manufacturer. *Flaked* cocoa constitutes the article simply ground to a paste in a suitable mill. *Granulated* cocoa is prepared by reduction to a coarse powder and covering the particles with a layer of sugar and starch. *Soluble* cocoa contains sugar as a diluting substance. *Carageen Moss, Iceland Moss,* and *Lentils* are used as special agents for incorporation, and the cocoas bear the name of the agent prefixed. To produce the low-priced forms of cocoa, more or less of the husk is ground up with the kernel, and sundry cheap diluting articles are also used for admixture.

The preparations of cocoa in which sugar is employed as the diluting article require no preliminary boiling or cooking for use. The addition of boiling milk or water suffices. Those, however, in which some kind of starchy substance has been used for admixture need boiling to properly liquefy and bring them into a homogeneous state for drinking.

Chocolate constitutes a superior form of prepared cocoa. It is made upon an extensive scale in France, where its manufacture has attained a high state of perfection. Forming as it does an article of luxury, much care is bestowed on its preparation. The seeds, after being sifted and picked, are gently roasted till the desired aroma is developed. They are then allowed to cool, and afterward lightly crushed and winnowed to separate the husk from the kernel. Different sorts of cocoa seeds are mixed—the more aromatic, for instance, with the more oily—for the purpose of improving the product. The cocoa is next ground by suitable machinery to a perfectly even paste. The grinding is effected by revolving rollers over a heated iron plate, which maintains the fatty matter of the seed in a liquid state, and thus allows a thin paste to be formed. During the process of grinding, sugar is incorporated with the cocoa to the extent of from one-third to an equal part of its weight, and just before completion an aromatic, as vanilla, cinnamon, or whatever the taste may direct, is added to give the flavor required. The final process consists in running the liquid paste into moulds; and, as cooling takes place, it becomes solid and hard.

The *husks* rejected in the manufacture of chocolate and cocoa are frequently sold to the poor, who boil them in water and obtain a wholesome beverage therefrom.

Cocoa is characterized and distinguished from tea and coffee by the large amount of fatty and albuminous matters it contains, these principles averaging as much as about 50 and 20 per cent. respectively in the unmanufactured article.

The chief constituents of cocoa are:

First.—A volatile oil, to which it owes its aroma, and which is produced during the process of roasting. The amount of this oil is very small.

Second.—Theobromine. resembles theine and caffeine, but is not identical with them. It is found to contain a larger proportion of nitrogen. All analyses agree upon this point, although the results of different chemists are not strictly in accord in the proportion of nitrogen assigned to each. The following selected analysis may be given as an illustration of the relative ultimate composition:

	Theobromine. (Woskresensky.)	Theine. (Mulder.)
Carbon, ...	46.33	49.48
Hydrogen, ...	4.55	5.37
Nitrogen, ...	35.38	28.52
Oxygen, ...	13.74	16.63
	100.00	100.00

Although not identical with theine and caffeine, it has been found by Strecker that theobromine may be made to yield caffeine. Theobromine, in fact, conjoined with methyl, produces caffeine, so that caffeine has been regarded as a methylated theobromine. The quantity of theobromine present in cocoa amounts to about 2 per cent.

Third.—Fatty matter, known as cacao butter. This constitutes a firm fat, and, unlike most other fats, keeps without becoming rancid on exposure to air. It amounts to about half the weight of the cocoa.

Fourth.—Albuminous matter. About one-fifth part of cocoa is composed of this.

Fifth.—Starch.

The following, according to Payen's observations, represents the average composition of cocoa of good quality deprived of husk and not submitted to roasting:

Composition of Cocoa (Payen).

Cacao butter, ...	48 to 50
Albumen, fibrine, and other nitrogenous matter, .	21 to 20
Theobromine, ...	4 to 2
Starch, with traces of sugar, ...	11 to 10
Cellulose, ...	3 to 2
Coloring matter, aromatic essence, . . .	traces.
Mineral matter, ...	3 to 4
Water, ...	10 to 12
	100 100

Looked at dietetically, cocoa possesses, though in a milder degree, the properties of tea and coffee; but it stands apart from these articles in the high nutritive power which its composition gives it. Containing, as pure cocoa does, twice as much nitrogenous matter, and twenty-five times as much fatty matter as wheaten-flour, with a notable quantity of starch and an agreeable aroma to tempt the palate, it cannot be otherwise than a valuable alimentary material. It has been compared in this respect to milk. It conveniently furnishes a large amount of agreeable nourishment in a small bulk, and in South America cocoa and maize-cakes are used by travellers, and form a food several days' supply of which is easily carried.

Chocolate and the various preparations of cocoa are usually consumed with milk; and, taken with bread, will suffice, in the absence of any other kind of food, to furnish a good repast. A preparation of cocoa and condensed milk is made and sold in closed tins by the Condensed Milk Company. Thus preserved, the admixture is ready for use at any time, requiring only the addition of water.

Whilst possessing highly nutritive properties, its richness in fat renders cocoa heavy and oppressive to a delicate stomach. It is therefore apt to disagree with the invalid and dyspeptic.

The remarks that have been made regarding the nutritive capacity of chocolate and prepared cocoa do not apply to cocoa nibs in the manner they are used. In the former case the entire article is consumed; whereas in the latter only a decoction of the coarsely crushed seed is employed, and this contains but a portion only of its constituents. Indeed, the decoction of the nibs forms a beverage holding a closely analogous position to tea and coffee.

Fictitious cocoas.—In the United States the earth-nut, ground-nut, or pea-nut (*Arachis hypogæa*), a kind of oily, underground pea, is roasted and converted into a spurious form of cocoa, and also largely grown for the table and for the production of oil. In Spain, also, the root of the *Cyperus esculentus*, or earth chestnut, is roasted and used as a substitute both for coffee and chocolate. Neither of these products contain any theobromine.

Coca.—There is yet another article belonging to the group under consideration remaining to be spoken of, which must not be confounded on account of its approaching similarity of name with that which has just been described. The leaves of the *Erythroxylon Coca* are employed in South America for furnishing a beverage which is consumed in the same way as tea, coffee, and cocoa. In Bolivia and Peru they are used by the natives for chewing, and are said to produce powerful effects upon the system. In Europe they have been sometimes administered as a medicinal agent. They contain a nitrogenized crystallizable principle called *cocaine*, which closely agrees in its chemical relations, and is identical, it is asserted, in its physiological action, with theine, caffeine, guaranine, and theobromine. In the *British Medical Journal*, vol. i., p. 510, 1874, there is to be found a communication by Dr. Alexander Bennett upon the properties of this principle, and it has been made the subject of investigation (*vide British Medical Journal*, vol. ii., 1874) by the Committee of the British Medical Association for investigating the antagonism of medicines.

ALCOHOLIC BEVERAGES.

There are several beverages derived from various sources in use which contain alcohol. The starting-point of all is a vegetable product in which starch or sugar is present. Fermentation is either allowed to occur spontaneously, as in the case of wine; or else set up by the addition of a ferment, as in that of beer. In this artificial way only is it that alcohol is developed, and whilst the beverages containing it all agree in exerting the same kind of stimulating action on the system, they differ in their effects in other respects, according to the associated constituents that may happen to be present. Their chief properties are due to alcohol, but their other constituents must by no means be regarded as playing an unimportant part.

The position held by alcohol in an alimentary point of view has been discussed in a previous part of this work (*vide* p. 82 *et seq.*). It will be there seen that much divergence of opinion has prevailed upon the prime question, whether alcohol is to be regarded as possessing any alimentary value or not. It will suffice here to refer the reader to what has already been mentioned, and to state that the weight of evidence appears to be in favor of the affirmative. A small portion seems undoubtedly to escape from the body unconsumed, but the main part of the alcohol that may be ingested is lost sight of, and presumably from being turned to account in the system. In the next few pages the general effects of the alcoholic beverages will be spoken of, preparatory to attention being given to their separate consideration.

Apart from any effect due to oxidation or consumption within the system—apart, in other words, from any direct alimentary application—the liquids of the class under consideration exert a marked influence upon the functions of the body. Taken in moderate quantity they increase the activity of the circulation. The heart beats more rapidly. The pulse becomes not only more frequent, but at the same time fuller. The arteries dilating allow the blood to flow more freely to the capillaries, thus leading to turgescence of the small cutaneous vessels, and accounting for the flushing of the face that is noticeable. It has been affirmed that the temperature is lowered. Dr. Parkes, however, from his recent thermometric observations, remarks that there is but little change induced in the temperature of the axilla and rectum of healthy men, but that what change occurs is in the direction of increase. The warm blood from the interior circulating more freely over the surface, imparts a temporary glow to external parts, but the outside is warmed at the expense of the inside. The amount of urinary secretion is increased, the appetite augmented, digestion promoted, the nervous system stimulated, and the mental faculties exhilarated. In moderate quantities, in short, observation shows that the alcoholic beverages act as a general stimulant.

It has been asserted that alcohol diminishes tissue-metamorphosis, and economises the consumption of material in the body. Amongst his other inquiries, Dr. Parkes has given attention to this point of consideration, and failed to observe the production of any alteration of importance in the elimination of nitrogen—a phenomenon which may be taken as a measure, other circumstances being equal, of tissue-destruction. It appears unlikely, in the face of the chemical results, he remarks, " that it can enable the body to perform more work on less food, though, by quickening a failing heart, it may enable work to be done which otherwise could not be so. It may thus act like the spur in the side of a horse, eliciting force, though not supplying it." A discrepancy exists in the results of the experiments of different authorities upon the elimination of carbonic acid, and upon this point precise data obtained by the improved method of investigation adopted at the present day are wanted.

Dr. Parkes has submitted to direct investigation the question whether the effect of alcohol is to increase or diminish the facility with which work is performed. In one of his series of observations ("Proceedings of the Royal Society," vol. xx., p. 412, 1872), a soldier passed a period of three days performing a certain amount of work without the use of brandy; and, after three days of rest, another period of three days' work with twelve ounces of brandy *per diem*, administered in four-ounce doses, at 10 A.M., 2 P.M., and 6 P.M. This man was requested to observe as closely as he could whether he did the work better with or without the brandy. He commenced the brandy period, it is stated, with the belief that the brandy would enable him to perform the work more easily, but ended with the opposite conviction. The work performed was chiefly done in the two hours immediately succeeding each dose of brandy. The two hours' work after the first four fluid ounces appeared to be accomplished equally well with and without the brandy. The man, it is said, could tell no difference except, to use his own words, " the brandy seemed to give him a kind of spirit which made him think he could do a great deal of work, but when he came to do it he found he was less capable than he thought." After the second four ounces of brandy, at 2 P.M., he felt hot and thirsty, but on the first two days thought he worked as well as on the water days. On the third day, however, the report says that he had palpitation of the heart, and was surprised to find that he was obliged to stop from time to time because of his breathing not being so good. The third four fluid ounces of brandy, taken at 6 P.M., produced on all three days very marked narcotic effects. The account given is that "immediately after taking it he became heavy, felt the greatest indisposition to exert himself, and could hardly refrain from throwing down his spade and giving up his work. He worked with no vigor, and on the second evening thought his muscular power decidedly lessened. On the third evening it was raining; he could not dig, but took walking and running exercise under cover. On attempting to run, he found, to his great surprise, as he is a particularly fast and good runner, that he could not do so. He had palpitation, and got out of breath, and was obliged to stop."

The experience of this man harmonizes with the advice that is given by guides and others who are in the habit of undertaking the ascent of mountains. Spirits, they say, take away the strength from the legs, and should, therefore, be avoided during a fatiguing expedition.

Some further evidence has also recently been published by Dr. Parkes, upon the subject under consideration, drawn from the experience of the Ashanti campaign of 1874.* In the introduction to the report he says, "The first effect of alcohol, when given during a march in a moderate dose (for example what is equal to one fluid ounce of absolute alcohol) [the amount contained in about 2½ fluid ounces of ordinary spirits] is reviving, but this effect is transient. As shown both in the report and in the first appendix, the reviving effect goes off after, at the utmost, two

---

* Report on the Issue of a Spirit Ration during the Ashanti Campaign of 1874. Churchills, 1875.

and a half miles of additional march, and sometimes much before this ; then the previous languor and sense of exhaustion not only return, but are sometimes more intense; and if alcohol is again resorted to, its effects now are less satisfactory. Its reviving power is usually not so marked, and its peculiar anæsthetic and narcotizing influence can often be distinctly traced. The men feel heavy, dull, disinclined to march, and are less willing and cheerful."

Surgeon Kynsey, in relating his personal experience, said, "Some of the marches between the Prah and Coomassie were very long, and as we got far up the country and near the enemy, although the actual length of the march was short, still it extended over a great many hours. On a few of these occasions I was induced to try, from excessive fatigue, the effects of a little spirit, with the following result. At first the fatigue seemed to me to be less; I felt decidedly better. But as I marched on, and the effects of the spirit disappeared, I felt decidedly less able to march, and the sense of fatigue became much more intensified, so much so that I never took the smallest portion of spirit during a march but I regretted doing so."

Sergeant Perrin was of opinion that "if the rum [the form of spirit-ration issued] had been given on the march itself it would have done no good, only harm. His reason for saying so was that on two or three occasions on the march one of the doctors gave him a glass of grog; the effect was reviving for a quarter of an hour, and after that he felt a great deal more languid than he did before."

Whilst the general testimony resulted in condemnation of the employment of spirits as a restorative *during* the fatigue of marching, the evidence on the other hand went strongly to show that, issued after the day's fatigue was over, the spirit-ration exerted a beneficial reviving effect, and afterward induced an increased feeling of warmth accompanied by the promotion of sleep. Upon these points Corporal Hindley, who had been always a temperate man and never in the habit previously of taking spirits, expressed himself as follows:—"Had two rations of rum (a ration equal to 2¼ fluid ounces) on the way to the Prah, taken in the evening just before going to bed. Thought it useful; when there was no issue, felt chilly and cold at night; felt warmer when he had taken the rum, and slept better; had no doubt about feeling warmer and sleeping better.. On the next day felt no ill-effects from the rum."

The writings of Dr. Anstie and Dr. Parkes agree in assigning about 1 fluid ounce of absolute alcohol, which is equivalent to 2 to 2½ fluid ounces of ordinary spirits, as the limit of moderation for a dose, or the quantity that can be disposed of in the organism of an adult male without producing any perceptible injurious effect upon the bodily functions. Up to this quantity its action, as already described, is that of a stimulant; but beyond, it begins to exert a narcotizing influence, and, when taken to excess, a more or less profound state of narcotism, as common observation but too abundantly testifies, may be induced. The effects now witnessed upon the general system are no longer those of a stimulant, but exactly the reverse, and hence to describe its action in large doses it may be spoken of as a depressant and narcotic.

It has been stated that, when consumed in moderate quantity, the alcoholic beverages appear to encourage the appetite and promote digestion. Taken in excessive quantity, however, nothing with greater certainty destroys the appetite and impairs digestion.

Popular belief sanctions the practice which is adopted by many of swallowing a mouthful of brandy or some other neat spirit after partaking of an indigestible article of food. Now, alcohol consumed in this way, by stimulating the mucous membrane of the stomach, and exciting an increased flow of gastric secretion, is calculated in reality to afford assistance to digestion, in harmony with the traditional idea that is entertained and that experience may be assumed to have suggested. Should it be introduced, however, in larger quantity into the stomach, an opposite result is to be looked for. The alcohol now, by virtue of the amount present, will throw down the nitrogenous digestive principle—pepsine—in a solid form, and so destroy the energy of the solvent juice. Thus, whilst a small quantity, by its stimulant action, may assist digestion, a large quantity stops it, and accounts for the rejection of food in an undigested state that is frequently noticed to occur after the too free indulgence in alcoholic liquids at or after a meal.

The effects of strong alcoholic liquids taken repeatedly to a prejudicial extent are well known to the practical physician. By direct contact it acts upon the stomach, and leads to a destruction of its secreting tubules. Nothing with such certainty impairs the appetite and the digestive power as the continued use of strong alcoholic liquids. From the stomach the alcohol is absorbed, and with its distribution through the system it interferes with nutrition, and leads to a general textural deterioration. Upon certain organs, however, its effects are more manifest than upon others. The liver, kidneys, and nervous system, for instance, very strikingly suffer, a diseased state being set up, which forms a distinctly recognizable source of death. Nothing, indeed, as a rule, with greater certainty leads to premature death than alcoholic intemperance, and the managers of insurance offices are well acquainted with this fact.

It has been mentioned that one of the immediate effects of the ingestion of alcohol is turgescence of the small cutaneous vessels of the face, producing the flushed appearance that is noticeable. A frequent repetition of this condition leads ultimately to its permanent establishment, and thus accounts for the well-known visage acquired by the Bacchanalian.

I have been hitherto referring to the action of alcohol *per se*, and in *spirits* we have little or nothing, it may be considered, besides this action to deal with, except, perhaps, in the case of hollands and gin, which possess diuretic properties, due to the flavoring agent (juniper) added. In the primary fermented liquids, however, there are associated ingredients which give rise to the production of modified and additional effects upon the system. The beverages, for instance, which are rich in saccharine and extractive matters, as particularly stout, porter, and the heavier ales, possess a nourishing and fattening power which does not belong to a simple alcoholic liquid. Such beverages also are apt to occasion headache and gastric derangement, or what falls under the denomination of biliousness, in those who lead a sedentary mode of life, whilst a lighter and purer alcoholic drink may be found to agree. Again, gout appears to be the offspring, not of a simple alcoholic liquid, but of alcohol in combination with saccharine and extractive matter; for observation shows that it is not the spirit, but the beer and port wine drinker that is especially liable to become the subject of the disease. As alcohol alone is not the source of gout, neither, it may be said, are the saccharine and extractive matters without the alcohol. It seems as though these solid, imperfectly fermented matters underwent, under the influence of the presence of alcohol, a defective assimilation in the system, and so gave rise to the development of the morbid products, which form the source of the chief manifestations of the disease.

BEER.—Beer consists of a fermented infusion of malt flavored with hops, and is a beverage of great antiquity. Barley is moistened with water, and allowed to germinate to a certain extent. It is then placed upon a kiln, where it is exposed to heat and dried, and the amount of heat employed determines the kind of malt produced. Pale malt, which is used for brewing ale, is dried at a temperature below 140°. Porter and stout derive their color from malt that has been dried at a higher temperature; and malt, called high dried, patent, or black malt, is specially made for employment as a coloring agent by roasting the grain in cylinders, in the same manner as coffee.

The object of malting is the conversion of the starch of the grain into dextrine and sugar. This in part occurs during the process of germination, the change being effected by the action of a nitrogenous principle of the nature of a ferment, which is known as diastase, and which is developed during germination. Kiln-dried malt, however, yields a larger amount of saccharine extract than that which has been allowed to dry spontaneously in the air; hence the conversion is still carried on during the exposure to heat in the kiln. Still unchanged starch remains, but the requisite conditions are present for the completion of the change during the preliminary part of the brewing process.

Brewing consists of three operations. In the first place, an infusion of the malt is obtained. This is then boiled with hops, and the product is afterward made to undergo fermentation.

The malt after being crushed, is placed in the *mash tun*, and water at a temperature of about 160° Fahr. is poured upon it. The two are well stirred together, and subsequently left covered over for a few hours. This operation is called *mashing*, and the liquid which results from it, *sweet wort*. The water takes up the saccharine matter contained in the malt, and, under the influence of the heat and moisture, the diastase acts upon the unchanged starch existing, and completes its conversion into sugar. Indeed, the diastase present is capable of effecting the transformation of a much larger amount of starch into sugar than that which the malt itself contains; and hence a certain quantity of unmalted barley or other grain can be utilized in making a "wort" for fermentation. The excise regulations of England do not permit the use of unmalted grain for brewing, but by distillers it is largely employed. In Belgium, potato starch, it seems, is somewhat extensively used in brewing, upon the principle explained, in the place of grain. The saccharine quality of the wort may be also increased by the addition of sugar itself, and a prepared sugar (probably grape-sugar) is sold to brewers for this purpose, and is considered by them to give improvement to the beer.

The wort, which has a marked sweet taste, is next transferred to a copper, and boiled with the appropriate quantity, according to the kind of beer intended to be produced, of hops. By this, the liquid acquires the aromatic bitterness belonging to beer, and the effect of the hops seems further to exert a preservative influence over the product. The liquid is now drawn off and strained from the hops, and placed in shallow *coolers* for the temperature to be lowered as quickly as possible. Refrigeration is also sometimes further aided by special measures for the purpose. When sufficiently cooled, the concluding process is performed, which consists of adding yeast, and allowing fermentation to occur. The addition

16

of yeast is not indispensable, for fermentation, it is found, will occur without it, but a considerably longer time is required. On this account it is usual to start the fermentation with yeast, and by the end of a few hours signs of the commencement of the process are visible, and within three or four days' time it is over. In the absence of yeast it requires a day or two for fermentation to commence, and a fortnight or three weeks to be completed, but the resulting beer is said to have a more vinous flavor than ordinarily brewed beer, and to keep longer without becoming sour.

By the process of fermentation the sugar of the wort is converted into alcohol and carbonic acid—the latter escaping, and the former giving to the beer its intoxicating property. When the process is over, the fermented liquid is either allowed to clarify spontaneously, or the suspended matter is carried down by the use of *finings*. It is lastly stored and allowed to ripen.

Scrupulous attention requires to be paid to all the minor points connected with the art of brewing. The quality of the beer and its power of keeping not only depend on the amount and quality of the materials used, but equally as much on the skill and care with which the several steps of the operation of brewing are carried out. The composition of the water used exerts a more or less marked influence on the product. The spring water of Burton-on-Trent is well known to stand in high repute for the pale and bitter ales which are now so largely consumed, and it is supposed that the sulphate of lime contained in it aids in clarifying and producing a bright and clear liquid.

Several varieties of beer are prepared. The term *ale* is applied to that which is made from pale malt. Vastly different qualities are sold, depending upon the amount of malt and hops employed: the former giving strength in alcohol, the latter in bitterness. Formerly the strong alcoholic ales were chiefly in request, but latterly the popular taste has changed, and it is now a light, bitter ale which is held in the highest esteem. This was first especially prepared for the Indian market, and hence the name of *Indian pale ale*, by which it is known in addition to that of *bitter ale*. Great care and attention require to be bestowed on the manufacture of this beverage, and on account of its clearness and brightness, and its delicate color and taste, the best materials only can be employed. Its richness in the aromatic-bitter principle of the hop gives it its predominant character, but at the same time, whilst containing a moderate amount of alcohol, the quantity of extractive matter is low, and fermentation has been carried to an extent to render it comparatively free from sugar. *Porter* is prepared from and is dependent for its strength on pale malt, but high dried malt is added to communicate color and flavor. It is looked upon as more easy of digestion and assimilation than ale of a corresponding quality. *Stout* constitutes a beverage of the same nature as porter. Its chief characteristic is the large proportion of extractive matter that is present. What is called *London Cooper* is generally understood to represent a mixture of stout and porter, but a distinct beer, occupying an intermediate position between the two, is also brewed and sold under this denomination.

Beer contains the following ingredients: water, alcohol, sugar, dextrine and other allied substances, nitrogenous matter, traces of fatty matter, aromatic, bitter, and coloring principles, saline matter, variable quantities of carbonic and acetic acids.

The alcohol, sugar and its allies, and the bitter principle, form the constituents which give to beer its characteristic properties.

The alcohol varies in different kinds of beer from 1 or 2 to about 9 or

10 per cent. by volume. The following is the proportion according to the analysis of Brande, the amount referring to alcohol of the sp. gr. 0.825 at 60° Fahr., which consists of 89 per cent. of absolute alcohol and 11 per cent. of water:

	Alcohol, sp. gr. 0.825, per cent., by measure.
Burton ale, ...	8.88
Edinburgh ale, ...	6.22
London ale (average), ...	6.20
Brown stout, ...	6.80
London porter (average), ...	4.20
London small beer (average,, ...	1.28

Adopting mean numbers, a pint (20 ounces) of beer will contain about one ounce of alcohol (Parkes).

The amount of solid extractive matter derived from the malt (chiefly sugar and other carbohydrates) varies from about 4 to 15 per cent. It is lowest in the bitter and highest in the strong and sweet ales and stout. Subjoined are the results of special analyses of certain beers for malt extract and alcohol:

	Malt extract, per cent.	Alcohol, per cent.	Analyzed by
Barclay & Perkins' London porter, .	6.0	5.4	Kaiser.
London porter, ...	6.8	6.9	Balling.
Burton ale, ...	14.5	5.9	Hoffmann.
Scotch ale (Edinburgh), . . .	10.9	8.5	Kaiser.

An imperial pint of good porter yields in general about an ounce and a half of extract (Brande).

Beer is a refreshing, exhilarating, nutritive, and, when taken to excess, an intoxicating beverage. Its nutritive properties are due to the extractive matter, consisting principally of carbohydrates, which it contains, and observation sufficiently testifies that beer which is highly charged with extract exerts a decidedly fattening influence. Its bitter principle renders it a stomachic and tonic. A light beer well flavored with the hop is calculated to promote digestion, and may be looked upon as constituting one of the most wholesome of the alcoholic class of beverages. It is not all, however, who can drink beer without experiencing inconvenience. In the case of persons of a bilious temperament, also with dyspeptics, and sometimes others, it is apt to excite headache, heaviness, and other sensations which fall under the popular designation of "biliousness." The stronger beers, taken continuously in excess, induce a full and plethoric state, and are liable, particularly if conjoined with sedentary habits, to result in the accumulation of defectively oxidized products, as uric acid, etc., in the system, and so lead to the developement of gout.

CIDER, PERRY.—These form fermented beverages, derived respectively from the juice of the apple and the pear. Fruit that is not fit for eating, on account of its acid, bitter, or rough taste, may be made use of for their manufacture. The fruit is crushed to a pulp, and this is subjected to pressure for the extraction of the juice. The amount of juice yielded nearly equals half the weight of the pulp employed. The juice contains the elements required for starting fermentation, and on exposure to air at the appropriate temperature the formation of alcohol takes place,

a froth collecting on the surface and a sediment subsiding. This constitutes the most delicate part of the operation, and upon the manner in
which it is conducted depends, in a great measure, the quality of the product. If allowed to proceed too far, the process passes into the acetous
fermentation, and the liquid becomes sour and thin, and if not far enough
the product is thick and unpalatable. The fermentation, by rights, should
lead to a spontaneous clarification. When a pale product is required the
pulp is submitted to pressure immediately after crushing. If the pulp be
left for some hours it undergoes a change, which leads to a coloration of
the juice. The fruit should be taken at its maximum richness in saccharine matter, and for this it should be gathered when ripe, and afterward
stored away for a month or six weeks, to allow it to mature.

Cider and perry are closely analogous liquids, but have a different
flavor. The following represents the percentage of spirit in the samples
that were examined by Brande:

	Alcohol, sp. gr. 0.825 at 60° F., per cent., by measure.
Cider, highest average, ...	9.87
Ditto, lowest do., ...	5.21
Perry, average of four samples, ...	7.26

In some localities cider and perry are consumed as the common drink,
taking the place of beer elsewhere. They constitute agreeable, wholesome, and refreshing stimulating beverages when in a perfectly sound
condition. Their proneness, however, to undergo the acetous fermentation renders it necessary that they should be drunk with caution, for in a
sour state they are apt to occasion colic and diarrhœa with those who are
not in the habit of constantly taking them.

WINE.—The term wine, when employed alone, is understood to signify the fermented juice of the grape. The word, however, is also used
in a more comprehensive way, being applied to the fermented liquids obtained from fruits generally, and likewise other vegetable products. But,
thus employed, a prefix is attached expressive of the source of the article,
as, for instance, with *orange* wine, *rhubarb* wine, *ginger* wine, *parsnip*
wine, *honey* wine, etc. It is only to the fermented juice of the grape
that the succeeding remarks are intended to refer.

Wine constitutes a beverage that appears to have been known from
the earliest periods of history. Until toward the close of the seventeenth
century the greater portion of the wine consumed in England was derived
from France. In consequence of the hostilities that then broke out between the two countries, a duty was for a time imposed on French wines
of so heavy a nature as to be almost prohibitory to their introduction.
Political influences were now also directed toward encouraging the importation and consumption of port, and soon the wines of Portugal assumed
the place that had been previously occupied by those of France. As
regards sherry, this is shown to have been well known in England in the
seventeenth century, by a work, published in 1619, entitled "Pasquil's
Palinodia, and his Progresse to the Taverne, where, after the survey of
the sellar, you are presented with a pleasant pynte of Poeticall Sherry."
The author extols sherry, against which "no fiery red-faced claret," he
says, can stand. Much of the "sack" formerly in use appears to have
been sherry, and this is corroborated by the following quaint lines taken

from the above-mentioned work, which contain also an allusion to several other drinks:

> "Strong hoop'd in bonds are here constrain'd to tarry,
> Two kinsmen neere allyde to sherry sack,
> Sweet Malligo, and delicate canary,
> Which warme the stomacks that digestion lacke."

> "The broth with barley sodden,
> Compares not with this licker,
> The drayman's beere is not so cleere,
> And foggy ale is thicker:
> Metheglin is too fulsome,
> Cold cyder and raw perry,
> And all drinks stand with cap in hand,
> In presence of old sherry.
> Then let us drinke old sacke, old sacke, boyes,
> Which makes us blythe and merry."

The import duties have always largely influenced the consumption of wines, and previous to 1861 no distinction was made between the light wines of France and Germany and the strong wines of Spain and Portugal. This necessarily told seriously in a commercial point of view against the former on account of the difference in character belonging to the two classes of wines; for not only do the stronger go farther, but a bottle when opened may be kept and gradually drunk instead of spoiling unless immediately consumed. In consequence of the altered tariff introduced by Mr. Gladstone, the year 1861 will in all probability be hereafter looked upon as forming an important era in the history of wine consumption in England. Great changes have even already been produced by the more equitable adjustment of the import duty which admits light wines at a lower rate than the strong. All wines containing less than 26 per cent. of proof spirit (and this will include all *natural* wines—that is to say, wines which constitute simply the fermented juice of the grape, without any addition of spirit) are now admitted at 1s. per gallon; while if containing above 26 per cent. the wine is regarded as belonging to the class of brandied or *fortified* wines, and is charged with the higher duty of 2s. 6d. per gallon, the maximum strength allowed being 42 per cent. of proof spirit—a strength which may be looked upon as fairly including all beverages that can justly lay claim to the title of wine. Liquids containing over the 42 per cent. are regarded as falling within the category of spirits, and are thereupon taxed at a much higher rate.

On account of the free trade which has thus been opened out by the present arrangements of the duties on wines, a large number of formerly unknown varieties of natural wines now find their way, to the advantage it may be considered of the public, from different countries into England, and afford an extensive choice even to the consumer of moderate means. Although falling under one generic name, these products of different countries present wide differences in their general characters and properties. Now, constituting as it does an article which is capable of affording valuable therapeutic aid, and called upon as the medical practitioner so frequently is to advise which kind of wine is the most suitable for his patient, it becomes necessary that he should possess, as a part of his professional knowledge, information that will enable him to give a judicious recommendation—indeed, it is scarcely too much to say that for those who practice amongst the well-to-do classes, an acquaintance with the distinctive virtues of the various wines to be met with around us is as essential to his success as a knowledge of the properties of the several drugs. The subject is 'an extensive one, but I will endeavor to treat it in as concise a manner as is consistent with due regard to the claims of explicitness.

Our starting-point is the grape. A few words are, therefore, necessary upon the nature of this fruit. It is a succulent berry, provided with a thin but tough enveloping structure or skin, which fulfils the office of confining the central juicy substance and preserving it from contact with the air.

The skins of some grapes are colorless or yellow, whilst others are impregnated with a deep blue coloring matter, from which the color of red wine is derived, for this, like other vegetable blues, becomes reddened in the presence of an acid. Chemistry shows that in both varieties of grape the skins contain a considerable amount of astringent matter under the form of tannic acid, and likewise a certain quantity of a waxy material which may be looked upon as evidently designed by its intercepting action on the passage of water to protect the fruit from the influence of wet on the outside and impede the escape of moisture from within.

The pulp or central fleshy part of the grape constitutes an organized structure comprising a mass of delicate vesicles holding the juice of the fruit. Thus, instead of being loose and free to run out when the berry is cut in half, the juice is retained in receptacles which require to be broken up before it is in a position to escape. It is this which necessitates the process of crushing, either by treading or the agency of machinery, which is had recourse to for procuring the juice as the first step in the manufacture of wine.

Except in a particular variety, named the *tintilla* or *teinturier* grape, the fleshy part of the fruit is devoid of color, or only possesses a faint yellowish or pinkish tint, although the skin may be deeply colored. The fresh juice, therefore, of the red and black presents the same appearance as that of the white grape. The coloring matter of the husk, indeed, as it exists in the fruit, is in a fixed or insoluble state, and it is only after the juice has fermented that it possesses the power of dissolving it out so as to lead to its presence in wine. In the above-named exceptional variety, however, the berry is pervaded throughout with coloring matter in a dissolved state, and thus the juice is dyed with it like that of the elderberry and black currant. The vine in question is specially cultivated, it is said, in some localities to be employed for increasing the color of wines obtained from other grapes.

Imbedded in the substance of the pulp are the little hard masses constituting the seeds, and known as the pips or stones. These, unlike the pulp, but like the husk, are rich in astringent matter, which gives rise to the rough taste that is perceived when they are crunched between the teeth. Chemistry shows that they also contain a certain amount of fatty matter.

As the grape-stalks are frequently placed in the fermenting vat together with the fruit, it may be mentioned that these, like the husks and stones, contain tannic acid, and thus help to give astringency to a wine into the preparation of which they have been allowed to enter.

Such is the constitution of the fruit which forms the basis of the variety of products comprehended under the term wine. Now, of the variation existing in the article under consideration, a part is dependent, it is true, upon the process of manufacture, but a part also is attributable to the characters of the grape employed. It is not difficult to realize that the differences existing in the qualities of the fruit should exert their influence upon the article obtained from it. The variety of vine, the soil upon which it is grown, the particular surroundings of the locality, the general climate of the place, the climate peculiar to the year, and the degree of ripeness of the fruit, all produce their modifying influence and tell upon the character of the wine. Ordinarily the juice of the grape is devoid of any decided fragrance, and the aroma of the wine is developed during fermentation and from the changes occurring as time advances after bottling; but in some instances — and the muscat grape affords a noticeable example — the fruit possesses a pronounced aroma which is communicated to the wine obtained from it.

The constituents of the grape which produce the most prominent influence upon the character of a wine are the acids and sugar, and these vary in amount to a very marked extent under different circumstances.

As already mentioned, tannic acid is encountered in the husks, pips, and stalks. This gives the quality of roughness or astringency to a wine. It does not exist in the juice. The acids met with here are malic and tartaric, the former preponderating in proportion in the unripe, the latter in the ripe fruit. As the fruit advances to maturity the amount of acid originally present undergoes diminution, and notably of the two acids, the malic. This ensues (in common with what occurs during the ripening of fruit in general) as a result of the influence of the light and heat of the sun. With this diminution of acidity an increase takes place in the amount of sugar; and thus, as sour fruit becomes sweet, its acquired absence of sourness must not be entirely attributed to loss of acids, for the increase in the amount of sugar will have the effect, according to its extent, of covering or concealing the taste of acidity.

The amount of free acid present in the juice of grapes produced by different countries, and in different seasons, varies from about 0.3 to 1.5 per cent., reckoned under the form of tartaric acid. For the production of good wine it is said that the proportion should not exceed about 0.5 per cent. From what has been stated, it will readily be understood that it is especially in the more northern wine-producing localities, as, for instance, the Rhine and Moselle districts, that the disadvantage arising from an excess of acidity is most experienced. A great deal of uncertainty, dependent upon the character of the season, is here found to exist. It is only in good years, indeed, that the grapes sufficiently ripen to give rise to a thoroughly satisfactory product, and in bad years they may remain too sour in some places to yield an acceptable wine. The proportionate amount of acid is sometimes artificially diminished by diluting the juice and adding sugar. Thus, a larger yield of less acid wine is afforded, but at the expense of quality in other respects, as the general constituents of the juice are thereby thrown out of their proper relation.

Of all the constituent elements of the grape, the sugar must be looked upon as holding the position of first importance, because it is the basis of fermentation, and without it there could be no production of wine. Chemists enumerate several varieties of sugar, and recognize differences in their chemical and physical properties, and also to some extent in their composition. The kind of sugar met with in the grape is named after the fruit itself, and also called glucose. This, however, admits of further differentiation, and, instead of one absolutely identical form of sugar being present, two modifications are found to exist. The one is susceptible of crystallization, and crystallizes, indeed, into the little, hard, granular masses that are to be met with in raisins which have been kept for some time.

It also has a right-handed rotatory influence over polarized light, and for this reason has received the name of dextrose. The other is non-crystallizable, and from possessing the power of turning the ray of polarized light to the left has been styled lævulose. Both of these forms of sugar constitute well-known modifications obtainable from a variety of other sources beside the grape. They are both susceptible of undergoing fermentation, and otherwise, indeed, agree in manifesting the same chemical behavior.

The amount of sugar present in grape-juice is subject to very extensive variation. It may range, it is said, between about 10 and 30 per cent. As with the acids, but in an inverse manner, the quantity is significantly influenced by climate and season. Whilst under the power exerted by the rays of the sun the sourness of fruit disappears, the quality of sweetness becomes developed, and in proportion to the heat of the climate and season so is the degree of sweetness attained. Hence, it is to the grape grown in hot countries, as Spain, Portugal, Madeira, Italy, Cyprus, etc., that we must look for the largest amount of sugar. The effect of different summers is most conspicuous in cooler climates, and, as will readily be understood, it is especially toward the fall, or when the grape is ripening, that the character of the season produces the greatest influence on the amount of saccharine matter. Upon the full ripening of the grape will depend the quality of the wine, but quality and quantity, it may be remarked, by no means necessarily go together, for in some years the yield may be large and the quality bad, whilst in others the reverse may hold good. For the production of good wine the grape-juice, it is stated, must contain not less than about 20 per cent. of sugar.

A warm and, it may further be said, a dry summer is propitious, then, for wine-production; and to obtain wine that best combines body, freedom from undue acidity, and a rich, vinous flavor, we must look to those countries where the grape acquires the fullest ripeness, and contains a maximum of sugar and minimum of acid and watery element. In some districts, indeed, for the production of the choicest wines, as for instance the Château d'Yquem in the Sauterne district, the bunches are left on the vines and the berries gathered separately as they successively attain the fullest ripeness. Tokay, which is renowned for its luscious and full vinous character, is even prepared from grapes that have been allowed to remain on the vine till the early frosts have set in, and till they have undergone a certain amount of desiccation, by which the juice has acquired a higher concentration. It is only in the case of white wines, however, that this fullest ripeness or over-ripeness is allowed to be attained. In the case of the red wines it is necessary for the sake of color that the grapes should be gathered earlier; for, as will be seen further on, the solution of the coloring matter of the husk is effected by the free acid of the juice in combination with the alcohol developed during fermentation, and the less the quantity of acid the less the amount of coloring principle taken up.

It has been stated that sugar is a necessary constituent of grape-juice in relation to wine-production, because it forms the fermenting principle. There is yet another essential ingredient, viz., the ferment, or principle to excite fermentation. This consists of nitrogenous matter under the form of albumen, and is usually deposited as lees during the process of fermentation. Properly fermented wine retains but little nitrogenous matter. Imperfectly fermented wine retains more, and thus becomes liable to spoil from the tendency to further change which its presence gives rise to.

The astringent matter, however, which is present in red wines exerts a certain amount of counteracting influence by its preservative and precipitating effects.

The first step in the manufacture of wine after the grapes have been gathered, is to crush them, in order that the juice may be liberated from its containing vesicles. The process was formerly accomplished by the operation of treading, but is now chiefly effected by the aid of rollers. Care is taken to avoid crushing the pips and stalks, as too much astringent matter, etc., would otherwise become taken up. So long as the juice is contained within the grape, and is thus protected from contact with the air, it is not observed to undergo fermentation. With the expressed juice, on the other hand, and to this the term "*must*" is applied, fermentation soon sets in under exposure to an appropriate temperature. No ferment is required to be added; the nitrogenous matter present supplies what is wanted for starting the change as soon as it is brought into contact with the atmosphere. It is evidently the exclusion of air by the skin which prevents fermentation from occurring whilst the juice is contained within the fruit.

The process of crushing having been accomplished, the juice is either at once expressed and fermented alone, or else the whole is fermented together for a while, and then expression performed. In the former case, whether black or white grapes are used, a non-colored and non-astringent product is the result; in the latter, astringent matter is taken up from the skins and stones, and from the stalks also when these are allowed to be present. Coloring matter likewise is dissolved out, so as to produce a dark-colored wine, when colored grapes have been employed. The color of the liquid becomes gradually deeper as fermentation proceeds, in consequence of the exercise of the solvent power which is enjoyed by the newly developed alcohol in combination with the pre-existing acid. The watery juice of the grape simply impregnated with its acid fails to touch the coloring matter. Directly alcohol, however, is present, it becomes taken up, and with it also astringent matter is dissolved; for the two so far comport themselves alike in this respect and accompany each other, that the rule may be laid down, the deeper the color the rougher the flavor of a wine. When contact with the skins has been sufficiently prolonged for the desired color and astringency to be communicated, the fermented liquor is separated from the "*mark*" by expression. The "*mark*," or expressed residue, still contains a quantity of coloring matter and other vinous substances, and sometimes a spurious wine is made from it by mixing it with a solution of sugar and allowing fermentation to occur.

The fermenting stage varies in duration according to the prevailing temperature. In warm localities it may be over in two or three days, whilst in cooler districts it may last considerably longer. As it commences, the "must" becomes more turbid than it was originally, and appears to be in motion from the ascent, in little bubbles, of the carbonic acid gas which is generated. The temperature of the liquid increases, and a froth collects on the surface, due to the escaping gas. After the process has acquired its maximum activity, and has begun to quiet down, the contents of the fermenting vat require to be stirred up, so that all the elements may be brought into fresh contact. Happily for our personal satisfaction, this is now, certainly in all large establishments, effected by mechanical means, but formerly the revolting practice prevailed of men in a naked state entering the vats for the purpose, and it was thought that the temperature of the body was useful in promoting fermentation. It is stated that several men thus employed have in the course of time been killed by the carbonic acid gas accumulated above the surface of the fermenting liquid.

The character of a wine is materially influenced by the temperature at which fermentation takes place, and this happens to be allowed to remain dependent on that which chances to belong to the locality and season; hence, partly, the source of the variation noticeable in the wines of different countries and years.

By active fermentation, for instance, at a high temperature, a disappearance of sugar occurs before time has been permitted for the development of bouquet and flavor. The vinous elements become exhausted or destroyed, and the resulting wine is thin and poor, and, after quickly maturing, shows signs of possessing defective lasting power. This defective lasting power is advanced as a justification for the custom that has arisen of "fortifying," or adding spirit to the wine produced from hot countries, as Spain, Portugal, Madeira, and the Cape. It is well known that the wines which we receive from these countries are in a "fortified" state, whilst those derived from cooler countries, as France, Germany, etc., contain no added spirit, and thereby constitute "natural" wines. In the former, after the fermentation has advanced to a certain point, the spirit is added to check its further progress before the saccharine matter is wholly exhausted. Through the saccharine and extractive matters thus left, the wine possesses a body and fruitiness which would have been lost had fermentation been allowed to continue undisturbed; and out of such body and fruitiness are generated those choice vinous qualities which become slowly developed as the liquid matures.

In France, Germany, Hungary, etc., where a cooler climate prevails, fermentation occurs with less rapidity, and is allowed to proceed until it comes to a spontaneous termination. Here, then, the transformation of saccharine matter is permitted to go on until it is quite or nearly lost, and, in consequence, there is produced a drier or less fruity wine, and one which takes less time to mature. With wines of this class also, a stronger bouquet or aroma is developed, either as a result simply of the slower fermentation or of the more acid quality of the grape, for the free acid is concerned in combination with the alcohol in the formation of the ethereal products which contribute to furnish the aroma. The Rhine and Moselle districts, which are amongst the most northern of wine-producing localities, yield wines that are particularly characterized by the amount of aroma they possess, and it is here, as previously stated, that the grape contains the largest proportion of acid.

Notwithstanding fermentation may have advanced to a complete exhaustion of the saccharine matter, the amount of alcohol produced does not nearly equal that found in the "fortified" wines. It suffices for preserving the wine whilst in closed casks and bottles, but not for giving it the power enjoyed by the other variety of keeping when opened and brought into contact with the air. Should it happen, further, through lowness of temperature or otherwise, that fermentation has not proceeded with sufficient activity or to a proper extent, a wine devoid even of lasting properties in cask and bottle will be produced, on account of the incomplete exhaustion and precipitation of the ferment.

Looking at the influence that is evidently exerted by the temperature at which the process of fermentation is carried on, it is somewhat surprising that means have not been yet devised and had recourse to for securing a fixed condition, and thus rendering the operation independent of the local circumstances that may happen to prevail.

As time proceeds, and fermentation diminishes in activity, the liquid begins to grow clearer by throwing down a sediment called "*lees.*" This consists of exhausted ferment, with other organic substances and cream of tartar. The latter is deposited on account of its sparing solubility in spirit, and is therefore proportionate to the amount of alcohol developed. The wine is now racked off from the "*lees*" into casks, to prevent the acetous fermentation setting in. Here vinous fermentation still continues slowly, and more sediment of the same nature as before subsides, the cream of tartar belonging to it being thrown in a crystalline form, and constituting what is known as "argol." Again the wine is racked and transferred to other casks; and the process is repeated, it may be, two or three times more. Much depends upon the care and attention bestowed upon these rackings of the wine performed during the first year; and another point that equally requires to be looked after is filling up the casks as occasion requires, to compensate for the loss occurring from soakage and evaporation, and prevent an empty space existing. The wine, during this storage, is undergoing changes which result in the ultimate development of its special flavor, bouquet, and other vinous properties, as the stage of maturation advances.

The empty casks which receive the wine in the process of racking are usually fumigated prior to use by burning some sulphur (a brimstone-match is sometimes used) within them, with the view of exerting a preservative effect.

One more step remains to be described. Wine is usually subjected to the finishing operation of "*fining.*" This is effected by the addition of an agent like the white of egg or isinglass, which, undergoing precipitation by the action of the wine, leads to the suspended impurities being entangled and carried down. By being thus clarified, wine is not only from its clearness and brightness rendered more pleasing to the eye, but, through the separation of the floating organic matter, acquires increased keeping power.

It appears to be the prevailing custom in Spain, Portugal, and the south of France to dust the grapes over previous to being crushed with plaster-of-Paris, which consists of burnt gypsum or sulphate of lime. Sometimes the plaster is added to the must instead. The object of this practice, which is styled "plastering," is not intelligible, but it has the effect of leading to an alteration of the saline constitution of the wine, which certainly there is no ground for regarding as beneficial. Chalk or carbonate of lime would have the effect of neutralizing or removing acidity, but not so the sulphate of lime. This substance leads to the removal, by precipitation in combination with lime, of the greater part of the tartaric acid, but it gives in its place an equivalent amount of sulphuric acid, which, combining with potash, furnishes the sulphate of potash in substitution for the natural cream of tartar of the wine. A "plastered" wine thus contains more sulphuric acid than is naturally yielded by the grape, and through this it may be recognized by the analyst. Dr. Hassall's analyses corroborate the statement made by Dr. Thudichum, that all the sherries imported into England are "plastered." Marsala and Madeira have been found by Dr. Hassall to be in a corresponding state to sherry.

In the case of champagne and other sparkling wines, a supplemental operation has to be performed to give them their effervescent character.

After having been fermented in the usual way, the wine is allowed to remain till the following spring to become bright and clear. It is then bottled and dosed with a concentrated solution of sugar. This leads to a second fermentation occurring within the bottles, and from the carbonic acid gas this time being prevented from escaping, the special quality belonging to the wine is acquired. During the process the wine throws down a further sediment, which is collected at the neck of the bottle, the bottles being inverted for the purpose. By an operation which is called " disgorging," the sediment is permitted to be blown off, and the bottles finally are securely corked and wired. After the lapse of a little time the wine becomes ready for use. For the better classes of champagne the dosing is made not simply with a solution of sugar, but with what is styled "liqueur." This consists of a specially fine-flavored wine mixed with sugar, and generally also brandy. The champagnes for different countries are dosed in such a manner as to produce the kind of wine, as to sweetness or dryness, suited to the market.

We have now reached the point for the consideration of wine itself. It has been seen that fermentation constitutes the essential part of the process attending its production, and the two constituents of the grape-juice which are directly concerned in the occurrence of this phenomenon are sugar and albuminoid matter—or the fermentescible body and the ferment. The main and indispensable change, then, connected with the conversion of grape-juice into wine, is the disappearance of sugar and its replacement by alcohol. There are many minor changes secondarily induced by or consequent upon the phenomenon of fermentation, and although these may only occur to an insignificant extent, yet their influence is great upon the character of the wine.

Under a chemical point of view, wine is a complex product containing components which are in part derived directly from the grape; in part owe their source to fermentation; and in part spring from the changes which occur during the process of maturation. A knowledge of its chemical composition may be spoken of as affording useful information regarding its general characters, besides revealing the existence of sophistication. At the same time, however, too much stress must not be laid on the results furnished by chemical analysis. It is true that the more prominent qualities are dependent upon the extent to which the leading constituents exist, and this information chemistry can supply, but there may be differences in the character of wines of the utmost importance in relation to marketable value, and no clue to them shall be afforded by the figures of the analyst. The palate and the stomach form the true guide for settling whether a wine is choice and good. "The stomach," says Dr. Druitt, "is the real test-tube for wines, and if that quarrels with it, no chemical certificate or analysis is worth a rush."

It would be out of place to enter minutely into the chemistry of wine, but something requires to be said upon the subject, and its leading constituents will be examined in the following order: Alcohol, sugar, astringent matter, coloring matter, extractive matter, acids, ethers, and volatile oil.

Although chemistry displays the existence of the above-enumerated principles in wine, yet in its action upon the system it may be considered that we have not to deal with the separate and independent effects of these principles, but with those of a liquid in which the ingredients are so amalgamated, incorporated, or blended together, as to produce a homogeneous whole. For example, if we look to alcohol, which constitutes its most influential component, the effects of a certain amount of this principle, as it is contained in wine, are not identical with those of the same amount diluted to an equal extent with water. The alcohol appears to become blended with the other ingredients, and in this state to exert a somewhat modified action upon the system. One of the advantages, and perhaps the chief, which wine derives from keeping, is probably attributable to this blending of its constituents. It is well known to acquire a uniformity of flavor by age, which stands in contrast to the crudeness and the mixed tastes belonging to it in a new state. Even made-up wine may, in the course of time, lose much of its objectionable nature, and become passable by acquiring an amalgamated condition.

Alcohol.—This forms the most potent ingredient of wine, being that which gives to it its intoxicating properties. Besides holding the position named, it must also be looked upon as playing an important part in relation to the article itself, on account of the preservative influence it exerts.

The special object attained by fermentation is the production of this principle, and unless extraneously added during the preparation of the wine, its amount is dependent on that of the sugar primarily contained in the fermenting liquid. One atom of grape-sugar becomes resolved into two atoms of alcohol and two of carbonic acid (new notation). This, looking at the formulæ of the bodies, is equivalent to saying that from 180 parts, by weight, of dry grape-sugar, 92 parts of alcohol are produced—in other words, every two parts of sugar yield about one of alcohol.

With this information it is easy to determine what should constitute the range of alcoholic strength of a natural wine. For example, reckoning that grape-juice contains, in accordance with what has been previously mentioned, from 10 to 30 per cent. of sugar; that all the sugar undergoes fermentation; and that none of the alcohol is lost, an alcoholic strength will be given of from (about) 5 to 15 per cent. by weight, which corresponds with about 10 to 30 per cent. of proof spirit. Theoretically, therefore, a natural wine should not contain more than 30 per cent. by weight of proof spirit, but, practically, it will not contain so much; for, apart from the whole of the sugar being transformed solely in the one direction, there must needs be a reduction of strength to some extent by the loss of alcohol occurring by evaporation during the process of fermentation.

Natural wine, it may be stated, rarely contains more than 22 per cent. *by volume* of proof spirit. The ordinary range is from 18 to 22. The maximum strength allowed by the English Government for the lower rate of import duty is 26 per cent., and this, it may be considered, is sufficiently high to include all natural wines. Indeed, independently of the amount of saccharine matter in the juice, the extent of alcoholic strength is limited by the action of the alcohol generated, for directly a certain quantity is present a check is put upon the further progress of fermentation, and the excess of sugar remains unfermented. Thus, although the juice may have been artificially sweetened by the addition of sugar, or the proportion of sugar increased by the partial desiccation of the grapes or the evaporation of the juice, only a limited alcoholic strength can be acquired as the result of fermentation. It may further be remarked that, as the presence of a certain quantity of alcohol puts a stop to the progress of fermentation, so does the existence of sugar beyond a certain proportion interfere with its commencement. There is a limit, in other words, to the strength of a saccharine liquid that can be thrown into fermentation.

The "fortified" wines contain, upon an average, about 34 or 36 per cent. by volume of proof spirit. These wines, which include such as port, sherry, Madeira, etc., reach us from the warmer wine-producing countries. After fermentation has advanced to a certain point, spirit is added, and thus further change is stopped, and the wine acquires, by virtue of its increased alcoholic strength, a keeping power under exposure to air which is not enjoyed by the unfortified product. The fortified class is allowed by the English customs a range of alcoholic strength of from 26 to 42 per cent. of proof spirit, and the maximum limit may be looked upon as fairly including all liquids that can justly lay claim to the title of wine.

From what has been stated, it will be seen that the relative average strength of natural and fortified wines may be represented by saying that the former kind contains about one-fifth and the latter one-third of its bulk of proof spirit; or, expressing it in a more familiar way, about five glasses of the natural and three glasses of the fortified wine contain the equivalent of one glass of brandy.

By keeping in cask, wine increases in alcoholic strength. This is to be accounted for by wood being more easily penetrated by water than by alcohol. Thus it happens that water is lost by evaporation from the outside of the cask in larger quantity than the alcohol, and the wine is left in a more concentrated condition.

The process for ascertaining the amount of alcohol in wine is very simple. It consists in distilling over, say half, from a given quantity, adding distilled water to the product to bring it to the same measure as that of the wine employed, and then taking the sp. gr. From this may be learnt, by the tables published, the percentage of alcohol present.

Besides the formation of alcohol, the process of fermentation is attended with the production of small amounts of glycerine and succinic acid. These principles thus constitute ingredients, to a small extent, of wine, but they cannot be regarded as of any significance.

Sugar.—Some wines are free, or nearly free, from sugar, while others contain varying amounts, the condition depending upon the extent to which fermentation has been carried. In natural, thoroughly fermented wines, as claret, Burgundy, hock, etc., there may be none, or, if any, only an insignificant quantity. In fortified wines, on the other hand, as port, sherry, Madeira, etc., more or less sugar is usually found, on account of fermentation having been artificially checked by the added spirit before the process was over. As these wines are kept, however, the amount undergoes a gradual diminution from some kind of metamorphosis occurring other than that of fermentation. Although a fortified wine, there are some kinds of sherry to be met with which are free, or next to free, from sugar. In what are classified as sweet wines, as, for example, Tokay, Constantia, Malmsey, Lachryma Christi, Tent, Malaga, etc., the quantity of sugar may amount to as much as 20 per cent. Here the process of fermentation is impeded by the large amount of sugar originally present in the "must," owing to the grapes having been allowed to become to a certain extent dried before being employed—indeed, some of these products possess a distinct, raisin-like flavor.

The natural wines which are characterized by sweetness are of low alcoholic strength, for in proportion as sugar is retained, so is there a diminished production of alcohol. Sweet and strong are therefore irreconcilable qualities in a natural state, and if combined imply the existence of added spirit.

Whatever sugar is present ought to be found in the state of grape-sugar, but the analytical examination of wine sometimes displays the existence of cane-sugar. It is especially with cheap sherries that this is noticeable, and it affords unmistakable evidence of adulteration.

Astringent matter.—The astringent matter of wine consists of tannic acid, and is derived from the skins, stones, and stalks of grapes. The white wines, which are prepared from the expressed juice of grapes only, are free from astringent matter. In the manufacture of the red wines the skins and stalks of the grapes are allowed to remain in the fermenting vat, and, as a consequence, astringent matter is taken up. Sometimes, also, a part of the astringent matter met with in wine is derived from the oak cask in which it has been kept.

On account of their freedom from astringent matter, the white wines possess a more delicate taste than the red. In red wines the amount of astringent matter at the commencement may be so great as to render them almost undrinkable. On keeping, however, the tannic acid becomes deposited in association with albuminous and coloring matters and bitartrate of potash (cream of tartar), and forms the crust which is observed to collect. At first the crust settles coarsely and thickly, but year by year the deposit becomes less and less, and at length may assume the shape of thin, filmy flakes, which, floating in the wine, produce what is known as "beeswing." With this deposition of crust the wine loses its hard taste and becomes soft and mellow, and according to its roughness to begin with, so will be the length of time required for maturing. As soon as it ceases to deposit it no longer improves by keeping, but commences, in fact, to deteriorate. By virtue of its effect in combining with and carrying down the albuminous matter of wine, and thereby preventing any further change, tannic acid must be looked upon as exerting a preservative influence.

A brown, humus-like substance, which has been named *apothema* by Berzelius, gradually undergoes formation as a product of the oxidation of tannic acid. This substance is not quite insoluble in wine. Enough is dissolved to give the yellow or tawny color belonging to port wine which has lost its other coloring matter by age. It is the source of the color which the skins of white grapes acquire in conversion into raisins.

Coloring matter.—Much variation exists as regards the color of wines. Some are pale to an extent to be almost colorless, whilst others are more or less deeply colored, the color passing either through shades of yellow and brown or red and blue.

Except in the case of the teinturier grape, the juice of grapes is colorless, and hence, when wine is made from the juice alone, or with the exclusion of the husk from the fermenting vat, the product is nearly colorless, no matter whether white or black grapes have been employed. Full ripeness of the grape adds a little to the tint, and on this account the champagne grape is not allowed to attain a maximum state of maturity, as paleness is considered a desirable quality for the wine to possess. If in preparing light-colored wine from white grapes the skins are allowed to be present during fermentation, a deeper colored product is obtained than from the juice alone, and this passes through a darker shade of yellow toward brown as age advances, owing to the gradual oxidation of tannic acid, and its conversion into apothema, as already explained. It is further a common practice, as with dark-colored sherries, for instance, to artifically color them in the following manner: the "must" obtained from very ripe grapes is evaporated in large pans till a deep brown sirupy liquid is obtained, a part of the sugar being caramelized during the process. This is added to the wine till the required shade of yellow or brown is produced. Sometimes even the coloring is effected by the direct addition of caramel or burnt sugar, but this is liable to communicate a bitter taste, and thereby injure the natural flavor of the wine. Pale wines frequently acquire a certain amount of color through being kept in oak casks.

The red wines derive their color from the husks of black grapes. These contain the coloring matter in an insoluble form, and thus the juice escapes being impregnated with it. Although insoluble in the fresh juice, it, however, undergoes solution when in contact with the fermented juice, the *rationale* being that the presence of alcohol in combination with the acids of the juice gives rise to the production of a liquid possessing a solvent power which the original aqueous liquid did not. As, then, alcohol becomes developed in the mixture of husks and fermenting juice, the coloring matter is taken up.

The coloring matter under consideration is primarily blue, and like other kinds of vegetable blue is reddened by an acid. Thus it is that as the acidity of the grape diminishes during the process of ripening, the color changes from red to dark blue. In wines the color also varies according to the amount of free acid present. This may be exemplified by adding an acid to a wine possessing a bluish black color. It will be observed to become sensibly reddened. If afterward some ammonia should be poured in, the color will be restored. Wines presenting a decidedly red tint may be rendered bluish black by means of the same agent.

It is well known that red wines become paler as their age increases. This arises from the coloring matter being deposited with the progress of formation of the crust. The astringent and coloring matters indeed closely follow each other. As the red color disappears, so the yellow, which is common to both red and white wines, becomes more visible: in the first place because it is less obscured, and next because it is gradually heightened by the conversion of tannic acid into apothema. In this way the production of the tawny color of old port is accounted for.

It is stated that the *teinturier* grape is specially cultivated in some localities for furnishing coloring matter to wine. It will be remembered that the juice of this grape is deeply stained, like that of the black currant, elderberry, and some other fruits. Foreign agents, as black cherries, bilberries, and particularly elderberries and logwood, it is also asserted, are frequently used for supplying color; and by their agency, white wines, it is further alleged, are sometimes dyed for the purpose of being sold as red.

Extractive matter.—In addition to the sugar, and the astringent and coloring matters which have been described, there are some undefined solid organic principles present in wine which are classified as "*extractives.*" The whole of these solid ingredients grouped together comprise what is understood as forming the "body" of wine. When the amount of solid matter is large, it is chiefly due to the presence of sugar.

Acids.—Wine always contains more or less free acid. The acids, malic and tartaric, existing in the grape exist also in its fermented juice, and moreover the alcoholic may be followed to some extent by the acetous fermentation, especially in poor wine, and thus lead to the presence of a proportionate amount of acetic acid. Leaving out of consideration the production of this latter acid, the extent of acidity of a wine will depend upon that of the grape from which it has been manufactured. There may be no perceptible acid taste when fermentation has not been fully carried out, on account of the sugar thereby present disguising it; but whenever fermentation has been completed some amount of acidity is recognizable, because the whole of the sugar has been converted into alcohol, and there is nothing to cover or conceal the acids which naturally existed to a greater or less extent in the grape. The taste therefore affords no criterion of the real acidity of a wine. A sweet wine, indeed, may contain considerably more acid than one which, through being dry, presents a certain degree of recognizable acidity.

As might naturally be inferred from what has been stated, it is the wines derived from the coolest wine-producing localities, as, for instance, particularly the Rhine and Moselle districts, which contain the largest proportion of acid. Where the climate is such that the grape is apt to fail in attaining full ripeness, undue acidity is a common defect, and special measures, which are uncalled for in warmer and more congenial localities, may require to be had recourse to, to give the wine a suitable character for drinking. Sometimes sugar is added to the wine itself to cover its acidity, and thereby render it palatable. Sometimes the " must " is diluted to reduce its percentage acidity, and then sweetened in order that it may yield by fermentation the requisite alcoholic strength. A wine manufactured in this way, whilst being provided with the ordinary amount of alcohol, will contain—leaving out of consideration the acids—a relative deficiency of the other vinous elements. Sometimes the undue acidity is removed by direct neutralization with the carbonate of lime or soda. A process ingeniously suggested by Liebig effects the separation of a portion of the acid by precipitation as cream of tartar. To the wine some neutral tartrate of potash is added, which combines with its free tartaric acid, and carries it down as the comparatively insoluble bitartrate or cream of tartar.

The effect of fermentation is to some extent to lead to a reduction of acidity. A portion of the tartaric acid belonging to the fruit exists in combination with potash under the form of bitartrate. Now this salt is very much less soluble in an alcoholic than in an aqueous liquid. Hence in proportion as alcohol is present the salt becomes thrown down, and being an acid salt a reduction of acidity is thereby effected. It collects inside the cask, and is known as "argol." The deposition also proceeds after the wine is bottled, and helps to give rise to the sweetness and mellowness acquired by keeping. In the case of the red wines, it falls in company with the astringent and coloring matters, and thus contributes to the production of the crust. In the case of white wines, it takes the form of colorless crystals, which may be seen adhering to the cork and lying in the bottle, looking something like powdered glass.

A great deal of unnecessary stress has been attached to the question of the amount of free acid in wine in relation to the production of acidity of stomach. The wines containing the smallest amount of acid are such as sherry, marsala, and port; whilst hock, moselle, light claret, and some Greek wines may be spoken of as standing at the opposite end of the scale. But, because these latter contain the most acid, they are not thereby rightly to be shunned on the score of greater liability to produce acidity. Indeed, experience shows that it is not acids which particularly favor the production of acidity of stomach, but in reality articles containing sugar, and especially where the sugar is in an unstable condition, as it is in wine, and thence more prone to undergo the acid fermentation. Nothing, in fact, is more productive of the trouble in question than the concoction which is retailed out under the name of sherry at many eating and drinking establishments, and which analysis shows to contain a considerable quantity of sugar. The presence of a moderate amount of acid does no harm; on the contrary, it may afford assistance to digestion. The

17

wine, however, should not be sufficiently sour to be disagreeable to the palate, and the kind of sourness which is to be regarded as decidedly objectionable is that arising from the acetous fermentation. A wine which has acquired sourness from such a source is no longer sound, and apt, if drunk, to occasion general derangement of the alimentary canal.

Ethers and volatile oil.—These constitute the source of the special flavor and aroma of wine, and give to it the distinctive characters it possesses. They doubtless contribute to produce a portion of the exhilarating effects it exerts, for the exhilarating power of a given quantity of wine cannot be wholly accounted for by the alcohol it contains. The value of a wine is more determined by the quality and amount of these ingredients than by its alcoholic constituent.

Some wines—muscat forms a striking example—possess an aroma which excites a reminiscence of the fresh fruit, and is in fact derived directly from the grape. It is probably due to an essential oil, and is increased in quantity by increasing ripeness of the fruit. Wines possessing it are called "aromatic wines." Besides this kind of aroma, which belongs only to the product derived from certain grapes, wine possesses an aroma which is peculiarly vinous, as it arises out of the results of fermentation. This becomes more pronounced as the wine ages in bottle. It is occasioned by the development of ethereal products, through the reaction of the acids and alcohol upon each other. It constitutes the "bouquet" of wine, and is met with in greater quantity in wine made from grapes which have not arrived at full ripeness; hence its predominance in the productions of the cooler wine-growing localities, as particularly the Rhine and Moselle districts. *Œnanthic ether* is the name which has been applied by Liebig and Pelouze to the chief ethereal product belonging to wine. It is obtainable only in exceedingly minute quantity; but, possessing a very strong vinous smell, a small amount goes a long way.

The flavoring of wines is carried on upon an extensive scale to suit the market of the country to which they are sent. Choice wines are reserved and added year by year to a stock which is kept expressly for use as a flavoring medium. Wines are also blended so as to furnish through successive years a product of the same flavor, strength, and appearance, independently of the variation that may belong to different vintages.

Cette, Marseilles, and Bordeaux are notorious places for "doctoring" wine. Cette in particular bears an unenviable name on account of the undisguised manner in which the fabrication of wine is carried on. By the skill acquired in the art of imitation, an article to represent a wine of any character or age can be supplied to order at a few hours' notice.

Wines are generally named after the locality producing them. In the description that will now be given of their respective characters, it will be convenient to group the products of different countries together under separate heads. Each country yields a wine possessing distinctive features of its own. The wines may be of the same character, but there is a flavor peculiar to each, which is readily perceptible. The product of one country which, as a wine, may be quite as good as or even better than that of another, may nevertheless be held in less repute because it does not conform with a conventional idea founded upon what the palate has been accustomed to.

Whilst wines differ considerably in their drinkable characters, each should possess a clean, sound, and simple taste. It should give an idea of unity in contradistinction to the mixed tastes belonging to a made-up article; and there should be an absence of anything indicating change or fermentescibility. The impression produced upon the palate by tasting alternately in succession a pure and a sophisticated wine is exceedingly striking, and brings out strongly the mixed character of the latter.

A good wine promotes the appetite, exhilarates the spirits, and increases the bodily vigor. It should have body or substance (which is different from alcoholic strength), and give rise to a sense of satisfaction instead of leaving a craving, empty, or hungry feeling such as is produced by a thin and sour drink.

As regards their general characters, wines are spoken of as: Natural or light, fortified or strong, red, white, sweet or fruity, dry or thoroughly fermented, full-bodied, thin, acidulous, astringent, and sparkling.

French wines.—The natural wines of France, which formerly constituted the principal wine consumed in England, and which from political considerations were for a considerable time displaced by the fortified wines of Portugal, have been latterly advancing into more general use · amongst us, especially since the alteration of the import duty in 1861. Clarets, Burgundies, and Champagnes are productions of France with which every one is acquainted. Besides these natural wines, a strong or fortified wine (Roussillon is an example) is produced in the south of France, which approximates in character to the wines of Portugal.

Clarets are derived from the Bordeaux district. They constitute red wines, and of the several varieties the best known are such as *Lafite, Latour, La Rose, Margaux, Mouton, Pauillac, St. Julien, St. Emilion,* etc. Some of the above brands bear the prefix of *Château,* this being applied to the wine made from the vines which grow immediately around the château of the producer, in contradistinction to that derived from the surrounding properties. White wines are also supplied from the Bordeaux district. They comprise such as *Sauterne, Vin-de-Grave, Bursac,* and an exceedingly choice production, the *Château d'Yquem.* The clarets, or red Bordeaux wines, contain no added spirit. Their alcoholic strength averages from 18 to 20 per cent. of proof spirit. Being fully fermented, they are rendered more or less free from sugar, and constitute, therefore, dry wines. They are light, agreeable, and refreshing to drink, have a delicate, fragrant odor, and a slightly rough or astringent taste, without, in good wine, any unpleasant acidity. The white wines of the Bordeaux class, like white wines generally, are finer flavored, and have a more delicate perfume and less astringency than the red. The Château d'Yquem is a specially choice, full-flavored wine, with a particularly luscious character, due to the richness in saccharine matter of the grape from which it is made, acquired by being allowed to remain on the vine till over-ripe before being gathered.

With the moderately exhilarating and the other properties that the clarets possess, they form an exceedingly valuable kind of stimulant, both for the healthy and the sick. There is scarcely any condition in which they are calculated to disagree. They form a most suitable beverage for persons of a gouty or rheumatic disposition, and also for the dyspeptic. It may be said that they are not prone to turn sour upon the stomach themselves, nor to cause other articles to become sour; neither do they provoke headache nor derangement in those who are subject to bilious disorders.

Burgundies are derived from the southern districts of the central parts of France—that portion of France, it may be said, which is most propitious to the growth of the grape. As with Bordeaux wine, so with Burgundy, both red and white varieties are produced. Of the red, *Clos de Vougeôt, Chambertin, Romanée, Volnay, Pommard, Beaune,* and *Macon* form well-known brands; and of the white, *Chablis, Pouilly, Meursault,* and *Montrachet.*

The wines of the Rhone districts, consisting of such as *Côte Rôtie, Hermitage* red and white, and *Beaujolais* (which has risen rapidly into notoriety as a reasonable priced wine during the last ten or twelve years), are generally classed with Burgundies.

In character Burgundy is a richer, fuller-bodied, or more generous wine than claret. With a choice aroma and strong wine flavor, it possesses a trace of bitterness. To appreciate its qualities to the fullest extent, it should be served in the middle of dinner, with the roast meat or game. Therapeutically, it is a valuable agent where poverty of blood or an ill-nourished state of the system exists. In such cases it is decidedly to be preferred to claret. An idea prevails that, unlike claret, Burgundy encourages the development of gout. This may be so with a very sumptuous wine presenting an approximation to port, but there is reason to think that the charge is unfounded in the case of the ordinary Burgundies that are supplied for use.

Beaujolais may be ranked as occupying a place between Burgundy and claret. Whilst wanting the fulness of body of the former, it is a rather stouter wine than the latter.

Champagnes are the produce of several parts of France, but the most renowned brands are derived from the department of the Marne—Reims forming the centre of the district on the northern, and Epernay that on the southern side of the river. They are classified as sparkling and still, and sweet and dry, and the better qualities are distinguished by the name of the producer. Amongst well-known and favorite brands may be mentioned those of *Roederer, Pommery and Gréno, Moet, Clicquot, Jules Mumm, Giesler,* and *Perrier Jouet.* In good wines the carbonic acid is so incorporated with the liquid as to escape slowly, or "creamily" as it is termed, when the bottle is opened.

Champagne, whilst only possessing the alcoholic strength of natural wines (Griffin's analysis of a sample showed 18 per cent. of proof spirit), is characterized in its effects upon the system by the rapidity of its action as a stimulant and restorative. As it acts more rapidly and strongly, so its effects also pass off more quickly. It may be described as a volatile stimulant, with a more transitory action than other beverages of the alcoholic class. It is a useful wine for exciting the flagging powers in cases of exhaustion. It also has a tendency to allay irritability of the stomach, and in some cases of vomiting may be found to be retained when other stimulants are rejected. Unless in a good sound state, however, there is scarcely any wine that is so calculated to upset the stomach. To give it effervescence sugar is added after its introduction into the bottle, for the purpose of inducing a second fermentation, and until this fermentation is complete the wine must be looked upon as in a state of change, and thereby apt to excite changes of the food within the stomach, which tend to interfere with the natural course of digestion. Unless the elements of the wine, also, are in proper relation and of proper goodness, it is apt to acquire ascescent and obnoxious properties, from the vinous passing into the acetous fermentation.

Besides Champagne, France produces other sparkling wines, the most notable of which are sparkling Burgundies, both white and red; a sparkling Hermitage; and also a wine closely resembling and often doing duty for Champagne, which is produced on the banks of the Rhone, and styled *St. Peray.*

The south of France, in the neighborhood of the Pyrénées, is the seat of production of quite a different kind of wine from the varieties that have been referred to. The wine in question, of which *Roussillon* and *Masdeu* furnish examples, belongs to the fortified class. It forms a French representative of the red wines of Portugal, but does not nearly come up to them in quality, and has something of the Burgundy or claret character about it. It sometimes passes under the names of Burgundy Port and French Port. In Thudichum and Dupré's analytical table the alcoholic strength of Roussillon stands at 36.2 per cent. of proof spirit.

German wines.—With the exception of what is known as *Hambro' sherry* (a low-priced fortified wine of, as its name implies, a sherry-like nature), which is not grown, but fabricated at and shipped from Hambro', the German wines form natural products. They are of light alcoholic strength, and are characterized by their marked and peculiar aroma or fragrance, and their acidulous nature. These properties render them grateful and refreshing to drink, as well as an excitant of the appetite. They thus form a specially appropriate beverage at the commencement of dinner. On account of the northern situation of the country, and the variation in the climate of different years, they exhibit a wider range of difference in quality according to the season (a hot and dry season being that which is most propitious) than the products of more southern latitudes. Notwithstanding the greatest care in the process of manufacture, a want of brightness characterizes the wines of Germany. Hence the custom of drinking them from colored glasses, the effect of which is to conceal from view that which might displease the eye.

The German wines produced on the banks of the Rhine generally pass in this country under the name of *hock*. They are mostly white, and the best known and most esteemed varieties are such as *Johannisberg*, *Steinberg*, *Rüdesheim*, *Marcobrunn*, *Rauenthal*, *Hockheim*, and *Nierstein*. *Assmannshäuser* represents a red variety of hock.

The wines produced on the banks of the Moselle agree in their general characters with hocks or Rhine wines, but they are somewhat more acid in taste, and have less body. Excellent sparkling wines are made both in the Rhine and Moselle districts.

Hungarian wines.—In general character the wines of Hungary may be said to resemble those of France more closely than those of any other country. With the exception of Tokay, which has long been prized amongst us as one of the choicest of wines, they were but little known in this country previous to the notice they received at the International Exhibition of 1862. Since then they have risen rapidly in public estimation, and now meet with an extensive consumption. They are good specimens of a light or natural wine, with a distinctive flavor of their own. Both red and white wines are produced, and the varieties are sufficiently numerous to present to the uninitiated a somewhat perplexing list of names. Of the red wines, the *Carlowitz* is the best known in England. It possesses good body, a full alcoholic strength for a natural wine, a slight astringency, and freedom from saccharine matter. It may be said, indeed, to constitute a generous wine of its class, and in this respect may be compared to Burgundy. Next to Carlowitz, *Ofner*, perhaps stands in highest estimation. The white wines are specially characterized by their softness and richness of grape flavor. The *Ruster* and

Edenburg are good and exceedingly agreeable-drinking wines. But *Tokay* far excels them all, and holds, in fact, a unique position. It is one of the most universally famed of wines, and always commands a price which places it only within reach of the wealthy. It is made of the juice which flows spontaneously from the finest over-ripe grapes. It ranks amongst the sweet wines, but with its sweetness it possesses " an exceedingly rich, aromatic, mouth-filling wine-flavor" (Druitt). It is usually drunk as a delicacy toward the end of dinner, but may be advantageously recommended for rousing the powers and giving life to the enfeebled invalid.

Greek wines.—These wines are less known in England than those which have been as yet referred to. A somewhat numerous list is presented for selection. They constitute natural wines, with a high alcoholic strength for their class. The white are clean, fresh, and agreeable-drinking, whilst the red have fulness and roughness belonging to the better kinds, with some degree of tartness in the cheaper kinds. Like other stout wines they undergo marked improvement on being kept. *Kephisia, St. Elie, Noussa, Patras, Thera,* and *Santorin* form representatives of dry wine, whilst *Vinsanto, Lachryma Christi,* and *Cyprus* constitute Greek products of the sweet wine class.

Italian wines.—A few wines reach this country from Italy. The red wines are full-colored, full-bodied, and dry, with a decided quality of roughness. White *Capri,* named from the rocky island standing at the entrance of the Bay of Naples which yields it, is an exceedingly refreshing, wholesome, and pleasant-drinking light wine, particularly for summer use. A sparkling *Asti* is imported, but, probably owing to defective preparation, it lacks stability and brightness. Although much drunk and favorably thought of in Italy, it cannot compete with the other sparkling wines placed at our disposal in England.

Australian wines.—Australia promises to stand high as a wine-producing country, possessing the favorable conditions it does for the growth of the grape, and starting as it has done with the careful manufacture of a pure article. Both red and white wines are imported into England from more vineyards than one, and it may be said of the best that they are rich, full-bodied, agreeable-drinking wines, without hardness or acidity. Whilst of the nature of Bordeaux and Burgundy, they have an aroma which is peculiarly their own, and which gives them a character distinct from the products of other countries.

Port and other wines of Portugal.—Port, like the wines of hot countries in general, as sherry, Marsala, Madeira, and Cape, belongs to the fortified class. Spirit is added after fermentation has advanced to a certain point, to check its further progress, and give the wine increased keeping power. Thus, a wine of an alcoholic strength averaging about 36 per cent. of proof spirit is produced, instead of about 20, as with the natural or unfortified varieties. If made without being fortified, the produce of Portugal presents a close resemblance in character to Burgundy, but wine of this sort is not to any notable extent exported for the English market, on account of its alleged want of sufficient keeping power for transport.

Port is a wine which possesses when new a considerable amount of saccharine matter, which gives it a marked fruity character. In the first place, the grapes, from the warm climate in which they are grown, acquire a sweetness which is not attained under exposure to a less amount of heat; and next, as has been mentioned, fermentation is stopped before the sugar has become exhausted. The wine is also rich in astringent and other extractive matters, and thus possesses, as it is termed, a full body. By keeping, the astringent in conjunction with the coloring matter becomes gradually deposited under the form of crust. The saccharine matter also undergoes transformation, and in this way the wine loses its rough, sweet, and fruity taste, and acquires what is known as the character of dryness. There is no wine which improves more by keeping than port. From possessing a roughness or harshness and confusion of flavors which may be absolutely unpleasant to the palate, it tones down in the course of time to a pure, mellow, and homogeneous liquid. Not only are some of the objectionable elements deposited, and the others blended or incorporated together, but, by the reaction of the acid and alcoholic principles upon each other, ethereal products become developed which give the aroma or bouquet that forms so choice a feature belonging to the ripened or matured wine.

It is a common practice amongst dealers to mix different sorts of port with the view of meeting the taste of the consumer, and it must be admitted that some of the most pleasant-drinking wines are produced in this way. It is said to be only in certain years that a wine is good enough to stand alone, and when so allowed to remain it is called a "vintage wine."

Port stands pre-eminent amongst wines as a full, rich, and strength-giving stimulant. It is of great service in enfeebled states of the system, and particularly during convalescence from fever and other debilitating diseases. Its astringency gives it a special value where there is also diarrhœa to control. For everyday use, while suiting many, it is far too heavy for others. By dyspeptics, the gouty, persons suffering from attacks of bilious or sick headache, and those passing urinary red sand it should, as a rule, be shunned. Drunk in excess it tends to induce a plethoric state, and there can be little doubt that not only is it an excitant of gouty attacks where the gouty disposition exists, but that the gouty habit may be developed through its influence. It seems to be the presence of imperfectly fermented matter in association with the spirit—and the same holds good with regard to other alcoholic beverages—that gives it its pernicious properties in relation to gout.

Port, some years back, was largely consumed amongst the upper classes as an after-dinner wine. At the present time its place may be said to be taken by claret, and, whatever the cause, it is now rare in society to come across men who admit that port agrees with them. If not drunk so much, however, amongst the upper classes, there has been no falling off in its consumption in England; and this, because it now finds its way into the houses of small tradesmen, and others, where formerly it was unknown.

A limited quantity of white wine reaches us from Portugal. *Bucellas* is a white Portuguese dinner wine, which, a short time since, met with a somewhat extensive consumption, but is now seldom heard of. *Lisbon*, also, is a white wine derived from Portugal. *White port* is likewise to be obtained, but is not often come across.

Sherry and other Spanish wines.—Under the generic name of sherry are included the ordinary white wines of Spain. The heat, dryness, and equality of the climate give advantages which render Spain a most successful wine-producing country. Sherry has long held a high position in public estimation as a wholesome and clean-drinking wine. Like the other products of hot countries it is subjected to the addition of spirit, and its alcoholic strength is about the same as that of port. Unbrandied sherry is often advertised, but the wine in an unfortified state is only exceptionally imported into England and consumed.

Several kinds of sherry are met with, varying in color, body, and taste. There are the pale, golden, and brown; and some are thin and dry, whilst others are full-bodied and rich. Naturally, the wine is pale, but to suit the market, color and body are given by the addition of "must" (grape juice) which has been evaporated down until it has assumed the condition of a thick and dark-colored syrupy liquid. This, as may be inferred, not only adds to its color and fulness, but also modifies its taste.

Certain sherries are characterized by distinct names, as, for instance, *Amontillado*, *Vino di Pasto*, *Montilla*, and *Manzanilla*. These are all dry wines, and are often found free or almost free from saccharine matter. Genuine Amontillado has a choice dry, nutty flavor, and Manzanilla a decided bitterness.

A pure and dry sherry may be said to constitute one of the most wholesome liquids for general use of the fermented class. It is devoid of astringency, and has not the strength-giving properties of port, but forms a wine that may be drunk when other wines disagree. There are some dyspeptics who complain of its producing acidity, but, as a rule, it is borne well, alike by those who suffer from dyspepsia and gout. A pure dry wine, however, must be selected for consumption.

The product known as *Hambro' sherry* is a made-up article. Hamburg is not a wine-growing but a wine-fabricating locality. Much of the cheap sherry sold, and a great portion of that supplied at refreshment-rooms and public-houses, is derived from this source. It is this which often brings sherry into disrepute by occasioning acidity, headache, and other symptoms of gastric derangement; and on account of the term Hambro' having acquired a character of reproach, the article is sometimes named after the river instead of the town, and thence styled *Elbe sherry*.

There are various sweet wines derived from Spain. *Malaga* is a sweet luscious wine of low alcoholic strength. *Paxarette* is another wine of an allied nature. *Rota Tent*, which is chiefly used in England for sacramental purposes, is also a sweet wine, with a low percentage of spirit. *Sack* is a name of antiquity as applied to wine. The sack of Shakespeare is believed to have been a Spanish wine which held the place of our sherry. The sack of the present day belongs to the group of sweet wines, and is brought chiefly from Madeira, and Palma, one of the Canary Islands.

A considerable quantity of *red wine* is likewise now imported from Spain. It is known as *Tarragona*, or Spanish port, and possesses the advantages of being a low-priced, sound, and full-bodied wine. It may be spoken of as forming the best substitute for port that is furnished.

Marsala.—This forms a Sicilian wine, which has attained considerable repute, and is largely consumed in this country. It is used in the same way as sherry, for which it constitutes a good, moderate-priced substitute. A price that will procure a good Marsala will only purchase an indifferent sherry, and there is much truth in the remark that for persons of moderate means it is far better that they should drink a good Marsala than a bad sherry. It is rather a full-bodied wine, not so free from saccharine matter as a dry sherry, and of about the average alcoholic strength of wines of the fortified class.

Madeira.—This is one of the choicest of the fortified wines. The amount produced can never pass beyond certain limits, on account of the restricted area of the island for the growth of the vine; and, latterly, from the severity with which the vine disease prevailed, its production had almost ceased altogether, for nothing less than rooting up the old plants and replacing them with new was necessitated. Time will be required for these new plants to arrive at a state of perfection, but, from the accounts that are given, the yield of wine is satisfactorily increasing, and the island promises soon again to become a flourishing wine-producing country.

Madeira is characterized by the fulness of its body and the choiceness of its aroma. It is a wine which, like port, greatly improves by keeping, and its mellowness is found to be further increased by transport to a hot country and back. Hence the practice of shipping Madeira to the East Indies and back, and it is probable to the effects of the heat and agitation that the improvement is due.

The wine known as *Malmsey* is supposed to have taken its name from Malvasia, a small island in the Archipelago. It was formerly derived from that and other islands, viz., Cyprus and Candia in the Archipelago, as well as the peninsula of Morea. The Malmsey wine now met with mostly reaches us from Madeira. It is a sweet and luscious wine made from grapes grown under a hot sun and allowed to hang on the vines till partially withered. As is well known, historical report says that the Duke of Clarence, brother of Edward IV., on being condemned to die, and being allowed, from his position, to choose the manner of death, selected drowning in a butt of Malmsey.

Cape or South African wines.—Formerly, when colonial were admitted at a lower duty than foreign wines, these were introduced on an extensive scale, but now that they do not enjoy this advantage they are not much heard of. The productions in question reach us as cheap imitations of port, sherry, and Madeira; but there is one Cape wine of wide renown, viz., *Constantia*, which stands upon its own merits, and ranks high in public estimation as a sweet or luscious wine.

MISCELLANEOUS FRUIT AND OTHER WINES.—Wine is made not only from the grape, but also from the juice of various other kinds of fruit, and likewise from the juice of other parts of plants containing sugar. Orange wine, currant wine, plum wine, gooseberry wine, and many others, for example, are derived from fruits; whilst palm wine, maple wine, parsnip wine, etc., are derived from other vegetable products. Each possesses distinctive characters of its own. None will bear comparison for purity and choiceness of flavor with the fermented liquid derived from the grape. It is not deemed necessary to devote space to their special consideration.

Mead or *Metheglin* is a wine prepared from honey and water. It is a fermented liquid of great antiquity in England, but is not much consumed now. It is rarely to be met with, indeed, except amongst the peasantry in certain localities. It is of moderate alcoholic strength, and of variable sweetness, according to the amount of unfermented honey remaining. By keeping, it improves and acquires a peculiar fragrance.

SPIRITS.—Spirits are the product of distillation of fermented liquids, and have as their base the alcohol which is formed during the process of fermentation. Fermented liquids have been known from the earliest periods of antiquity, but it was not till the twelfth century that the method of obtaining spirit by distillation was discovered by Abucasis. As the alcohol passes over, it is accompanied by other volatile products, and thus the odor and flavor of the spirit vary with the source from which it is obtained. This applies to the product of first distillation, and accounts for the well-known difference that is noticeable in the various spirits, such as brandy, whiskey, rum, etc., that are supplied for use. By repeated distillation, or rectification as it is termed, the alcohol may be separated from the other principles through their difference in volatility, and made to lose the identity that belonged to the original spirit. It clings, however, very tenaciously to water, and can only be separated from this associate by admixture with an agent, as pearlash (carbonate of potash), quicklime, etc., which has a strong affinity for it, and holds it back whilst the alcohol distils over. It is in this way that pure or abso-. lute alcohol is obtained, a liquid having a sp. gr. at 60° Fahr. of 0.794, and, therefore, being considerably lighter than water.

Pure or absolute alcohol, which has been referred to, is only employed for chemical purposes. What is called *rectified spirit* consists of alcohol with 16 per cent. of water, the mixture having a sp. gr. of 0.838 at 60° Fahr. *Proof spirit* consists of an admixture of alcohol and water in nearly equal proportions, viz., 49 parts by weight of the former, and 51 of the latter, and has a sp. gr. of 0.920 at 60° Fahr. Both these latter are used for making the tinctures of pharmacy.

Proof spirit is taken in England as the Government standard for levying the Excise and Customs duty. According to the proportion of alcohol and water, so will be the sp. gr., and tables have been framed showing the relation between the two, and thus enabling the strength of the spirit to be determined when the sp. gr. has been ascertained, which is usually done by means of an instrument called the *hydrometer*. With a larger proportion of alcohol than exists in proof spirit the sp. gr. is lowered, and the spirit is said to be *over proof*, whilst conversely with a less proportion it is raised, and the spirit is said to be *under proof.* From the ascertained sp. gr. can be learnt, with the aid of the tables supplied, how much per cent. either *over* or *under* proof a spirit may be; and in this way, with a given duty per gallon for proof spirit, the charge to be levied, reckoned at a proportionate rate, can be calculated for spirits of any other strength. It is necessary, however, that the spirit under examination should consist only of alcohol and water; and, where any foreign matter is present, its separation must be effected by distillation, and the bulk of the distilled product raised to that of the original liquid by the requisite addition of distilled water, just as requires to be done for ascertaining the alcoholic strength of a simple fermented liquid, like wine, beer, etc.

Spirits as they reach the consumer, whilst presenting a certain range of variation, may be said to be of *about* the strength of proof spirit, or to consist, in other words, of about equal parts of absolute alcohol and water.

Brandy.—Brandy (a corruption from the German *Branntwein*, French *Brandevin*, burnt wine, or wine subjected to the influence of heat) is the name applied to the spirit procured from the distillation of wine. Its quality varies with the kind of wine from which it is obtained, and the care with which the process of distillation is carried out. It is chiefly white wine that is used, on account of its yielding a more delicate and agreeable flavored spirit than red. The most esteemed brandy is that which is made in France, and the districts of Cognac and Armagnac are more renowned than any others for the quality of the product. As first distilled, like other spirits, brandy is a colorless liquid. By keeping in an oak cask it acquires a pale-sherry tint from the tannic acid which it extracts. Dark brandies are artificially colored with caramel. The flavor and aroma of brandy are due to the œnanthic ether and other volatile products belonging to wine which pass over with the alcohol and water in the process of distillation. As with wine, from which it is derived, the flavoring principles become modified and the brandy improved by keeping. Thus it is that old Cognac possesses a delicacy of flavor which does not belong to new. When first imported it is generally 1 or 2 per cent. over proof, but its strength decreases by storage in cask. As sold, it may be as much as 10 or 15 or more per cent. under proof. Brande places the average strength of brandy at 42 per cent. *by measure* of absolute alcohol.

Brandy occupies the first place in public estimation of all the ardent spirits. Its purity and the delicacy of its flavor give it the position that it holds, and render it suitable for selection in any case where, either dietetically or therapeutically, a spirit is required. It is a popular remedy for sickness, diarrhœa, exhaustion, spasms, and for correcting indigestion, or stimulating the digestion of an indigestible article of food. Burnt brandy is often specially useful in protracted sickness, and will be sometimes found to be retained when other articles are rejected.

Rum.—In the West and East Indies, molasses, the skimmings from the sugar boilers, etc., are mixed with water, fermented, and subsequently submitted to distillation. The distilled product is afterward colored with partially burnt sugar, and constitutes rum. Rum is a spirit that improves greatly—acquiring a fine, mellow, soft flavor—by keeping. Its alcoholic strength is about the same as that of brandy. Jamaica rum is considered the best. Sliced pine-apples are sometimes placed into puncheons containing the finer qualities of rum, and the product is known as *pine-apple rum.*

Whiskey.—The term whiskey is stated to be a corruption of the Celtic word *usquebaugh*—water of life. The article constitutes one of the corn spirits, but, unlike gin, is derived from the malted grain. It is usually made from malted barley. The peculiar flavor which it possesses is due to the effect of kiln-drying upon the grain, and during this process the nature of the fuel employed produces its influence on the character of the product, the use of peat and turf fires giving the smoky aroma which is looked upon as a desirable product. As with brandy and rum, whiskey is a spirit which greatly improves by keeping, a soft and mellow taste being thereby communicated to it. If the flavor be not objected to, whiskey may be used in precisely the same way as brandy, with which it closely corresponds in alcoholic strength. Scotland and Ireland are the countries that are famed for the production of whiskey. A difference exists in the flavor of the products of the two countries, but when of good quality they may be regarded as of equal repute and utility.

Gin, Geneva, Hollands, or Schiedam.—The spirit comprehended under these names was originally, and, for some time, wholly, imported into this country from Holland. It is a corn spirit, derived chiefly from unmalted grain, which, after distillation, is purified by the rectifier, and subsequently flavored, principally with juniper berries. The name *Geneva* is derived from *Genièvre,* the French for the juniper plant and berries, and this by corruption has been shortened into *gin.* When the manufacture of Geneva, or gin, was started in England, the Dutch spirit fell under the designation of *Holland Geneva, Hollands,* and *Schiedam,* the latter being derived from the export town of that name.

In the preparation of gin the fermented liquid is distilled, as in the case of the other spirits, but, instead of the process being allowed to stop here, the distillate is subjected to rectification by re-distillation. The object is to obtain a perfectly pure and neutral spirit as a basis for the addition of the flavoring agents. Besides common alcohol, there is a small amount of *amylic alcohol,* or *oil of potato spirit—fuselöl* of the Germans—developed during fermentation. Possessing, as this principle does, a strong acrid taste and nauseous odor, it forms a contaminating ingredient which it is considered advisable to get rid of. It happens to be of a less volatile nature than common alcohol, and hence, on redistillation the process can be so conducted as to leave it behind in the still. The spirituous liquid thus left also contains other impurities, and goes under the name of "*faints.*" To convert rectified corn-spirit into gin, it is flavored with juniper and various aromatics. Oil of turpentine, according to what is stated, is also sometimes used. As sold by the rectifier, the strength is about 20 per cent. under proof (it is not allowed by law to be sent out stronger than 17 per cent. under proof), but the retailers afterward dilute and generally sweeten it. Thus sweetened it becomes "*cordial gin,*" and also passes under the name of "*Old Tom.*"

On account of the juniper belonging to it, gin possesses diuretic properties to an extent not enjoyed by the other spirits. Age does not improve it in the same manner as it does brandy, rum, and whiskey.

Several other spirits are in use in different parts of the world. It will suffice to mention here that *arrack* is the name given to the spirit obtained from a fermented infusion of rice, and also from *toddy* or *palm wine;* that *koumiss,* which has been lately extolled as useful in the treatment of consumption, is procured in Tartary from fermented mare's milk, and latterly also has been made in this country from cow's milk artificially sweetened; and that *robur,* or *tea-spirit,* the latest novelty in spirits, consists of ordinary spirit flavored with tea. With regard to this last, it may be said that a special value is claimed for it as a spirit by its introducer, but, looked at physiologically, it is composed of agents which exert antagonistic effects upon the animal system.

LIQUEURS.—Liqueurs constitute distilled spirituous liquids, sweetened and flavored with various fruits and aromatic substances. They are not much used except as stimulants at the end of dinner. Some of them are employed as appetizing agents. Their variety is great, but only the best known will be referred to here, and it will suffice simply to mention the principles to which they owe their flavor.

Curaçoa has an aromatic bitter taste which is due to orange-peel. *Noyeau* is flavored with the kernels of the peach and apricot, sometimes with those of the cherry, and sometimes with bitter almonds. *Maraschino* derives its flavor from cherries. *Kirschwasser* also owes its properties to the cherry. Cherries are bruised and allowed to ferment. The stones are cracked and the kernels broken and used as well. Distillation is afterward performed. *Chartreuse* was originally prepared in a monastery bearing this name in France. In 1864 the Pope prohibited the monks from any longer making it for sale, and, as the recipe was not published, the Chartreuse which is now sold is a different liqueur from the original. *Parfait amour* contains a number of aromatics. In a recipe for it the following are enumerated: lemon-peel, cinnamon, rosemary, cloves, mace, cardamoms, and orange-flower water. *Anisette* is flavored with aniseed and coriander. *Kümmel* is the principal liqueur of Russia, and consists of sweetened spirit flavored with cumin and caraway-seeds. *Absinthe* differs from the above in being a bitter liqueur. It consists of a sweetened spirit flavored with wormwood, and is generally drunk diluted with water before a meal to stimulate digestion and excite a flagging appetite. It is, perhaps, one of the most treacherous and pernicious for habitual use of all the liquids of the alcoholic class. *Bitters* are likewise used in a similar way, and receive their flavor from various bitter agents—most commonly from angostura-bark, orange-peel, or angelica-root and seeds.

CONDIMENTS.

Condiments consist of seasoning or flavoring agents. Without being strictly alimentary substances, they nevertheless play no insignificant part in the alimentation of man, and prove of service in more ways than one. Their first effect is to render food more tempting to the palate, and thereby increase the amount consumed. We are guided in the choice of food by taste and smell, and that which agreeably affects these senses excites the desire for eating. Condiments are employed for this special purpose, and thus a flagging appetite receives a stimulant. Through their aromatic and pungent qualities they also assist digestion, the *modus operandi* being by promoting the flow of the secretions, and increasing the muscular activity of the alimentary canal. In some cases they may be further useful by serving to correct injurious properties that may belong to an article of food.

Standing in the position they do, it is not considered necessary to give a special description of the various condiments. A somewhat extensive group of them exists. One, viz., salt, is simply of a saline nature. It is the most universally employed of all. Some, as vinegar, lemon-juice, pickles, and capers, owe their virtue to acidity. Others owe it to their pungency, as, for example, mustard, pepper, cayenne, ginger, curry, and horseradish. Others, again, form an aromatic group of condiments, which includes such as cinnamon, nutmegs, cloves, allspice, vanilla, mint, thyme, fennel, sage, parsley, onions, leeks, chives, shallots, garlic, and some others. Besides these, there are various sauces of artificial production which are employed to give zest for food by their flavor.

THE PRESERVATION OF FOOD.

THE preservation of food has been practised from time immemorial. The ancient processes, however, resolved themselves into such as simply drying, salting, etc. Food thus preserved only imperfectly represents the article in the fresh state; but in the present age of progress the art has not been allowed to stand still, and methods are now had recourse to by which both animal and vegetable foods are preserved in such a way as to be susceptible of being kept for an indefinite period, and then being almost equal in quality to what they were originally. With the improvements that have taken place, a new trade has been established, which has rapidly grown into significance, and promises to prove of the deepest importance to the human race. Food is now being utilized that was formerly wasted, because it exceeded the requirements of the district, and it was not known how it could be rendered available in distant parts. In Australia and South America, particularly, the amount of animal food procurable far surpasses the wants of the inhabitants, and it has been the practice to sacrifice the animals for their wool, skins, fat, and bones, which formed exportable commodities. The processes that have been invented, now permit the meat to be preserved and to be transported in a fit condition for taking the place of fresh food elsewhere; and, with the facility of transit that exists, countries where food is scarce may be supplied from those where abundance prevails, whatever the distance intervening between the two. The art of preserving food has been brought to a sufficient state of perfection for this to be realized, but, at the same time, it must be admitted that there remains room for improvement, and, doubtless, with advancing experience, improvement will follow. Much attention, indeed, is being given to the matter, and it may be looked upon as forming one of the most important questions of the day.

The object in view is to check the change which spontaneously occurs when food is exposed to ordinary conditions. I need not enter here into the theoretical considerations that have been broached regarding the precise cause of this change, which we speak of as decomposition and putrefaction. Suffice it to state that there are three conditions essential to its occurrence. These are the presence of, 1st, warmth; 2d, moisture; and, 3d, air. The exclusion of either of these conditions will prevent the occurrence of decomposition, and thus we are supplied at once with three means of preserving food, viz., 1st, by the influence of cold; 2d, the removal of moisture, or drying; and 3d, the exclusion of air.

There is still another principle of action that can be brought to bear, and this is, 4th, the influence of certain chemical agents. The effect of these is (whether by destroying or rendering inactive the germs contained in the air supposed to excite decomposition, or whatever else their *modus operandi*) to render the article resistant to the operation of the ordinary influences.   Each of these principles of action will be cursorily referred to.

1. *Cold.*—At the freezing-point molecular change is entirely checked, and as long as they remain in a frozen state, organic substances are maintained in a state of preservation for an indefinite time.   In illustration of this, it may be mentioned that the guides at Chamounix are ready to relate to visitors the circumstance that human remains, belonging to members of an Alpine party killed by an avalanche whilst making the ascent of Mont Blanc in 1820, Were disclosed in a perfectly fresh state in 1861 and 1863 at the foot of the Glacier des Bossons, five and one-half miles from the seat of the accident.   Immersed in the glacier, they were gradually brought down by its continual descent to the point where they were discovered, which is where the glacier is progressively melting away in correspondence with its advance.

Cold is very extensively employed as a preservative agency.   Ice is now largely used by fishmongers, and other dealers in perishable animal foods, to enable them to keep their stock in a fresh condition.   The ice-chest is also considered almost a necessary appurtenance, certainly during the summer months, for preserving food in large establishments.   In ocean-going passenger-steamers, meat is preserved on a large scale by introduction into an ice-room or chamber.   An attempt has just been made to bring meat over in a frozen state from Australia.   The experiment failed from the cold not having been properly sustained on the voyage, but there is no reason that the process should not be susceptible of being successfully carried out, so far as the act of preservation is concerned. The question of expense, however, will have to form an element of consideration, and experience must decide whether any serious deterioration of the article arises from the complete freezing that is necessary.   Meat that has been frozen is subsequently less resistant to change than before, and butchers in this country take steps to avoid allowing the frost in very cold weather to affect the contents of their shops.

2. *Drying.*—Preservation by drying is applied to both animal and vegetable foods.   The practice is one of great antiquity, and it allows a number of articles of ordinary consumption to be kept in a state always ready for use.   Latterly it has been artificially applied to potatoes and other vegetables, as well as some fruits, and with such success that, after being properly soaked and cooked, they closely approach, both in appearance and taste, the fresh articles, and thus furnish a very fair substitute for them where circumstances do not permit them to be obtained.   It does not answer so well for animal substances, although a quantity of food (both meat and fish) preserved in this way is to be met with.   The drying here leads to more or less loss of the natural flavor, and an unpleasant taste is apt to be generated.   Under the name of *charqui,* beef which has been cut into strips or slices, and dried, is imported from South America. *Pemmican,* which was formerly so extensively used by Arctic voyagers, consists of dried and pulverized meat mixed with fat.   It presents a large amount of nourishment in a small space.

3. *Exclusion of air.*—This is the principle upon which food is now being extensively preserved, to some extent for home use, but chiefly for transport from one locality to another.   It is imperfectly carried out in the domestic operation of covering potted-meat with a layer of melted butter or some other kind of fat.   Some articles also are preserved by immersion in oil.   The bottled and tinned provisions represent a more perfect application of the process.   The food is introduced into a suitable bottle or

tin, and, after having been heated so as to drive out the air by the generation of steam, the opening is closed and hermetically sealed in order to prevent any subsequent re-entrance from without.   When properly performed, the efficacy of the process is such, that after the lapse of many years the provisions have been found in a perfectly good and sound condition.   It is applied to both animal and vegetable articles of food.

The fruit and vegetables preserved in bottles and tins permit us to obtain the representative of the fresh article at all seasons of the year and in all localities, and so closely does the preserved approach in character the fresh fruit or vegetable, that there is little discoverable difference between the two.

Every variety of meat and soup, and also fish, lobsters, etc., are now to be obtained in a preserved state, and importation upon a very extensive scale has lately been carried on into this country from Australia and elsewhere.   An important branch of trade has, indeed, sprung up during the last few years in this department of commerce, which is rapidly increasing, and promises ultimately to attain enormous dimensions.   The plan of preserving that is generally adopted is described in an Australian journal to be as follows:

The meat-preserving establishments are so situated as to combine, as fully as may be found possible, proximity to a well-supplied cattle market, with facilities for the shipment of the finished product.   Whenever practicable, grazing paddocks are provided adjacent to the works, in which to keep the stock purchased until required for use.   The animals are slaughtered, skinned, and dismembered.   From the slaughter-house the meat is removed on tramways, or by sliding it along suspended from iron bars, to the "boning-room," where the process of meat-preserving properly commences.   Expert butchers, paid by the piece, here take the meat in hand, and, taught by long practice and stimulated by the desire to earn large wages, perform their work with surprising skill and rapidity.   Their duty is to cut the meat from the bone and remove superfluous fat; and so thoroughly is the work done, that a hungry dog, it is stated, would have to turn over a large number of bones before it could obtain a dinner from the minute shreds of meat adhering to them.   The meat is now conveyed to the kitchen, and here it is in the first place cut into suitable pieces for tinning, and weighed.   In some establishments it is then partially cooked, generally by means of steam; in others it is put into the tins in a raw state, with the addition of a little salt.   Usually a surplus allowance of a few ounces, the number varying according to the size of the tin, is made for the loss that occurs in cooking.   Sometimes some rich gravy, extracted from portions of meat which are not suitable for tinning, is added to each tin.   The tops are then soldered on, a small hole being left in the middle of each.   This is one of the most critical operations in the whole process, since everything depends on the tins being air-tight, and the most skilful tinsmiths are employed to perform it.   The canisters, arranged in numbers together on a perforated tray, are next lowered into a bath containing a saturated solution of chloride of calcium, and there allowed to remain immersed to within an inch or two of their tops, at a gradually increasing temperature, until the contents are cooked, and all atmospheric air is expelled through the small orifice in the top.   The hole is then closed with solder, and the canister subjected to a short, thorough immersion in the heated solution, the temperature of which considerably exceeds that of boiling water.   All that now remains is to cool, clean, test, and paint the canisters.   After removal from the heated bath they are placed in cold water, cleaned, and then transferred to the testing-room. This is an artificially heated room, in which they are allowed to remain for a period of six days. Should there be the slightest leak in the solder of the tin, the defect will show itself within this time by the bulging out of the ends, due to the generation of gas as the result of decomposition occurring within. The canisters that stand the test are, lastly, painted, labelled, and packed for exportation. As long as their contents remain good they give signs of the absence of putrefactive gases by the depression of the surface caused by the condensation ensuing after the process of hermetically sealing.

Meat preserved in this way sustains no loss of its nutritive capacity, and it possesses the pecuniary advantage of being free from bone. The material is there with its proper aptitude for digestion. The only objection is, that through the heat employed to ensure its preservation it is brought into an over-cooked condition. It is probably impossible, in depending only on heat, to escape from this objection, for experiments on the putrefactive process show that not only is it necessary to exclude all air containing active germs, but the germs must be destroyed that are in contact with the article itself, and it requires a high temperature to accomplish this result.

Milk may be preserved by the same method, but when treated in the ordinary state the disadvantage arises of the butter separating and not being afterward miscible with the liquid. To overcome this objection the milk is concentrated to a thickish consistence, and is also mixed with sugar. In this state it will keep for some time after the tin is opened.

4. *Preservation of food by the use of antiseptics.*—There are several agents that are employed for this purpose. Salt is one of the most common, and nitre is frequently associated with it. The effect of a saline, however, is to depreciate the nutritive value of the article by extracting the soluble constituents, and by also hardening the texture, so as to render it difficult of digestion. Syrup, alcohol, and vinegar form other agents in common use as preservatives. After being to some extent salted, certain kinds of meat and fish are often subjected to smoking. The empyreumatic vapor with which they become penetrated possesses a strong antiseptic capacity, which greatly promotes their power of keeping.

The analysis of brine shows that the process of salting must materially diminish the nutritive value of meat, for it is found to contain a large portion of the ingredients of its juice. Not only does the contraction which ensues cause the infiltrating liquid to be driven out, but the liquefied salt tends further to draw out by osmosis its diffusible organic and saline constituents. Liebig estimates the loss of nutritive value as amounting to one-third or even one-half. Soaking salted meat in water removes its saltness, but cannot, of course, restore the nutritive principles that have been lost.

From experience it has been learnt that salted and dried food cannot be used continuously for a lengthened period without impairing the health. The well-known effect is the development of a cachectic state which manifests itself under the form of what are called scorbutic affections.

18

PRINCIPLES OF DIETETICS.

THE physiological properties of the various alimentary principles, looked at individually, were considered in a former part of this work; they here require to be spoken of collectively in reference to the maintenance of life.

It happens that an article, viz., milk, is produced by the operations of nature for the special purpose of sustaining life during an early period of the existence of the mammalian animal. Such an article may be taken as affording a typical illustration of natural food. Now we find, on looking to its composition, that it contains the following alimentary principles:

Nitrogenous matter (caseine principally, and in smaller quantity some other forms of albuminoid matter).

Fatty matter (butter).

A carbohydrate (lactine).

Inorganic matter, comprising salines and water.

The egg, also, stands in an analogous position. As all the parts of the young animal are evolved from it, it must needs represent the material, or contain the suitable principles, for the development and growth of the body, and the same groups of principles are to be recognized that exist in milk, although in the case of one of them it is only present to a somewhat minute extent. 1st, nitrogenous matter is largely present, under the form of albumen, both in the white and yolk; 2d, oily matter is contained in the yolk; 3d, saccharine matter, a principle belonging to the carbohydrate group, is to be detected; but only, it must be mentioned, to a sparing extent, in which respect the composition of the egg differs notably from that of milk; 4th, inorganic matter, consisting of salines and water, completes the list, and for the saline matter required, that belonging to the shell is drawn upon as the process of incubation proceeds. As Liebig has pointed out, there is an insufficiency of mineral matter in the soft contents of the egg for the development of the skeleton and other parts of the chick, but the shell forms a store of earthy matter which gradually becomes dissolved by the phosphoric acid generated through the oxidizing influence of the air upon the phosphorus existing amongst the contents of the egg. By the occurrence of this process the shell becomes thinner and thinner as incubation, or development of the chick, advances.

We thus see that in these products, which are specially designed in the economy of nature for the development and nutrition of animal beings, it is a combination of principles that is present. This may be therefore taken as suggestive that such a combination is needed, and experiments upon alimentation have abundantly proved it to be the case. It is not this or that alimentary principle which can be separated artificially from others that will suffice for sustaining life, but different principles associated together, just as we find them in the productions of nature. As objects of nature ourselves, it is the productions of nature that form our appropriate food. We are so framed as to depend for existence upon natural productions, and unless we are supplied with such a combination of principles as is met with in natural productions, defective nutrition results.

It was formerly thought that the nitrogenous principles ought to be capable of sustaining life, seeing that they not only represent what is wanted for administering to the nutrition of the body, but through their carbon and hydrogen can also contribute toward heat-production, and it excited surprise when it was discovered experimentally that animals perished of inanition, exactly as if they had been deprived of all food, when confined exclusively to these principles. Tiedemann and Gmelin found that geese were starved upon an abundant supply of white of egg, but it is especially to the researches of the Paris Gelatine Commission that we are indebted for a comprehensive survey of the subject.

The labors of this Commission were instigated with the view of determining whether the gelatinous extract from bones could properly supply the place of meat, particularly as food for the poor. It had been asserted that such was the case, and the investigation was undertaken by a commission appointed by the Academy of Sciences of Paris and named the Gelatine Commission. After nearly ten years, it is stated, of uninterrupted research, the report was sent in by Magendie in the name of the Commission. The question which the Commission primarily undertook to decide was : *Whether it was possible, economically, to extract from bones an aliment which alone or mixed with other substances could take the place of meat;* but the inquiry led on to the study of the nutritive properties of the alimentary principles in general. The conclusions arrived at by this Commission form simple expressions of well-ascertained facts, and therefore, unlike many physiological conclusions, stand uncontroverted by the experience of the thirty years which have elapsed since the report was drawn up.* They are of sufficient interest and importance to lead me to introduce them here. They run as follows :

First.—It is not possible by any known process to extract from bones an aliment which, either alone or mixed with other substances, can take the place of meat.

Second.—Gelatine, albumen, and fibrine, taken separately, nourish animals but for a very limited period, and only in a very incomplete manner. In general they soon excite an insurmountable disgust, so that the animals rather die than partake of them.

Third.—These same alimentary principles, artificially reunited and rendered agreeably sapid by seasoning, are taken more readily and for a longer period than when in a separate state ; but they have no better ultimate influence on nutrition, for the animals that eat them, even in considerable quantities, end by dying, with all the signs of complete inanition.

Fourth.—Muscular flesh, in which gelatine, albumen, and fibrine are united according to the laws of organic nature and associated with other matters, as fat, salts, etc., suffices, even in very small quantity, for complete and prolonged nutrition.

---

* Comptes Rendus des Séances de l'Académie des Sciences, tome 13me, p. 282. Paris, 1841.

Fifth.—Raw bones can do the same, but the quantity consumed in the twenty-four hours must be very much larger than in the case of meat.

Sixth.—Every kind of preparation, such as decoction with water, the action of hydrochloric acid, and particularly the transformation into gelatine, diminishes, and seems even, in certain cases, almost completely to destroy the nutritive quality of bones.

Seventh.—The Commission, however, is unwilling at present to express an opinion upon the employment of gelatine associated with other aliments, in the nourishment of man. It believes that direct experiment can alone throw light upon this subject in a definite ·manner. It is actively occupying itself with reference to the point, and the results will be made known in the second and last part of the report.

Eighth.—Gluten extracted from wheaten or maize flour satisfies by itself complete and prolonged nutrition.

Ninth.—Fats taken alone sustain life for some time, but give rise to an imperfect and disordered nutrition, fat accumulating in all the tissues, sometimes in the state of oleine and stearine, sometimes in that of almost pure stearine.

Looking at the above conclusions, the one which refers to gluten (eighth) stands in opposition to the others. Surprise is expressed in the report, and it does seem surprising, that whilst other isolated alimentary principles failed in sustaining life, gluten should be capable of affording perfect nourishment for animals; nevertheless, it is stated that animals were kept upon it for three months without interruption, and presented throughout this period all the signs of excellent health. The explanation suggested in the report for this discordant and unexpected result is that the gluten employed did not form a pure alimentary principle, but retained some starch and other non-nitrogenous matter. Doubtless, also, there must have been mineral matter likewise present, for it would be inconsistent from what we now know, that life should be maintained for a lengthened period in the absence of this constituent of food. Under this view the discordancy becomes reconciled, the result observed being attributable to a mixture of substances being in reality consumed, instead of a single alimentary principle.

The Paris Commission having found that gelatine taken alone failed to nourish animals, a Commission of the Institute of Amsterdam undertook to determine whether it increased the nutritive value of other aliments to which it might be added. Evidence was drawn in the same manner as had been done by the Paris Commission, from experiments conducted upon dogs, and the conclusion arrived at was that gelatine was not only of no nutritive value when taken alone, but was not made nutritive by combination with other substances.[*] This conclusion, which places gelatine in the position of a useless agent in an alimentary point of view is inconsistent with the now well-established fact that the ingestion of gelatine, like that of other nitrogenous principles, gives rise to an increase in the elimination of urea; for, as pointed out in a previous part of this work, with the production of urea from nitrogenous matter a hydrocarbonaceous compound is left, which is evidently susceptible of being turned to account as a force-producing agent in the system.

Some results obtained by Mr. Savory, it may be remarked, have been interpreted and quoted as showing that nitrogenous matter, combined only with the appropriate saline principles, suffices for the maintenance of

---

[*] Gazette Médicale, tome 12me, p. 176. Paris, 1844.

life. Thus, in "Kirke's Physiology," seventh edition, p. 259, it is stated: "Contrary to the views of Liebig and Lehmann, Savory has shown that, while animals speedily die when confined to non-nitrogenous diet, they may live long when fed exclusively with nitrogenous food." Again, Dr. Parkes ("Hygiene," third edition, p. 160) says: "For though the dog and the rat (Savory) can live on fat-free meat alone, man cannot do so." Bischoff and Voit found that dogs could be sustained on meat deprived of visible fat, and maintained at their full weight with but very slight variation, whilst Ranke, it appears, could not maintain himself in perfect nutrition on meat alone.

Now, with reference to these statements, it must be borne in mind that after the removal of the visible fat, flesh still contains a certain amount which is brought into view by analysis. It cannot be deprived of fat beyond 1 per cent., and in Savory's experiments on rats, the flesh (lean veal) employed was found to contain 1.55 per cent.* But, let us look into the particulars of the experiments, and see what they in reality prove.

In the first place, 1.55 per cent. of fat in meat means *rather over* 6 *per cent.* in the dry matter of meat, about three-fourths of fresh meat being made up of water.

In one experiment a couple of rats, which had been nearly brought to the verge of death by restriction to starchy matter and fat, were fed with bread and meat for four days, and then with meat alone. A week after commencing the meat their united weight was 9 oz. 1½ dr., and three weeks later 10 oz. 1 dr. Being now placed on a diet of meat, with non-nitrogenous food (starch and fat), a notable improvement occurred, for in three days' time they weighed 11 oz.; four days later 14 oz. 12 drs.; and a week later still, 14 oz. 4 drs.

In another experiment two rats, weighing 12 oz. were placed on an exclusive diet of lean meat and water. They remained healthy in appearance, but *steadily lost weight, and in a month's time weighed only 8¾ oz.* They were now placed on a miscellaneous diet, and in a week's time weighed 12½ oz.

In a third experiment two rats, weighing together 12 oz. 7 drs., were kept upon the meat diet exclusively. On the thirteenth day *one of the rats died*, the weight of its body being 2 oz. 8 drs., and that of the other 6 oz. 3 drs. The live one was still restricted to the same food, *and this died ten days later*, the weight of its body then being 5 oz. It is worthy of mention, as a passing remark, that two other pairs of rats which had been taken at the same time, one pair being fed on a non-nitrogenous diet and the other on a mixed diet, remained still alive.

I have entered into these particulars because the experiments in question, contrary to their true effect, have been referred to as invalidating the accredited doctrine—that to sustain life in an *efficient* manner there must be an admixture of the nitrogenous and non-nitrogenous alimentary principles. Before quitting the subject it is right to state that a hawk was kept for two months on the same meat food, and improved, it is asserted, in appearance and condition. No weights, however, are given, and the quantity of food consumed is not mentioned. With the 1.55 per cent. of fat in the fresh meat, forming rather over 6 per cent. of the dry material, a sufficiently notable amount of fat may have been ingested if the quantity of food consumed was large. It is not contended that heat or force-production generally is dependent solely upon the non-nitrogenous aliment supplied, for it is well known that the nitrogenous principles undergo metamorphosis into urea, and an oxidizable residue which is susceptible of utilization in that direction; but observation tends to show that, for the proper maintenance of nutrition (and it must be remembered that fat is a necessary agent in the accomplishment of the formative processes), the presence of *some* non-nitrogenous matter at least is needed in the food.

If the nitrogenous principles, from their capacity for yielding the requisite material for the construction and maintenance of the tissues, and likewise from their capacity for undergoing metamorphosis into urea and a hydrocarbonaceous product susceptible of appropriation to force-production, might appear theoretically sufficient, so far as organic matter is concerned, for the support of life, such even cannot be said with respect to the non-nitrogenous principles. These could not possibly be expected to suffice for maintaining life, as an element is missing which is wanted for the formation of the tissues. Experimental proof, however, has been adduced upon the point. Fat formed one of the articles subjected to investigation by the Gelatine Commission, and its inability to support life is shown amongst the conclusions that were arrived at. Boussingault also fed a duck on butter only, and found that it died at the end of three weeks of starvation. Butter, it is said, exuded from all parts of the body, and the feathers seemed as if they had been soaked in melted butter.

Sugar, gum, and starch were submitted to experiment by Magendie on dogs, and Tiedemann and Gmelin on geese; the animals became emaciated and more and more feeble, till they perished of inanition. Like experiments have since also been performed by others, and corresponding results obtained.

When fat is combined with other non-nitrogenous matter, emaciation is still one of the phenomena observed. In Mr. Savory's experiments on rats * fed on equal parts by weight of arrow-root, sago, tapioca, lard, and suet—a mixture found to contain only .22 per cent. of nitrogen—the animals underwent emaciation and died of inanition, fat having disappeared from the body, as occurs under complete privation of food. Notwithstanding this absence of fat from the body, the fur of the animals was observed to have presented a decidedly greasy appearance, just as though fat exuded from the skin, in correspondence with what Boussingault noticed in his experiment where a duck was fed exclusively on butter.

It may be inferred that nitrogenous matter is required not only for the formation of the tissues, but likewise for contributing, by the promotion of the requisite change, to the utilization of the non-nitrogenous principles, and, unless it exist in suitable amount in the food, these principles fail to pass on to their proper destination. It is known that the carbohydrates contribute to the formation and accumulation of fat; but, for this to take place, the concurrence of a due amount of nitrogenous matter is required. Boussingault's experiments on pigs showed that whilst potatoes alone did not suffice for fattening the animals, they grew fat with the addition of nitrogenous matter; and the presence of fat also in the food seems in some manner or other likewise to promote the transformation of the carbohydrates. Boussingault also found that the cow was insufficiently nourished on potatoes and beet-root alone, although given in very large quantity.

The question as to whether non-nitrogenous matter should enter into the composition of food has been sufficiently discussed already, but another question presents itself: Are both fats and carbo-hydrates necessary? If we look to the diets of different nations we almost invariably find that both these principles are represented. Still it is evident that fat alone will suffice for yielding the non-nitrogenous matter required for the support of life, for we find in certain parts of the globe that there are large numbers of persons who subsist, and maintain themselves in good health, exclusively on animal food, in which fat forms the only representative of non-nitrogenous matter. As to whether, however, the carbo-hydrates can similarly supply what is wanted, forms a question that is not so summarily to be disposed of. It is true there are some articles of vegetable food which are capable of sustaining life, and which, whilst freely containing a carbohydrate, contain a comparatively insignificant quantity of fat; but the presence of fat, as has been already mentioned, appears to be of service in promoting the metamorphosis of the carbo-hydrates in the system. It also exerts a favorable influence over the assimilation of nitrogenous matter and the processes of tissue formation and nutrition; and it may be said that there is strong reason to believe that the association of a certain amount of fatty matter with the carbo-hydrates is probably necessary for the maintenance of the organism in perfect health. The belief is further entertained that its deficiency is sometimes the source of the development of the tuberculous diathesis.

Inorganic matter, under the form of saline materials and water, is equally as essential for satisfying the requirements of life as the organic components of food. Although such saline materials and water do not appear to be individually concerned in the interplay of changes which form the source of the phenomena of life, they nevertheless enter as essential elements into the constitution of the textures and fluids of the body, and thus must needs be supplied, to an adequate extent to meet the requirements of nutrition and secretion, with the food from without.

Such form the principles that are required as components of food for the maintenance of the body in a healthy condition. But as yet I have only referred to the nature of the principles, and not to their amount. As regards the inorganic portion of food, it may simply be said that enough of the several principles encountered in the body must be supplied to meet the wants of nutrition and secretion. The organic portion, however, cannot be so summarily disposed of, and the question first arises: What relative proportion of nitrogenous and non-nitrogenous principles is best adapted for administering to the requirements of life?

It may be fairly concluded that the requirements as regards food vary with exposure to different conditions. According to the expenditure that is taking place, so, in a good scheme of dieting, should materials be supplied which are best calculated to yield what is wanted. Under exposure to hard labor and inactivity, and to a high and low external temperature, the consumption of material in the system differs, and the supply of food should be regulated accordingly. Notwithstanding the tenor of recent experiments as to mechanical or muscular work being obtainable from the oxidation of non-nitrogenous matter, general experience is to the effect that for the maintenance of a good condition nitrogenous matter is required in larger quantity under greater exertion than during a state of rest. The inhabitants of the colder regions also require to be more perfectly supplied with combustible matter than persons inhabiting warmer climates.

The laws of nature are such as to conduce to an adaptation of the supply of food to its demand. We are all conversant with the fact that exercise and exposure to cold—conditions which increase the demand for food—sharpen the appetite, and thus lead to a larger quantity of material being consumed; whilst, conversely, a state of inactivity and a warm climate tell in an opposite manner, and reduce the inclination for food. A badly fed laborer is capable of performing but a slight day's work, and a starving man falls an easy victim to the effects of exposure to cold.

Not only is there thus a correspondence between the amount of food required and the inclination for taking it, but, probably arising from the teachings of experience, we find the nature of the food selected in different countries to vary, and to constitute that which is most in conformity with what is needed.

For example, the dwellers in the arctic regions, besides consuming an enormous—even prodigious—quantity of food, partake of that kind which abounds in the most efficient form of heat-generating material, viz., oleagi-. nous matter. It is from the bodies of seals and whales, and such like sources, that the food of the extreme northerners is obtained. It is true the coldness of the climate will not permit the production and supply of the carbohydrates by vegetable growth, as occurs in low latitudes; but, if it did, they could hardly be consumed in sufficient quantity to yield the requisite amount of heat.

Sir Anthony Carlisle relates an anecdote from his experience amongst the arctic inhabitants: "The most northern races of mankind," he says, "were found to be unacquainted with the taste of sweets, and their infants made wry faces and sputtered out sugar with disgust; but the little urchins grinned with ecstasy at the sight of a bit of whale's blubber."

In the tropics, on the other hand, it is especially upon vegetable products—products largely charged with principles belonging to the carbohydrate group instead of fat—that the native inhabitants subsist. The succulent fruits and vegetables, says Liebig, on which the natives of the south prefer to feed, do not in the fresh state contain more than 12 per cent. of carbon. The blubber and train oil, on the other hand, which enter largely into the diet of the extreme northerner, contain, he remarks, from 66 to 80 per cent. of carbon.

For a temperate climate reason would suggest something between the two extremes as yielding the most suitable form of food, and custom, we find, has led to the selection of a mixed diet, which furnishes the combination of the two kinds of heat-producing principles.

It is, then, upon the principle of adaptiveness to the particular requirement existing that the diet should be made to conform. The performance of work was until recently believed, in accordance with Liebig's teachings, to have its source in the metamorphosis of nitrogenous matter. It was considered that muscular and nervous action resulted from an oxidation of muscular and nervous tissue, and that, according to the extent of action occurring, so was a supply of the nitrogenous alimentary principles demanded to replace the oxidized material. This gave to nitrogenous matter a special position in relation to the manifestation of nervomuscular activity, and Liebig measured the working value of food by the amount of what he styled the plastic elements of nutrition it contained. The following table was framed by him to show, upon this principle, the relative working value of various articles of food in common use. To bring the comparison to uniformity, the non-nitrogenous matter is all reckoned as starch. The relative value of fat and starch for heat-producing purposes may be reckoned from the amount of oxygen respectively required for the complete oxidation of the product, and it is found to stand in the ratio of 1 to 2.4. Thus, by a simple process of calculation, fat, when this form of non-nitrogenous matter exists in a given article of food, is easily reduced into its heat-producing equivalent of starch.

Liebig's Tabular Representation of the Relative Nutritive Value of Various Articles of Food.

	Plastic nitrogenous matter.	Non-nitrogenous calorifacient matter reckoned as starch.
Veal,	10	1
Hare's flesh,	10	2
Beef,	10	17
Beans,	10	22
Peas,	10	23
Fat mutton,	10	27
Fat pork,	10	30
Cow's milk,	10	30
Woman's milk,	10	40
Wheaten flour,	10	46
Oatmeal,	10	50
Rye,	10	57
Barley,	10	57
Potatoes,	10	86 to 115
Rice,	10	123

It has been previously shown in this work that there is now strong reason to believe that, in opposition to Liebig's view, the non-nitrogenous elements of food contribute, as well as the nitrogenous, to the production of muscular force, and, with this before us, nitrogenous matter ceases to hold the special value as a source of working power that was, till quite recently, assigned to it.

It was through the extension of the doctrine of the conservation of energy (which implies that force is readily transmutable from one form into another, but, like matter, not susceptible of being created from nothing, nor of being destroyed) to living bodies, combined with the results obtained by Fick and Wislicenus in their ascent of the Faulhorn (*vide* p. 45), that physiologists were led to entertain the view that is now held. Fick and Wislicenus proved that the oxidation of their muscular tissue, as measured by the amount of nitrogen voided with the urine, sufficed only for the production of a small proportion of the force expended in the accomplishment of the measured work performed. The only conclusion they could arrive at, therefore, was that muscular power originated from the oxidation of non-nitrogenous matter, of which their food exclusively consisted for a short time before and during the period of the ascent.

Experiments have since been performed by other observers, with corroborative results, and it may now be looked upon as a settled point that non-nitrogenous alimentary matter contributes, in a manner not before suspected, to muscular force-production.

As a sequel to this deduction, Professor Frankland * undertook the experimental determination of the force-producing value of various articles in common use as food. His results represent the actual force evolved by complete oxidation, under the form of heat, measured by means of the calorimeter. Now, heat and mechanical work are not only mutually convertible, but bear a fixed quantitative relation to each other. A certain amount of heat, in other words, is transformable into a definite amount of motive power capable of performing a fixed and ascertainable amount of mechanical work. Thus, by calculation, the value of a given article of food is easily represented in working power. It is in this way that the measure of working power has been deduced. Professor Frankland's table will be found annexed. In it the Continental weights and measures are employed.† The unit of heat is the amount of heat which will raise the temperature of 1 gramme (15.432 grains) of water 1° Cent. (1.8° Fahr.). A kilogrammetre of force is the representative of the power required to lift 1 kilogramme (2.2046 pounds avoirdupois) 1 metre (3.2808 feet) high. The value of the various articles mentioned in the list in units of heat is the result of direct observation, whilst that in kilogrammetres of force is obtained by calculation upon the basis of Mr. Joule's estimate, which represents the heat that will raise the temperature of 1 kilogramme of water 1° Cent. as equivalent to the mechanical power required to lift 1 kilogramme 423½ metres high, or, what is the same thing, 423½ kilogrammes 1 metre high.

---

* Philos. Mag., vol. xxxii., 1866.

† Expressed in English weights and measures it is the foot-pound, or the power required to lift one pound one foot high, which forms the unit of work, and 772 foot-pounds represent, according to Mr. Joule's estimate, the dynamic equivalent of 1° Fahr.—that is, the heat required to raise the temperature of one pound of water 1° Fahr. constitutes the equivalent of the power required to lift one pound 772 feet high. Kilogrammetres are convertible into foot-pounds by multiplying by 7.232; one kilogramme (2.2046 pounds avoirdupois) raised one metre (3.2808 feet) high equalling one pound raised 7.232 feet high.

Force-producing Value of One Gramme (15.432 *Grains*) *of Various Articles of Food* (Frankland).

NAME OF FOOD.	Per cent. of water present.	FORCE-PRODUCING VALUE.		
		In units of heat.	In kilogrammetres of force.	
			When burnt in oxygen.	When oxidized in the body.
Cod-liver oil, ...	—	9,107	3,857	3,857
Beef fat, ...	—	9,069	3,841	3,841
Butter, ...	—	7,264	3,077	3,077
Cocoa-nibs, ...	—	6,873	2,911	2,902
Cheese (Cheshire), ...	24.0	4,647	1,969	1,846
Isinglass, ...	—	4,520	1,914	1,550
Bread-crust, ...	—	4,459	1,868	—
Oatmeal, ...	—	4,004	1,696	1,665
Flour, ...	—	3,936	1,669	1,627
Pea-meal, ...	—	3,936	1,667	1,598
Arrow-root, ...	—	3,912	1,657	1,657
Ground rice, ...	—	3,813	1,615	1,591
Yolk of egg, ...	47.0	3,423	1,449	1,400
Lump sugar, ...	—	3,348	1,418	1,418
Grape-sugar (commercial), . .	—	3,277	1,388	1,388
Hard-boiled egg, ...	62.3	2,383	1,009	966
Bread-crumb, ...	44.0	2,231	945	910
Lean ham (boiled), ...	54.4	1,980	839	711
Mackerel, ...	70.5	1,789	758	683
Beef (lean), ...	70.5	1,567	664	604
Veal (lean), ...	70.9	1,314	556	496
Guinness's stout, ...	88.4	1,076	455	455
Potatoes, ...	73.0	1,013	429	422
Whiting, ...	80.0	904	383	335
Bass's ale (alcohol reckoned), . .	88.4	775	328	328
White of egg, ...	86.3	671	284	244
Milk, ...	87.0	662	280	266
Apples, ...	82.0	660	280	273
Carrots, ...	86.0	527	223	220
Cabbage, ...	88.5	434	184	178

In the foregoing table it will be seen that the working value is not the same where nitrogenous matter has to be dealt with, when oxidized in the body, as when burnt in oxygen. This arises from the occurrence of complete oxidation in the one case, and not in the other. Whilst with non-nitrogenous matters complete oxidation of the elements occurs within the body, as when burnt without, it is not so with nitrogenous matters. These in the system are only partially consumed, the nitrogen escaping under the form of urea, and carrying off a portion of the carbon and hydrogen in an imperfectly oxidized condition. This final product of animal consumption, therefore, possesses a certain amount of unexpended force (at least one-seventh of that originally belonging to the material), whereas the final products of burning in oxygen—consisting of free nitrogen, carbonic acid, and water—represent fully exhausted principles. It is of course assumed, in speaking of the force-producing value of articles consumed in the body, that this only refers to the material that is actually digested and utilized, which certainly as a rule is far from comprising the whole that is consumed as food.

Taking the force-value as given above, and reckoning, in accordance with Helmholz' calculation, that the animal system is capable of turning one-fifth of the actual energy developed by the oxidation of the food to account as external work, Professor Frankland has determined the weight and cost of various alimentary articles that would be required to raise the body-weight of a person of 10 stone, or 140 lbs., to a height of 10,000 feet.

Weight and Cost of Various Articles of Food that would Require to be Consumed in the System to Raise the Body of a Person Weighing 10 *Stone, or* 140 *Lbs., to a Height of* 10,000 *Feet* (Frankland).

Name of Food.	Weight in pounds required.	At price per pound.	Cost.
		s. *d.*	*s.* *d.*
Cod-liver oil,	0.553	3 6	1 11¼
Beef fat,	0.555	0 10	0 5½
Butter,	0.693	1 6	1 0½
Cocoa-nibs,	0.735	1 6	1 1¼
Cheshire cheese,	1.156	0 10	0 11½
Oatmeal,	1.281	0 2¾	0 3½
Arrow-root,	1.287	1 0	1 3½
Flour,	1.311	0 2¾	0 3¾
Pea-meal,	1.335	0 3½	0 4½
Ground rice,	1.341	0 4	0 5½
Isinglass,	1.377	16 0	22 0½
Lump sugar,	1.505	0 6	0 9
Commercial grape-sugar,	1.537	0 3½	0 5½
Hard-boiled eggs,	2.209	0 6½	1 2½
Bread,	2.345	0 2	0 4¾
Lean ham (boiled),	3.001	1 6	4 6
Mackerel,	3.124	0 8	2 1
Lean beef,	3.532	1 0	3 6½
Lean veal,	4.300	1 0	4 3½
Potatoes,	5.068	0 1	0 5¼
Whiting,	6.369	1 4	9 4
Apples,	7.815	0 1½	0 11¾
Milk,	8.021	5*d.* per quart	1 3½
White of egg,	8.745	0 6	4 4½
Carrots,	9.685	0 1½	1 2½
Cabbage,	12.020	0 1	1 0¼
Guinness's stout (bottled),	6¾ bottles.	10*d.* per bottle	5 7½
Bass's pale ale (bottled),	9 bottles.	10*d.* "	7 6

Looked at in the manner above represented, muscular work, like heat, in opposition to Liebig's theory, is derivable from the oxidation of non-nitrogenous as well as nitrogenous matter, and Professor Frankland's tables show that .55 lbs. of fatty matter will furnish the same amount of power as is obtainable from 1.3 lb. of flour, 1.5 lb. of sugar, 3.5 lbs. of lean beef, and 5 lbs. of potatoes. Traube even inverted the proposition of Liebig, and asserted, in the most decided manner, that the substances by the oxidation of which force is generated in the muscles are not the albuminous constituents of the tissue, but non-nitrogenous principles, viz., either fats or carbohydrates.

According to the foregoing table, wherein is mentioned the cost of the various articles of food required to be consumed to accomplish a given amount of work, it appears, viewing these articles purely in their capacity as force-producing agents by oxidation, that the same amount of work is obtainable from oatmeal costing 3½d.; flour, 3¾d.; bread, 4¾d.; and beef fat, 5½d.; as from beef costing 3s. 6½d., and isinglass, £1 2s. 0½d.

Taking all the facts at present revealed into consideration, we appear to be warranted in adopting the following terms of expression. It is in the first place admitted on all hands that food is the source from which muscular power is derived, and hence the supply of food should be in proportion to the amount of work that is performed. It was formerly thought that food must be converted into muscular tissue before it could be available for the performance of work which involved the origin of work from nitrogenous alimentary matter. The effect of recent investigation, however, is to show that it is not to an oxidation of muscular tissue that we are to look for the force produced. The muscles appear to stand in the position of instruments for effecting the conversion of the chemical energy evolved by the oxidation of combustible matter into working power. Fats and carbohydrates can furnish the combustible matter required, and, under ordinary circumstances, probably do largely, if not chiefly, supply it. Nitrogenous matter can do so likewise, but it has to undergo a preparatory metamorphosis for effecting the separation of nitrogen in a suitable form for elimination.

As pointed out in a previous part of this work (*vide* p. 41 *et seq.*), it is under the form of urea that the nitrogen of digested and absorbed nitrogenous matter mainly escapes. This body consists, besides nitrogen, of carbon, hydrogen, and oxygen, and the amount of oxygen is such as to leave a portion of the carbon and hydrogen in a combustible or oxidizable condition. In the escape of urea, therefore, there is a loss or waste of a portion of the force-producing power of the original nitrogenous principle, and, taking dry nitrogenous matter, as nearly as possible one-third passes off as urea. The remaining two-thirds form the available portion for force-production. But this residuary portion is made up in part of oxygen, and it is only in reality 50 per cent. of the original nitrogenous matter that consists of carbon and hydrogen in an oxidizable condition. Thus it is that, for force-production, nitrogenous matter is of less value than the fats and carbohydrates.

Observation shows that the results of experience fully accord with the teachings of science. In the case of navvies and other hard-working men the appetite is known by the employer to form a measure of capacity for work. A falling off of the appetite means, that is to say, a diminished capacity for the performance of work. A farmer, where wages were good, when asked, "how it was that he paid his laborers so well?" replied, "that he could not afford to pay them less, for he found that less wages produced less work." Indeed, one might just as reasonably expect that a fire would burn briskly with a scanty supply of fuel, or a steam-engine work with a deficient supply of coal, as that a man could labor upon a meagre diet. Men have also learned, where arduous work has to be performed, and similarly in cold climates where a large amount

of heat has to be produced—for the demand is the same in the two cases
—that the requirements are best met by a liberal consumption of fatty
matter, which is the most efficient kind of force-producing material, with
the food. The fat bacon relished and eaten with his bread by a hard-
working laborer yields, at a minimum cost, the force he forms the medium
for producing.

As thus considered, the non-nitrogenous alimentary principles appear
to possess a higher dietetic value than the nitrogenous, and when regarded solely in relation to capacity for force-production, there is no
doubt they in reality do so. But there is a further point to be looked at.
The physical development and maintenance of the body must be likewise
taken into account, and for this it is nitrogenous alimentary matter only
that can supply what is needed. Wherever vital operations are going
on, there exists nitrogenous matter. It is, indeed, through the instru-
mentality of nitrogenous matter that the operations of life occur. The
tissues which form the instrument of living action require to be constructed in the first instance; and next, to be constantly renovated, to
compensate for the loss by deterioration which is continually going on.
Thus, a demand for nitrogenous alimentary matter is created quite apart
from direct contribution to force-production; and, further, not only is
nitrogenous matter required for the construction and repair of the tissues,
but likewise to form a constituent of the secretions, for all secretions
which possess active properties owe them to the presence of a nitrogenous principle. Here, then, is an additional demand for nitrogenous matter, and it is to be remarked that as increased work leads to an increased
development of the tissues employed, and thereby an increased appropriation of nitrogenous matter, so it calls for an increased production of
secretions in consequence of the larger amount of food that has to be
prepared for consumption. In this way, theoretically, without contributing in a direct manner to force-production, the performance of work
may be looked upon as necessitating a proportionate supply of nitrogenous alimentary matter.

Practically, it is found that hard work is best performed under a
liberal supply of nitrogen-containing food. The reason probably is that
it leads to a better nourished condition of the muscles and of the body
generally. Under the use of animal food, which is characterized by its
richness in nitrogenous matter, the muscles, it is affirmed, are observed
to be firmer and richer in solid constituents than under subsistence upon
food of a vegetable nature. What meat is to man, corn, which of all
vegetable fodder contains the albuminates in the largest proportion, is
to the horse. Highly bred horses require richly nitrogenous food. The
Arab, says Donders, never lets his horse eat grass and hay to satiety.
Its chief food is barley, and in the wilderness it gets milk, and if great
effort is required, even camel's flesh. The horses which in Sahara are
used for hunting ostriches are kept nearly exclusively on camel's milk
and dried beans. In the case of our horses, too, he continues, it is well
known that to do heavy work they require more than grass and hay.
Corn is necessary to give strength and activity. Coachmen know that
"the oats must be in them." In order to perform hard work, horses
must have, not watery, but firm muscles, and the food which serves best,
—viz., the more richly nitrogenous—to produce such muscles, is afterward necessary to maintain their condition. As albuminous food produces firm muscles, so exercise makes them red. To sum up, science
intimates that a liberal supply of nitrogenous matter is necessary to pro-

duce and maintain muscles in a good condition for work, and the result of experience is to confirm it.

I have been speaking of food considered in relation to the performance of work, but it would be unphilosophical to look at it only in this light. The question should be viewed under a broader aspect, and the point really for the physiologist to discuss is under what combination of alimentary principles the highest state of development, both mental and physical, is attainable. If regarded as living for the mere performance of work, and looked at economically, man, it may be said, would bear an unfavorable comparison with a machine set in motion by steam. Mechanical work is under no form so costly as under that produced by muscular agency, and particularly by that of man. It has been calculated, it is true, (vide p. 5), that whilst, through the medium of the animal system, one-fifth of the power stored up in the food consumed is realizable as external mechanical work, the amount realizable from fuel is only one-tenth in the case of even the best constructed steam-engine, the remainder being dissipated or lost as heat. Thus far the animal machine is more economical of its force than the machine of artificial construction; but, on the other hand, the fuel (food) consumed in the former is very much more costly than that consumed in the latter. From this consideration human labor can never compete in economy with steam, and hence, as suggested by Donders, the worst use to make of a man is to employ him exclusively in mechanical work—a proposition which harmonizes with the increasing introduction of machinery in our advancing age of civilization. Letheby,* on the subject of the comparative costliness of food and fuel, says, "taking a steam-engine of one horse-power (that is, a power of raising 33,000 lbs. a foot high per minute) it will require two horses in reality to do the same work for ten hours a day, or twenty-four men; and the cost would be 10d. for the steam-engine, 8s. 4d. for the two horses, and just £2 sterling for the twenty-four men."

From what has preceded we may conclude that, with a supply of nitrogenous matter sufficient for the thorough development and subsequent maintenance of the body in good condition, the best materials for the production of working power, as well as heat, are the non-nitrogenous principles, and that of these the fats are more effective than the others.

Tables have been given of the relative amounts of the different alimentary principles requisite for the proper support of life, such tables having been framed either by ascertaining through observation the minimum upon which the body can be maintained in a healthy state, or by stopping the supplies from without and estimating the consumption of material occurring in the system from the outgoings found by examination to take place. The latter method must be discarded as fallacious. Existence under an absence of food fails to represent the natural state, and the outgoings fall short of their ordinary amount: a portion being naturally derivable from food-metamorphosis, as well as from the consumption of material by oxidation for life-manifestation.

The table given by Moleschott is generally accepted as furnishing a fair representation of a standard or model diet—that is, a diet containing the requisite combination of alimentary principles for just maintaining health in a person of average height and weight, under exposure to a temperate climate and a moderate amount of muscular work. It is as follows:

---

* Cantor Lectures "On Food," 1870, p. 109.

Alimentary Substances in a Dry State Required Daily for the Support of an Ordinary Working Man of Average Height and Weight (Moleschott).

Dry food.	In oz. avoir.	In grains.	In grammes.
Albuminous matter, ...	4.587	2,006	130
Fatty matter, ...	2.964	1,296	84
Carbohydrates, ...	14.250	6,234	404
Salts, ...	1.058	462	30
Total, ...	22.859	9,998	648

Thus, about 23 oz. form the quantity of dry, solid matter contained in this standard diet, and a fifth of it is composed of nitrogenous matter. If we reckon that our ordinary food contains, say 50 per cent. of water, these 23 oz. will correspond to 46 oz. of solid food in the condition in which it is consumed. To complete the alimentary ingesta, a further quantity of from 50 oz. to 80 oz. of water may be put down as taken, under some form or other, daily.

The dynamic or force-producing value of this daily standard diet amounts to 3,960 foot-tons.*

It must be distinctly understood that the above quantities are to be looked upon as yielding what is necessary for the support of life under medium conditions. The amount of material consumed in the body, and therefore the food required to compensate for the loss occurring, varies with the external temperature and the work performed. In speaking of a standard diet, the expression must not, therefore, be taken for more than it is really worth. It would be as absurd to look upon a certain diet as adjusted to the requirements of every particular case as to assign to a certain amount of coal the capacity, when consumed in a grate, of main-

---

* For calculating the dynamic value the experimental determinations of Frankland are used. These, as has been previously explained, were obtained by ascertaining with the calorimeter how much heat is evolved during the oxidation of a given quantity of a substance subjected to examination. The measured heat is then transformed into its equivalent of working power; and represented in kilogrammetres, or force required to raise a kilogramme one metre high (*vide* p. 282). The following are the figures given for the undermentioned alimentary articles which have been taken as representing the three groups of organic alimentary principles.

Force produced by the Oxidation of One Gramme (15.432 *Grains*) *as consumed within the Body.*

	In kilogrammetres.
Albumen (purified), ...	1,805
Fat (beef fat), ...	3,811
Starch (arrow-root), ...	1,657

Kilogrammetres are convertible into foot-tons (tons lifted one foot high) by multiplying by 00.32285. Below are given the figures representing the foot-ton value of an ounce.

Force produced by the Oxidation of One Ounce (437.5 *Grains*) *as consumed within the Body.*

	In foot-tons.
Albumen (purified), ...	165.20
Fat (beef fat), ...	351.56
Starch (arrow-root), ...	151.66

taining a room at a given degree of heat under varying states of external temperature; or, when consumed in a furnace, of enabling a locomotive to propel a train irrespective of its weight over a given number of miles.

Men are led by instinct to adjust the quantity of food consumed to the particular requirements existing, and it is well known that the appetite is sharpened by exposure to cold and under the performance of labor, and lessened by warmth and habits of inactivity.

Travellers have dilated on the large amount of food consumed by the inhabitants of cold as compared with that consumed by those of temperate and hot climates. Accounts are given which almost appear incredible regarding the enormous quantities of food devoured by dwellers in the arctic regions. Thus, Sir John Ross * states that an Esquimaux "perhaps eats twenty pounds of flesh and oil daily." Sir W. Parry,† as a matter of curiosity, one day tried how much food an Esquimaux lad, scarcely full grown, would consume if allowed his full tether. The food was weighed, and, besides fluids, he got through in twenty hours, 8¼ lbs. of flesh and 1¾ lb. of bread and bread-dust, and "did not consider the quantity extraordinary." Sir George Simpson,‡ from his travelling experience in Siberia, says: "In one highly important particular the Yakuti may safely challenge all the rest of the world. They are the best eaters on the face of the earth." Having heard more on this subject than he could bring himself to believe, he resolved to test the matter by the evidence of his own senses. He procured a couple of men who had, he states, a tolerable reputation in that way, and prepared a dinner for them consisting of 36 lbs. avoirdupois of beef and 18 lbs. of butter for each of them. By the end of an hour they had got through half of their allowance in Sir George Simpson's presence. Their stomachs at this time projected "into a brace of kettledrums." They were then left in charge of deputies, and Sir George was assured, on returning two hours later, that all had been consumed. He remarks that, after such surfeits, the gluttons remain for three or four days in a state of stupor, neither eating nor drinking, and meanwhile are rolled about, with a view to the promotion of digestion.

It is right to state that the arctic regions do not stand alone in affording examples of great excess in eating. Illustrations, for instance, have also been given of the performance of equally prodigious feats of gluttony by the inhabitants of other regions of the globe. The Hottentots and Bosjesmans of Southern Africa, where food is not really required to the same extent as in northern localities, are conspicuous, according to the records of travellers, for their gormandizing propensities. "The Hottentots," says Barrow,§ "are the greatest gluttons upon the face of the earth. Ten of our Hottentots ate a middling-sized ox, all but the two hind legs, in three days." Regarding the Bosjesmans, he says, "The three who accompanied us to our wagons had a sheep given to them about five in the evening, which was entirely consumed by them before the noon of the following day. They continued, however, to eat all night, without sleep and without intermission, till they had finished the whole animal. After this their lank bellies were distended to such a degree that they looked less like human creatures than before."

---

* Narrative of a Second Voyage in Search of a North-West Passage, p. 448. London, 1835.

† Second Voyage for the Discovery of the North-West Passage, p. 413. London, 1824.

‡ Narrative of a Journey Round the World during the Years 1841 and 1842, vol. ii., p. 809. London, 1847.

§ Account of Travels into the Interior of Southern Africa. 1801.

Apart from the evidence afforded by the above extraordinary revelations, the bodily experience of those engaged in arctic travelling is sufficient to display the necessity of a large consumption of food to enable resistance to be offered to the effects of exposure to cold. "He who is well fed," remarks Sir John Ross,[*] "resists cold better than the man who is stinted, while the starvation from cold follows but too soon a starvation in food. . . . . In every expedition or voyage to a polar region," he further observes: "at least if a winter residence is contemplated, the quantity of food should be increased, be that as inconvenient as it may. It would be very desirable, indeed, if the men could acquire the taste for Greenland food, since all experience has shown that the large use of oil and fat meats is the true secret of life in these frozen countries." Sir John Franklin [†] also states: "During the whole of our march we experienced that no quantity of clothing could keep us warm while we fasted; but on those occasions on which we were enabled to go to bed with full stomachs we passed the night in a warm and comfortable manner."

Turning now to the adjustment of food to the performance of work, it is mentioned by Liebig [‡] that the English navvies who were sent out during the Crimean war to make the Balaclava railroad consumed daily from 150 (5.291 oz.) to 159 (5.608 oz.) grammes of albuminate, and that the men in the Munich breweries, where the work is heavy, consume on an average 165 grammes (5.820 oz.) *per diem*, whilst the amount entering into the rations of the Bavarian and English soldier, in time of peace, is about 126 grammes (4.444 oz.).

Dr. Playfair § has collected and grouped the dietaries of persons engaged in various ways. His arrangement shows that there is in practice a correspondence between the amount of work performed and of food consumed. The dictates of experience are seen to be in harmony with the suggestions of science. In order to give a representation of the relative value of different dietaries the amounts of the nutritive principles require to be ascertained and set forth. This is the only way by which dissimilar diets can be brought to uniformity so as to allow of anything like an exact comparison being made.

Now, to ascertain the amounts of the alimentary principles contained in a given dietary, or to fix its dietetic value, the composition of the constituent articles requires to be known. Tables have been given by different authorities representing the composition of the various articles of food. No two tables, however, will be found exactly to agree. The composition, in fact, of an alimentary substance is in no case fixed and invariable. It is not surprising, therefore, that the results furnished by different analysts should vary. Taking, however, the figures of an established chemical authority as a basis of calculation, sufficient reliance may be placed upon the estimate yielded. It is true the amounts of nutritive principles worked out must not be looked upon as representative of anything like absolute precision; still they may be regarded as sufficiently near for all practical purposes. The following table is drawn from Dr. Liebig's work,|| with a few additions selected from a table compiled by Dr. Parkes.¶

* Op. cit.
† Narrative of a Journey to the Shores of the Polar Sea in the Years 1819 to 1822, p. 424. London, 1823.
‡ Lancet, vol. i., p. 5. 1869.
§ On the Food of Man in Relation to his Useful Work. Lecture delivered at the Royal Society, Edinburgh, and Royal Institution, London, April, 1865.
|| On Food, Cantor Lectures, 1st ed., p. 6. 1870.
¶ Practical Hygiene, 3d ed., p. 165.

Table Showing the Percentage Composition of Various Articles of Food.

(From a table furnished by Letheby, with additions marked thus (a) from one furnished by Parkes.)

	Water.	Albumen, etc.	Starch, etc.	Sugar.	Fat.	Salts.
Bread, ...	37	8.1	47.4	3.6	1.6	2.3
Biscuit,(a)	8	15.6	—73.4—		1.3	1.7
Wheat flour, ...	15	10.8	66.3	4.2	2.0	1.7
Barley meal, ...	15	6.3	69.4	4.9	2.4	2.0
Oatmeal, ...	15	12.6	58.4	5.4	5.6	3.0
Rye meal, ...	15	8.0	69.5	3.7	2.0	1.8
Indian corn meal, ...	14	11.1	64.7	0.4	8.1	1.7
Rice, ...	13	6.3	79.1	0.4	0.7	0.5
Peas, ...	15	23.0	55.4	2.0	2.1	2.5
Arrow-root, ...	18	—	82.0	—	—	—
Potatoes, ...	75	2.1	18.8	3.2	0.2	0.7
Carrots, ...	83	1.3	8.4	6.1	0.2	1.0
Parsnips, ...	82	1.1	9.6	5.8	0.5	1.0
Turnips, ...	91	1.2	5.1	2.1	—	0.6
* Cabbage, ...	91	2.0	—5.8—		0.5	0.7
Sugar, ...	5	—	—	95.0	—	—
Treacle, ...	23	—	—	77.0	—	—
New milk, ...	86	4.1	—	5.2	3.9	0.8
Cream, ...	66	2.7	—	2.8	26.7	1.8
Skim milk, ...	88	4.0	—	5.4	1.8	0.8
Buttermilk, ...	88	4.1	—	6.4	0.7	0.8
Cheese,(a)	36.8	33.5	—	—	24.3	5.4
Cheddar cheese, ...	36	28.4	—	—	31.1	4.5
Skim cheese, ...	44	44.8	—	—	6.3	4.9
Lean beef, ...	72	19.3	—	—	3.6	5.1
Fat beef, ...	51	14.8	—	—	29.8	4.4
Lean mutton,.	72	18.3	—	—	4.9	4.8
Fat mutton, ...	53	12.4	—	—	31.1	3.5
Veal, ...	63	16.5	—	—	15.8	4.7
Fat pork, ...	39	9.8	—	—	48.9	2.3
Green bacon, ...	24	7.1	—	—	66.8	2.1
Dried bacon, ...	15	8.8	—	—	73.3	2.9
Ox liver, ...	74	18.9	—	—	4.1	3.0
Tripe, ...	68	13.2	—	—	16.4	2.4
† Cooked meat, roast, no dripping being lost. Boiled assumed to be the same,(a)	54	27.6	—	—	15.45	2.95
Poultry, ...	74	21.0	—	—	3.8	1.2
White fish, ...	78	18.1	—	—	2.9	1.0
Eels, ...	75	9.9	—	—	13.8	1.3
Salmon, ...	77	16.1	—	—	5.5	1.4
Entire egg, ...	74	14.0	—	—	10.5	1.5
White of egg,.	78	20.4	—	—	—	1.6
Yolk of egg, ...	52	16.0	—	—	30.7	1.3
Butter and fats, ...	15	—	—	—	83.0	2.0
Beer and porter,.	91	0.1	—	8.7	—	0.2

* The nitrogenous matter in Dr. Parkes' table is put down as 0.2, but 2.0 is evidently meant
† Ranke's analysis.

Playfair's dietaries, to which reference has been made, will now be introduced. The food is brought into its equivalent in nutritive principles. I have calculated and appended to each the dynamic, or force-producing value according to the determinations of Frankland. The dynamic value must not be taken for more than it is really worth. It is scarcely necessary to state that the proper distinction must be kept in view between dynamic and nutritive value.

Subsistence diet.—This is drawn from certain prison dietaries; the diet of needlewomen in London; the common dietary for convalescents in the Edinburgh Infirmary; and the average diet during the cotton famine in Lancashire in 1862. The mean of these several dietaries gives a daily allowance of—

		Ounces.
Nitrogenous matter,	. . . . . .	2.33
Fat,	. . . .	0.84
Carbohydrates,	. . . . . .	11.69

Dynamic value * of daily allowance 2,453 foot-tons.

Diet of adult in full health, with moderate exercise.—The dietaries of the English, French, Prussian, and Austrian soldiers during peace are taken as the basis of this class. The mean of these dietaries stands as follows:

		Ounces.
Nitrogenous matter,	. . . . . .	4.215
Fat,	. . . .	1.397
Carbohydrates,	. . . . . .	18.690
Mineral matter,	. . . . . .	0.714

Dynamic value, 4,021 foot-tons.

Diet of active laborers.—To represent this class Dr. Playfair has placed together the dietaries of soldiers engaged in the arduous duties of war, viz., those of the English during the Crimean and Kaffir wars; the French during the Crimean war; the Prussians during the Schleswig war; the Austrians during the Italian war; the Russians during the Crimean war; the Dutch during the Belgian war; and those of the Federal and Confederate armies in the American war of 1860–65. The mean of the above gives the following quantities:

		Ounces.
Nitrogenous matter,	. . . . . .	5.41
Fat,	. . . .	2.41
Carbohydrates,	. . . . . .	17.92
Mineral matter,	. . . . . .	0.68

Dynamic value, 4,458 foot-tons.

In addition to the group just furnished, Dr. Playfair points to the dietaries of the Royal Engineers during peace, as affording a representation of the amount of food required by laboring men performing a fair, but not

---

* *Vide* note, p. 288.

an excessive, amount of work during the twenty-four hours. In this branch of the military service, he says, the men while in the depot at Chatham are actively occupied either in constructing field-works, or in pursuing their avocations as artisans, from which class of people they are selected. The actual amount of food consumed by 495 men belonging to different companies was carefully ascertained for twelve consecutive days and reduced to its dietetic value. The mean of all the returns came out as follows:

	Ounces.
Nitrogenous matter, ...	5.08
Fat, ·	2.91
Carbohydrates, ...	22.22
Mineral matter, ...	0.93

Dynamic value, 5,232 foot-tons.

Diet of hard-working laborers.—Dr. Playfair remarks that we do not possess many well-recorded examples of ordinary laborers' diets containing precise information as regards amounts. In those included in his table, however, the actual weight of food consumed was determined. They comprise the dietary of the English navvy engaged in the Crimea, and in the construction of the Rouen railway; of hard-worked weavers; of fully fed tailors; and of blacksmiths. With these are grouped the dietaries of the English and French sailor, and the mean given stands as follows:

	Ounces.
Nitrogenous matter, ...	5.64
Fat, ...	2.34
Carbohydrates, ...	20.41

Dynamic value, 4,849 foot-tons.

In the first and last of these dietaries nothing, it will be observed, is said of mineral matter. Reckoning, however, that an average amount is here supplied, the lowest of the foregoing series of dietaries will comprise between 15 and 16 oz. of dry food, and the highest a little over 31 oz. The amount of nitrogenous matter present stands in a varying proportion of from about the one-fifth to the one-sixth and a half of the whole.

The English soldier on home service, says Dr. Parkes, receives from Government one pound of bread and three-quarters of a pound of meat, and buys additional bread, vegetables, milk, and groceries. The nutritive value of his usual food is represented by Dr. Parkes to be as follows:

	Ounces.
Nitrogenous matter, ...	3.86
Fat, ...	1.30
Carbohydrates, ...	17.35
Mineral matter, ...	0.808

The supply of carbon in this diet, as calculated by Dr. Parkes, is 4,718 grains, and of nitrogen only 266 grains per diem.

The dynamic value, calculated in the same manner as in the case of the preceding dietaries, amounts to 3,726 foot-tons.

By Dr. Playfair* the nutritive value of the English soldier's diet is given as somewhat higher, thus:

						Ounces.
Nitrogenous matter,	.	.	.	.	.	4.250
Fat, .	.	.	.	.	.	1.665
Carbohydrates,	.	.	.	.	.	18.541
Mineral matter,	.	.	.	.	.	0.789

Dynamic value, 4,099 foot-tons.

According to Dr. Playfair† also, the nutritive value of the English sailor's fresh meat diet stands as follows:

						Ounces.
Nitrogenous matter,	.	.	.	.	.	5.00
Fat, .	.	.	.	.	.	2.57
Carbohydrates, .	.	.	.	.	.	14.39

Dynamic value, 3,911 foot-tons.

Workhouse dietaries, although applied to large numbers of people, and followed with scrupulous attention to weight and measure, fail to afford information of the kind required for advancing our position with reference to the point under consideration. They are framed particularly for the maintenance of the aged, the infirm, the sick, and the young. There are but few able-bodied people as inmates of these establishments, and the diet for this particular class is, perhaps, often fixed below what would be needed for a permanency, so that no encouragement may be offered to a prolonged stay being made. Moreover, although model dietaries are issued by the Local Government Board, the local authorities have the power to frame dietaries of their own, and provided they are considered to furnish sufficient food, sanction to their adoption is given. Thus it happens that in point of detail great diversity prevails within the different establishments throughout the country.

For the various county and borough jails the same liberty exists as in the cases of workhouses. Dietaries have been recommended by the Home Office for different classes of prisoners according to the duration of sentence, and to whether it is with or without hard labor, but it is left to the discretion of the county authorities to adopt them or to frame others of their own. The result is, that some have conformed whilst a larger number have not, and thus, again, there is much diversity to deal with. For long sentences the dietaries must necessarily be adequate to meet the requirements of life, but for short sentences the punishment of confinement is increased by a scanty allowance of food. For instance, in the recommendations from the Home Office, the daily allowance for prisoners sentenced for less than seven days without hard labor consists of 1 pound of bread and 2 pints of oatmeal gruel, made with 2 ounces oatmeal to the pint; and for over seven days and under twenty-one, of 1½ pounds of bread and 2 pints of. gruel. The nutritive value of the first-named diet stands thus—1.800 ounces of nitrogenous matter, .480 ounces of fat, and 10.712 ounces of carbohydrates; and of the second—2.448 ounces of nitrogenous matter, .608 ounces of fat, and 14.792 ounces of carbohydrates. For longer terms potatoes and meat are also allowed.

---

* On the Food of Man in Relation to his Useful Work, p. 11. Edin., 1865.
† Op. cit., p. 18.

In the Government convict * establishments the prisoners are all under long sentence, and uniformity is carried out in classes arranged according to occupation. This constitutes a rational principle of dieting. The health of the prisoners must be maintained, and the diet is such as has been found by experience to suffice for this end. On the other hand, upon the score of economy, and likewise that no unnecessary bodily comfort may be supplied, the food is reduced to as short an allowance as is found to be compatible with the preservation of health. These dietaries, therefore, should afford us illustrations of just the requisite quantity of food for supporting life under the performance of different amounts of labor. For these reasons I will introduce here the dietaries at the present time in use; and, for the purpose of comparison, give their calculated nutritive value founded on the composition of food according to the table furnished at p. 291.

The cocoa supplied consists of prepared cocoa, which is contracted for as such. It doubtless, like other forms of prepared cocoa, contains a certain admixture of starchy, or starchy and saccharine matter. I have taken the average of Hassall's results of the examination of various samples of prepared cocoa, and reckoned that it contains about 35 per cent. of carbohydrates in combination with the pure article, the composition of which is assumed to be in accordance with the analysis given by Payen.

The nutritive value of the meat is calculated from the analysis of cooked meat given by Parkes. The composition of cheese is also taken from the analysis furnished by Dr. Parkes, which represents a medium quality.

The shins are made into soup, and I have assumed that the whole of the animal matter is extracted from the bones. It was ascertained for me that the shins actually supplied consist upon an average of 59.57 per cent. of meat and 40.43 per cent. of bone. The meat is reckoned in accordance with the composition of lean beef (vide table, p. 291). As regards the bone, I found by observation that a fore and hind shin taken together and deprived of meat lost 15.29 per cent. of water upon being dried by exposure to heat until they ceased to lose weight. The dry bone is reckoned as consisting of one-third animal matter and two-thirds earthy, and the animal matter is calculated as of the same value as lean meat.

In the absence of a record of the analysis of onions they have been assumed to be of the same nutritive value as turnips—an assumption which, even if not precisely correct, cannot materially influence the calculated result.

---

* With convicts sentenced to hard labor the hours of labor, I notice, are made to vary in the summer and winter, being 10 hours 40 minutes per diem in the former, and 8 hours 55 minutes in the latter. Whether this arrangement has been designed in relation to food or for some other reason of prison management I do not know, but it stands in harmony with what is rational in a physiological point of view. Both the work performed and the heat produced must be represented by an equivalent of food, and under the arrangement before us the food which corresponds to the extra amount of labor demanded of the convicts in the summer, is free for appropriation to the production of the extra amount of heat necessitated in the winter. If the food were exactly adjusted to the requirements in the summer it would be insufficient for the accomplishment of the same amount of labor during the winter. To provide for the production of the extra amount of heat required in the winter there must be either an increase in the amount of food or a diminution in the amount of labor. The latter course in prison management is observed to be pursued.

Hard-labor Diet.

(Daily period of labor—summer, 10 hrs. 40 min.; winter, 8 hrs. 55 min.)

Weekly allowance.	Nitrogenous matter.	Carbo-hydrates.	Fat.	Mineral matter.	Total solid matter.
	Oz.	Oz.	Oz.	Oz.	Oz.	Oz.
Cocoa, ...	3.500	0.560	1.540	1.295	0.105	3.500
Oatmeal, ...	14.000	1.764	8.932	0.784	0.420	11.900
Milk, ...	14.000	0.574	0.728	0.546	0.112	1.960
Molasses, . . .	7.000	—	5.390	—	—	5.390
Salt, ...	3.500	—	—	—	3.500	3.500
Barley, ...	2.000	0.126	1.486	0.048	0.040	1.700
Bread, ...	168.000	13.608	85.680	2.688	3.864	105.840
Cheese, ...	4.000	1.340	—	0.972	0.216	2.528
Flour, ...	8.625	0.931	6.081	0.172	0.147	7.331
Meat(cooked,with-out bone or gra-vy), ...	15.000	4.140	—	2.318	0.442	6.900
Shins (made into soup), . . .	16.000	3.376	—	0.640	4.144	8.160
Suet, ...	1.500	—	—	1.244	0.030	1.274
Carrots, ...	2.000	0.026	0.290	0.004	0.020	0.340
Onions, ...	3.500	0.042	0.252	—	0.021	0.315
Turnips , ...	2.000	0.024	0.144	—	0.012	0.180
Potatoes, . . .	96.000	2.016	21.120	0.192	0.672	24.000
Total weekly allowance, . .		28.527	131.643	10.903	13.745	184.818

Light-labor Diet.

(Labor consists of oakum-picking, etc.)

Weekly allowance.	Nitrogenous matter.	Carbo-hydrates.	Fat.	Mineral matter.	Total solid matter.
	Oz.	Oz.	Oz.	Oz.	Oz.	Oz.
Cocoa, ...	3.500	0.560	1.540	1.295	0.105	3.500
Oatmeal, ...	14.000	1.764	8.932	0.784	0.420	11.900
Milk, ...	14.000	0.574	0.728	0.546	0.112	1.960
Molasses, ...	7.000	—	5.390	—	—	5.390
Salt, ...	3.500	—	—	—	3.500	3.500
Barley, ...	2.000	0.126	1.486	0.048	0.040	1.700
Bread, ...	145.000	11.745	73.950	2.320	3.335	91.350
Cheese, ...	4.000	1.340	—	0.972	0.216	2.528
Flour, ...	4.625	0.499	3.261	0.092	0.079	3.931
Meat(cooked,with-out bone or gra-vy), ...	12.000	3.312	—	1.854	0.354	5.520
Shins (made into soup), ...	12.000	2.532	—	0.480	3.108	6.120
Suet, ...	0.750	—	—	0.622	0.015	0.637
Carrots, ...	2.000	0.026	0.290	0.004	0.020	0.340
Onions, ...	3.500	0.042	0.252	—	0.021	0.315
Turnips, ...	2.000	0.024	0.144	—	0.012	0.180
Potatoes, ...	96.000	2.016	21.120	0.192	0.672	24.000
Total weekly allowance, . .		24.560	117.093	9.209	12.009	162.871

Industrial Employment Diet.

(Employment as tailors, shoemakers, weavers, etc.)

Weekly allowance.	Nitrogenous matter.	Carbo-hydrates.	Fat.	Mineral matter.	Total solid matter.
	Oz.	Oz.	Oz.	Oz.	Oz.	Oz.
Cocoa, ...	3.500	0.560	1.540	1.295	0.105	3.500
Oatmeal, ...	14.000	1.764	8.932	0.784	0.420	11.900
Milk, ...	28.000	1.148	1.456	1.092	0.224	3.920
Molasses, ...	7.000	—	5.390	—	—	5.390
Salt, ...	3.500	—	—	—	3.500	3.500
Barley, ...	1.000	0.063	0.743	0.024	0.020	0.850
Bread, ...	148.000	11.988	75.480	2.368	3.404	93.240
Cheese, ...	4.000	1.340	—	0.972	0.216	2.528
Flour, ...	8.625	0.931	6.081	0.172	0.147	7.331
Meat (cooked, without bone or gravy), ...	16.000	4.416	—	2.472	0.472	7.360
Shins (made into soup), . . .	8.000	1.688	—	0.320	2.072	4.080
Suet, ...	1.500	—	—	1.244	0.030	1.274
Carrots, ...	1.000	0.013	0.145	0.002	0.010	0.170
Onions, ...	3.000	0.036	0.216	—	0.018	0.270
Turnips, ...	1.000	0.012	0.072	—	0.006	0.090
Potatoes, ...	96.000	2.016	21.120	0.192	0.672	24.000
Total weekly allowance, . .	**25.975**	**121.175**	**10.937**	**11.316**	**169.403**

Penal Diet.

(For offenders against the prison laws. May be continued for three months. Also used every fourth day in the place of punishment diet where punishment diet is ordered for more than three days.)

Daily allowance.	Nitrogenous matter.	Carbo-hydrates.	Fat.	Mineral matter.	Total solid matter.
	Oz.	Oz.	Oz.	Oz.	Oz.	Oz.
Bread, ...	20.000	1.620	10.200	0.320	0.460	12.600
Oatmeal, ...	8.000	1.008	5.104	0.448	0.240	6.800
Milk, ...	20.000	0.820	1.040	0.780	0.160	2.800
Potatoes, ...	16.000	0.336	3.520	0.032	0.112	4.000
Total daily allowance, . .	**3.784**	**19.864**	**1.580**	**0.972**	**26.200**

Punishment Diet.

(Bread and water diet for the punishment of prisoners.)

Daily allowance.	Nitrogenous matter.	Carbo-hydrates.	Fat.	Mineral matter.	Total solid matter.
	Oz.	Oz.	Oz.	Oz.	Oz.	Oz.
Bread, ...	16.000	1.296	8.160	0.256	0.368	10.080

Representing the nutritive value of these diets in the same manner as that previously adopted, they come out as follows:

HARD LABOR DIET, *per diem.*

	Ounces.
Nitrogenous matter, ...	4.075
Fat, ...	1.557
Carbohydrates, ...	18.806
Mineral matter, ...	1.963

Dynamic value, 4,072 foot-tons.

LIGHT LABOR DIET, *per diem.*

	Ounces.
Nitrogenous matter, ...	3.508
Fat, ...	1.315
Carbohydrates, ...	16.727
Mineral matter, ...	1.715

Dynamic value, 3,577 foot-tons.

INDUSTRIAL EMPLOYMENT DIET, *per diem.*

	Ounces.
Nitrogenous matter, ...	3.710
Fat, ...	1.562
Carbohydrates, ...	17.310
Mineral matter, ...	1.616

Dynamic value, 3,787 foot-tons.

PENAL DIET, *per diem.*

	Ounces.
Nitrogenous matter, ...	3.784
Fat, ...	1.580
Carbohydrates, ...	19.864
Mineral matter, ...	0.972

Dynamic value, 4,193 foot-tons.

PUNISHMENT DIET, *per diem.*

	Ounces.
Nitrogenous matter, ...	1.296
Fat, ...	0.256
Carbohydrates, ...	8.160
Mineral matter, ...	0.368

Dynamic value, 1,541 foot-tons.

On comparing the hard labor diet with the collection of dietaries framed by Dr. Playfair (*vide* p. 292) it will be seen that it very closely conforms with the representative diet for full health and moderate exercise, and is considerably under that, particularly in nitrogenous matter, of active laborers. The industrial employment diet is of a rather higher nutritive value in each respect than the light labor diet. The penal diet, whilst containing less nitrogenous matter than the hard labor diet, surpasses it in carbohydrates and has about the same amount of fat. In force-producing value it holds the higher position of the two. The punishment diet would be inadequate for the support of life as a continuance.

Some extraordinary instances of subsistence upon a small amount of food—indeed the amount is so small as almost to excite suspicion with regard to its accuracy—are to be found recorded. A well-known case, remarks Dr. Carpenter, is that of Thomas Wood, the miller of Billericay, reported to the College of Physicians in 1767 by Sir George Baker, in which a remarkable degree of vigor is said to have been sustained for upward of eighteen years upon no other nutriment than 16 oz. of flour made into a pudding, with water, no other liquid of any kind being taken. In nutritive value 16 oz. of flour will represent 1.72 oz. of nitrogenous matter, 0.32 oz. of fat, and 11.28 oz. of carbohydrates.

A more striking instance still is that afforded by the case of Cornaro, a Venetian of noble descent, who lived in the fifteenth and sixteenth centuries, and attained an age of upward of 100. Impressed with the conviction that the older a man gets and the less amount of power he possesses the less should be the amount of food consumed, in opposition to the common notion that more should be taken to compensate for his failing power, he, at about 40 years of age, resolved to enter upon a new course, and betake himself to a spare diet and scrupulously regular mode of life, after having, as he says, previously led a life of indulgence in eating and drinking, and having been endowed with a feeble constitution and "fallen into different kinds of disorders, such as pains in my stomach, and often stitches, and spices of the gout, attended by what was still worse, an almost continual slow fever, a stomach generally out of order, and a perpetual thirst." He also did all that lay in his power "to avoid those evils which we do not find it so easy to remove. These are melancholy, hatred, and other violent passions, which appear to have the greatest influence over our bodies. The consequence was, that in a few days I began," he adds, "to perceive that such a course agreed with me very well; and by pursuing it, in less than a year I found myself (some persons, perhaps, will not believe it) entirely freed from all my complaints. . . . I chose wine suited to my stomach, drinking of it but the quantity I knew I could digest. I did the same by my meat, as well in regard to quantity as to quality, accustoming myself to contrive matters so as never to cloy my stomach with eating or drinking; but constantly rise from the table with a disposition to eat and drink still more. In this I conformed to the proverb which says that a man, to consult his health, must check his appetite. . . . *What with bread, meat, the yolk of an egg, and soup, I ate as much as weighed in all 12 oz. neither more nor less. . . . I drank but 14 oz. of wine.*"* Upon this scanty allowance Cornaro tells us he perseveringly subsisted; and he lived in possession of all his faculties to write a series of discourses at the respective ages of 83, 86, 91, and 95, directed toward urging others to follow a similar course. These discourses, which are imbued with vigor and vivacity, and contain many shrewd remarks on the subject of living, seem to have excited considerable attention at the time they appeared, and for many years afterward. A translation from the Italian original was published in London in 1768, from which the above extracts have been taken.

Reference has been made in the foregoing pages to the actual diets consumed under various conditions, and the value of these diets in alimentary *principles*. It will be instructive now to consider the *elementary* components of food in relation to the outgoing *elements* from the body. Regarded under this point of view, scientific data are afforded for showing

---

* The italics have been introduced by the author.

the combination of alimentary principles that is best adapted for administering in the most economical manner to the wants of the system. We
can ascertain, for instance, the amount of carbon and nitrogen escaping
from the body as products of destruction, and then with a knowledge of
the composition of food can define the precise kind and amount required
for compensation without any surplus on either side.

To assist in determining the amounts of different alimentary articles
required to be consumed to yield a given daily supply of nitrogen and carbon, a table has been furnished by Payen,* of which the following is a
copy, with the omission of such as have been deemed unimportant:

*Table, from Payen, showing the Quantity of Nitrogen and Carbon in 100
Parts of Various Alimentary Articles. Under the head of carbon is
included, not only this element, but likewise its equivalent of the hydro-
gen† existing in the compound in excess of what is necessary to form
water with the oxygen present.*

(Multiplying the figures representing the nitrogen by 6.5 gives the equivalent amount
of nitrogenous matter.)

	Nitrogen.	Carbon.
Beef, without bone, ...	3.00	11.00
Roast beef, ...	3.528	17.76
Bullock's heart, ...	2.831	16.16
Calves' liver, ...	3.093	15.68
Foie gras, ...	2.115	65.58
Calves' lights, ...	3.458	14.50
Sheep's kidneys, ...	2.655	12.15
Skate, ...	3.85	12.25
Conger eels, ...	3.95	12.60
Cod-fish, salted, ...	5.02	16.00
Sardines in oil, ...	6.00	29.00
Herrings, salted, ...	3.11	23.00
Herrings, fresh, ...	1.83	21.00
Whiting, ...	2.41	9.00
Mackerel, ...	3.74	19.26
Sole, ...	1.91	12.25
Salmon, ...	2.09	16.00
Pike, ...	3.25	11.50
Carp, ...	3.49	12.10
Gudgeons, ...	2.77	13.50
Eels, ...	2.00	30.05
Eggs, ...	1.90	13.50
Cow's milk, ...	0.66	8.00
Goat's milk, ...	0.69	8.60
Russian caviare, ...	4.49	27.41
Mussels (fleshy substance), ...	1.804	9.00
Oysters (fleshy substance), ...	2.13	7.18
Lobster (raw fleshy substance), ...	2.93	10.96
Lobster (soft internal substance), ...	1.87	7.30
Cheese, Brie, ...	2.93	35.00
Cheese, Gruyere, ...	5.00	38.00

* Substances Alimentaires, p. 488. Paris, 1865.
† A given quantity of hydrogen is equivalent to three times the amount of carbon
in capacity of appropriating oxygen under conversion respectively into water and carbonic acid.

	Nitrogen.	Carbon.
Cheese, Cheshire,	4.126	41.04
Cheese, Parmesan,	6.997	40.00
Cheese, cream,	2.920	71.10
Cheese, Roquefort,	4.210	44.44
Cheese, Dutch,	4.80	43.54
Cheese, Neufchatel, fresh,	1.27	50.71
Beans,	4.50	42.00
Beans, green dried,	4.46	46.00
Beans, Haricots,	3.92	43.00
Beans, dried, split,	4.15	48.50
Lentils,	3.87	43.00
Peas, dried, ordinary,	3.66	44.00
Peas, split, green, dried,	3.91	46.00
Hard wheat from the south,	3.00	41.00
Soft wheat,	1.81	39.00
Flour, Parisian white,	1.64	38.50
Rye flour,	1.75	41.00
Barley,	1.90	40.00
Indian corn,	1.70	44.00
Buckwheat,	2.20	42.50
Rice,	1.80	41.00
Oatmeal,	1.95	44.00
Bread, Parisian white,	1.08	29.50
Bread, household, stale,	1.07	28.00
Bread, household, new,	1.20	30.00
Potatoes,	0.33	11.00
Carrots,	0.31	5.50
Mushrooms, forced,	0.66	4.520
Truffles, black,	1.350	9.45
Truffles, white,	1.532	9.10
Chestnuts, ordinary,	0.64	35.00
Chestnuts, dried,	1.04	48.00
Gooseberries,	0.14	7.79
Figs, fresh,	0.41	15.50
Figs, dried,	0.92	34.00
Plums, dried,	0.73	28.00
Nuts, fresh,	1.40	10.65
Almonds, sweet, fresh,	2.677	40.00
Coffee, from infusion of 100 grammes (3¼ oz.),	1.10	9.00
Tea, from infusion of 20 grammes (308½ grains),	0.20	2.10
Chocolate, from 100 grammes (3¼ oz.),	1.52	58.00
Lard,	1.18	71.14
Butter, ordinary fresh,	0.64	83.00
Olive oil,	Traces.	98.00
Beer, strong,	0.08	4.50
Alcohol, absolute,	——	52.00
Spirits of wine,	——	27.00
Wine,	0.015	4.00

Dr. Parkes * sets forth the quantity of nitrogen and carbon contained in the typical alimentary principles, and remarks that the amount of the

* Hygiene, third ed., p. 166.

two elements present in a given diet may be thence calculated, presum·
ing its value in alimentary principles to have been ascertained. Thus, he
says:

> 1 oz. of water-free albuminate contains 69 grains nitrogen, 233 grains carbon.
> 1 oz.   "   fat contains 345.6 grains carbon.
> 1 oz.   "   carbohydrate (except lactine) contains 194.2 grains carbon.
> 1 oz.   "   lactine contains 175 grains carbon.

In employing this method it is necessary, in the first place, to ex·
tract, with the aid of the table at p. 291, the dry alimentary principles.
Then, with the use of the figures above given, the nitrogen and carbon
may be ascertained.

From the investigations that have been conducted, it appears that the
daily quantity of nitrogen required to compensate for the elimination oc·
curring under ordinary conditions of life may be said to range from about
250 to 350 grains (16 to 22½ grammes); and of carbon, from 4,000 to 6,000
grains (259 to 388½ grammes). Amongst badly fed operatives the
amounts upon which subsistence has been maintained have been observed
to be as low as about 170 grains (11 grammes) of nitrogen, and 3,600
grains (233 grammes) of carbon.

Taking Moleschott's model diet (vide p. 288), and applying Dr.
Parkes' method of calculation, the amounts of nitrogen and carbon come
out as follows:.

		Grs. Nitrogen.	Grs. Carbon.
4.587 oz. dry albuminate,	. . .	316	1068
2.964 oz. " fat,	. . . .	—	1024
14.257 oz. " carbohydrate,	. .	—	2768
Total	. . . .	316	4860

These amounts, it will be perceived, correspond with about the mean
of the usual range of ingested nitrogen and carbon mentioned above.

Let it be assumed, then, that 300 grains of nitrogen and 4,500 grains of
carbon are daily required. I will proceed to show, after the manner
adopted by Payen, * in what way these elements are most economically,
or with the least waste of material, supplied.

The ratio of the quantities named is as 1 to 16, which implies that six·
teen times as much carbon is required as nitrogen. In albumen the ratio,
on the other hand, is about as 1 to 3.5. Hence, if albumen alone were
supplied, in furnishing the 300 grains of nitrogen, there would only be
1,050 instead of the 4,800 grains of associated carbon; and conversely, if
the 4,800 grains of carbon were supplied, there would be 1,371 grains of
accompanying nitrogen, or rather more than 4½ times the amount re·
quired. In bread, following Payen's analysis, the ratio of nitrogen to
carbon is as 1 to 30. The amount of bread, therefore, that would yield
300 grains of nitrogen would contain 30 times the quantity or 9,000 grains
of carbon; that is, nearly double the amount required; and should an
amount of bread be consumed that would just suffice to yield the 4,800
grains of carbon, 160 grains, or only rather more than half the quantity
of nitrogen required, would be supplied.

From these considerations, it follows that neither bread nor albumen
are adapted for economically furnishing what is wanted, and what is true

---

* Substances Alimentaires, p. 483. Paris, 1865.

concerning these articles is equally so of others containing a preponderance of either carbon or nitrogen. It is upon a due admixture of the two that the principle of adjustment is founded; and as nitrogenous principles preponderate in animal food and the carbonaceous or non-nitrogenous in vegetable, we see that the teachings of science harmonize with the instinctive propensity which inclines man so universally to the employment of a mixed diet whenever the circumstances under which he is placed admit of its being obtained.

The following tabular arrangement will more forcibly illustrate the point in question.

Let meat be taken instead of albumen. In round numbers it contains 11 per cent. of carbon and 3 per cent. of nitrogen. 43,637 grains, or rather over 6 pounds, will thus yield 4,800 grains of carbon; 1,309 grains of nitrogen.

Bread contains, say 30 per cent. of carbon and 1 per cent. of nitrogen (Payen). Hence, 30,000 grains, or rather over 4 pounds, will yield 9,000 grains of carbon; 300 grains of nitrogen.

In the first case there is the requisite quantity of carbon and a surplus of 1,009 grains of nitrogen, which corresponds with 33,633 grains, or about 4¾ pounds, of meat; and in the second, the requisite quantity of nitrogen and a surplus of 4,200 grains of carbon, which corresponds with 14,000 grains, or 2 pounds of bread.

Suppose, now, that a suitable admixture of bread and meat be given, the result will stand as follows:

14,000 grs. (2 lbs.) of bread contain   4,200 grs. carbon, 140 grs. nitrogen.
5,500 grs. (about ¾ lb.) of meat contain 605 grs.   "   165 grs.   "

Total,   4,805   305

Hence from 2 pounds of bread and about ¾ pound of meat we can obtain a sufficient amount of both carbon and nitrogen; whilst rather over 6 pounds of meat and rather more than 4 pounds of bread, if taken singly, would be respectively required to satisfy the demand in the case of the two elements.

The train of reasoning here pursued is equally applicable to a combination of nitrogenous food with the non-nitrogenous principle—fat. By a proper adjustment of these articles the precise quantities of carbon and nitrogen required can be in a similar manner supplied without waste in either case.

PRACTICAL DIETETICS.

PROPER FOOD OF MAN.

UPON the supply of a proper quantity and quality of food, the maintenance of health and life is dependent. The records of this and other nations have from time to time afforded bitter evidence of how intimately disease and mortality are associated with the supply of food. *Plague, pestilence,* and *famine* stand associated together in the public mind, and, through an imperfect knowledge of the principles of dietetics, the most calamitous results have sometimes occurred from improper dieting amongst large bodies of men. The consideration of food thus becomes a matter of the deepest public importance. To its physiological contemplation the previous pages have been devoted, and now its practical bearings, both in relation to health and sickness, will form the subject of attention.

As has been already stated, it is to organic nature that we have to look for our supply of food, and we have found it to be derivable from both animal and vegetable products. Looking at the various animal organisms around us, it is noticeable that some are designed for subsistence upon an exclusively animal, others upon an exclusively vegetable, and others, again, upon a mixed diet.

Let us see what kind of food is best adapted for the support of man. It may be premised by saying that no animal possesses so great a power of accommodating itself to varied external conditions as man, and this is true of diet as well as of other things. Without this power the distribution of mankind over the surface of the globe must have been much more limited than it is. The difference of climate in different latitudes not only gives rise to different personal requirements as regards food, but likewise modifies the character of the alimentary products that are to be found; and it happens, as with other portions of the plan of nature, that the two are in harmony with each other. In illustration of this subject, I will here introduce a collection of extracts from various sources, representing the nature of the food consumed by the inhabitants of different parts of the globe.

Extracts from the Works of Various Authors Descriptive of the Kind of Food Consumed by the Inhabitants of Different Parts of the Globe.

ARCTIC REGIONS.—" The *Esquimaux* are mainly an animal-feeding people, and their food consists of the reindeer, musk-ox, walrus, seals, birds, and salmon. They will, however, eat any kind of animal food, and are fond of fat and marrow."—" Lubbock's Pre-historic Times," p. 485. 1869.

" Our journeys have taught us the wisdom of the *Esquimaux* appetite, and there are few among us who do not relish a slice of raw blubber or a chunk of frozen walrus-beef. The liver of a walrus (awuktanuk), eaten with little slices of his fat, of a verity, it is a delicious morsel. Fire would ruin the curt, pithy expression of vitality which belongs to its un-cooked juices. Charles Lamb's roast pig was nothing to awuktanuk. I wonder that raw beef is not eaten at home. Deprived of extraneous fibre, it is neither indigestible nor difficult to masticate. With acids and con-diments, it makes a salad which an educated palate cannot help relishing, and, as a powerful and condensed heat-making and anti-scorbutic food, it has no rival.

"I make this last broad assertion after carefully testing its truth. The natives of South Greenland prepare themselves for a long journey in the cold by a course of frozen seal. At Upernavik they do the same with the narwhal, which is thought more heat-making than the seal; while the bear, to use their own expression, is 'stronger travel than all.'

"In Smith's Sound, where the use of raw meat seems almost inevitable from the modes of living of the people, walrus holds the first rank. Cer-tainly this pachyderm, whose finely condensed tissue and delicate-perme-ating fat—oh! call it not blubber—assimilate it to the ox, is beyond all others, and is the very best fuel a man can swallow. It became our con-stant companion whenever we could get it, and a frozen liver upon our sledge was valued far above the same weight of pemmican."—"Kane's Arctic Explorations," vol. ii., pp. 15, 16. 1856.

THE GREENLANDERS.—"The choicest dish of the Greenlanders is the flesh of the reindeer. But as those animals have now become extremely scarce—and several of them are soon consumed by a hunting-party—they are indebted to the sea for their permanent sustenance: seals, fish, and sea-fowl. Hares and partridges are in no great estimation as delicacies. The head and fins of the seal are preserved under the grass in summer, and in winter a whole seal is frequently buried in the snow. The flesh, half-frozen, half-putrid, in which state the Greenlanders term it mikiak, is eaten with the keenest appetite. The ribs are dried in the air and laid up in store. The remaining parts of the seal, as well as birds and small fishes, are eaten, well boiled or stewed with a small quantity of sea-water. On the capture of a seal the wound is immediately stopped up, to pre-serve the blood, which is rolled into balls like forcemeat."—"Simmond's Curiosities of Food," p. 32. 1859.

THE ICELANDERS.—"The diet of the Icelanders consists almost solely of animal food, of which fish, either fresh or dried, forms by far the largest proportion. During the summer they have milk and butter in considera-ble abundance; but of bread and every other vegetable food there is the utmost scarcity, and among the lower classes an almost entire privation. . . . . As an effect of these circumstances in the mode of life of the Ice-landers, cutaneous diseases, arising from a cachectic state of the body, are exceedingly frequent among them, and appear under some of their worst forms. Scurvy and leprosy are common in the island, occurring es-pecially on the western coast, where the inhabitants depend chiefly upon fishing, and where the pastures are inferior in extent and produce. . . . Scurvy is observed to occur with greatest frequency at those periods when there has been a deficiency of food among the inhabitants, or when the snow and frost of the winter succeed immediately to a wet autumnal sea-son. For its cure a vegetable diet is employed, in as far as the circum-stances of the Icelanders will allow of such means. Fruits of every kind are altogether wanting to them; but some advantage is derived from the employment of the *Cochlearia* (*officinalis et Danica*), of the trefoil (*Tri-*
20

folium repens), of the berries and tops of the juniper (*Juniperus communis*), and of the *Sedum acre*, plants which are all indigenous in the island. Inflammatory affections of the abdominal viscera are likewise very common among the Icelanders, chiefly, perhaps, in consequence of the peculiar diet to which they are accustomed.

"The diet of the Icelanders likewise gives much disposition to worms, and the ascarides are observed to be particularly frequent."—"Mackenzie's Travels in Iceland," pp. 407–412. 1811.

SIBERIA.—Lower Kolyma.—"One of the women prepares the frugal dinner or supper, which usually consists of either fish or reindeer-meat boiled or fried in train-oil. As an occasional delicacy, they have baked cakes of fish-roe or of dried and finely-pounded muksuns, which are the substitutes for meal. . . . . Bread is everywhere rare. From the meal, which is so dear that only the rich can buy it, a drink is prepared called saturan."—"Wrangell's Expedition to the Polar Sea," p. 75. 1844.

The Jakuts.—"Their food consists of sour cow's milk and mare's milk, and of beef and horseflesh. They boil their meat, but never roast or bake it, and bread is unknown among them. Fat is their greatest delicacy. They eat it in every possible shape—raw, melted, fresh, or spoilt. In general, they regard quantity more than quality in their food. They grate the inner bark of the larch, and sometimes of the fir, and mix it with fish, a little meal, and milk, or by preference with fat, and make it into a sort of broth, which they consume in large quantities. They prepare from cow's milk what is called the Jakut butter. It is more like a kind of cheese or of curd, and has a sourish taste; it is not very rich, and is a very good article of food eaten alone."—"Wrangell's Expedition to the Polar Sea," p. 23. 1844.

NORTH AMERICAN INDIANS.—"The buffalo-meat, however, is the great staple and staff of life in this country [Mandan Village, Upper Missouri], and seldom, if ever, fails to afford them an abundant and wholesome means of subsistence. There are, from a fair computation, something like 250,000 Indians in these western regions, who live almost exclusively on the flesh of these animals through every part of the year."—"Catlin's Letters on the North American Indians," vol. i., p. 122.

INDIAN TRIBES OF THE INTERIOR OF OREGON.—"They all prefer their meat putrid, and frequently keep it until it smells so strong as to be disgusting. Parts of the salmon they bury under ground for two or three months, to putrefy, and the more it is decayed the greater delicacy they consider it."—"Wilks' U. S. Exploring Expedition, vol. iv., p. 452.

MEXICO.—"The Indians of New Spain—those, at least, subject to the European domination—generally attain to a pretty advanced age. As peaceable cultivators and inhabitants of villages, they are not exposed to the accidents attending the wandering life of the hunters and warriors of the Mississippi and of the savannas of the Rio Gila. Accustomed to uniform nourishment of an almost entirely vegetable nature, that of their maize and cereal *gramina*, the Indians would undoubtedly attain very great longevity if their constitutions were not weakened by drunkenness. Their intoxicating liquors are rum, a fermentation of maize and the root of the *Jatropha*, and especially the wine of the country, made of the juice of the *Agave Americana*, called *pulque*. This last liquor is nutritive on account of the undecomposed sugar which it contains. Many Indians addicted to *pulque* take for a long time very little solid nourishment. When used with moderation, it is very salutary, and, by fortifying the stomach, assists the function of the gastric system."—"Taylor's Selections from Humboldt's Works relating to Mexico," pp. 67, 68. 1824.

"The usual food of the laboring classes, throughout such states as I visited, is the thin cake of crushed maize, which I have described under the name tortilla; and it is remarkable that, notwithstanding the great abundance of cattle in many places, the traveller can rarely obtain meat in the little huts which he finds on his road. Chilis are eaten abundantly with the tortillas, being stewed in a kind of sauce, into which the cakes are dipped. A few fowls are at times to be seen wandering near the cottages, or some pigs rambling through the village, and the flesh of these creatures furnishes a feast on holidays."—"Lyon's Residence in Mexico," vol. ii., pp. 244, 245. 1828.

PAMPAS INDIANS.—"The Indians of whom I heard the most were those who inhabit the vast unknown plains of the Pampas, and who are all horsemen, or rather pass their lives on horseback. The life they lead is singularly interesting. In spite of the climate, which is burning hot in summer and freezing in winter, these brave men, who have never yet been subdued, are entirely naked, and have not even a covering for their head.

"They live together in tribes, each of which is governed by a cacique; but they have no fixed place of residence. Where the pasture is good, there are they to be found until it is consumed by their horses, and they then instantly move to a more verdant spot. They have neither bread, fruit, nor vegetables; but they subsist entirely on the flesh of their mares." —"F. B. Head's Journeys Across the Pampas," p. 120. 1828.

"The ground is the bed on which, from their infancy, they have always slept. The flesh of mares is the food on which they have been accustomed to subsist."—Ibid., p. 122.

Sir Francis Head, when crossing the Pampas, got tired at first with the constant galloping, and was forced to ride in a carriage after five or six hours on horseback. "But after," he says, "I had been riding for three or four months, and had lived on beef and water, I found myself in a condition which I can only describe by saying that I felt no exertion could kill me. Although I constantly arrived so completely exhausted that I could not speak, yet a few hours' sleep upon my saddle on the ground always so completely restored me, that for a week I could daily be upon my horse before sunrise, could ride till two or three hours after sunset, and have really tired ten and twelve horses a day. This will explain the immense distances which people in South America are said to ride, which I am confident could only be done on beef and water."—Ibid., p. 51.

GUACHOS.—"We find a people living between the twentieth and fortieth parallels of latitude, in the Argentine Republic, known as Guachos [the half-white inhabitants of the Pampas]. They are a mixed race of Indian and Spanish blood, who are employed at the ranchos or great cattle stations, and spend the greater part of their time on horseback, in hunting the half-wild cattle which roam over the wide grassy plains extending from the Atlantic coast to the foot of the Andes. . . . . These people live entirely on roast beef, with a little salt, scarcely ever tasting farinaceous or other vegetable food, and their sole beverage is maté, or Paraguay tea, taken without sugar."—"Odontological Society's Transactions," vol. ii. new series, p. 44.

THE NATIVES OF AUSTRALIA.—"Their food consists of fish when near the coasts; but when in the woods, of opossums, bandicoots, and almost any animal they can catch, and also a kind of *grub*, which they find in decayed wood. Sometimes they spear a kangaroo. They roast all the fish and animals on the ashes, skin and all, just as they catch them. When it is pretty well done they divide it amongst themselves by tearing it with their teeth and fingers, and, excepting the bones, they devour every part, including the entrails."—"Robert Dawson's Present State of Australia," pp. 67, 68. 1830.

"Amongst the almost unlimited catalogue of edible articles used by the natives of Australia, the following may be classed as the chief: All salt and fresh-water fish and shell-fish, of which in the large rivers there are vast numbers and many species; fresh-water turtle; frogs of different kinds; rats and mice; lizards and most kinds of snakes and reptiles; grubs of all kinds; moths of several varieties; fungi and many sorts of roots; the leaves and tops of a variety of plants; the leaf and fruit of the Mesembryanthemum; various kinds of fruits and berries; the bark from the roots of many trees and shrubs; the seeds of leguminous plants; gum from several species of acacia; different sorts of manna; honey from the native bee, and also from the flowers of the Banksia by soaking them in water; the tender leaves of the grass-tree; the larvæ of insects; white ants; eggs of birds; turtles or lizards; many kinds of kangaroo; opossums; squirrels, sloths, and wallabies; ducks, geese, teal, cockatoos, parrots, wild dogs, and wombats; the native companion, the wild turkey, the swan, the pelican, the leipoa, and an endless variety of water-fowl and other descriptions of birds."—"Eyre's Central Australia," vol. ii., pp. 250, 251.

NEW ZEALAND.—"In former times the food of the natives consisted of sweet potatoes, taro (Caladium esculentum), fern-root (Pteris esculenta), the aromatic berries of the kahikatea (Dacrydium excelsum), the pulp of a fern-tree (Cyathea medullaris) called korau or mamako, the sweet root of the Dracæna indivisa, the heart of a palm-tree (Areca sapida), a bitter though excellent vegetable, the Sonchus oleraceus, and many different berries. Of animals they consumed fishes, dogs, the indigenous rat, crawfish, birds, and guanas. Rough mats of their own making, or dog-skins, constituted their clothing. They were hardened against the influence of the climate by the necessity of exerting themselves in procuring these provisions, and by their frequent predatory and travelling excursions, which produced a healthy excitement, and with it an easy digestion of even this crude diet."—"Dieffenbach's Travels in New Zealand," vol. ii., pp. 17, 18. 1843.

Fish is the principal food of the inhabitants, and, therefore, the inland tribes are frequently in danger of perishing of famine. "Their country produces neither sheep nor goats, nor hogs, nor cattle; tame fowls they have none."

The vegetables eaten are fern-root, yams, clams, and potatoes.

They also eat dogs.—"Cook's First Voyage" (Hawkesworth, vol. iii., p. 447).

Roots of the fern are to the people what bread is to the inhabitants of Europe.

"The birds which sometimes serve them for a feast are chiefly penguins and albatrosses.—Ibid., p. 459.

THE NATIVES OF THE FRIENDLY ISLANDS.—"Yams, plantains, and cocoa-nuts compose the greatest part of their vegetable diet. Of their animal food, the chief articles are hogs, fowls, fish, and all sorts of shell-fish; but the lower people eat rats.

"Hogs, fowls, and turtle seem to be reserved for their chiefs."—"Cook's Third Voyage," vol. i., p. 397.

The Inhabitants of Otaheite.—"Their food consists of pork, poultry, dog's flesh, and fish; bread-fruit, bananas, plantains, yams, apples, and a sour fruit which, though not pleasant by itself, gives an agreeable relish to roasted bread-fruit, with which it is frequently beaten up."— "Wallis' Voyage," 1767 ("Hawkesworth's Voyages," vol. i., p. 483).

"I cannot much commend the flavor of their fowls, but we all agreed that a South Sea dog was little inferior to an English lamb; their excellence is probably owing to their being kept up and fed wholly upon vegetables."—"Cook's First Voyage" ("Hawkesworth's Voyages," vol. ii., pp. 196–199).

"Their common diet is made up of at least nine-tenths of vegetable food."

"Of animal food a very small portion falls at any time to the share of the lower class of people, and then it is either fish, sea-eggs, or other marine productions."—"Cook's Third Voyage," vol. ii., pp. 148 and 154.

Feejee Islands.—"What all voyagers have said of the cocoa-nut tree we found to be true, only, instead of its uses being exaggerated, as some have supposed, they are, in my opinion, underrated. A native may well ask if a land contains cocoa-nuts, for if it does he is assured it will afford him abundance to supply his wants."—"Wilkes, U. S. Exploring Expedition," vol. iii., p. 334.

Tanna (one of the New Hebrides).—"The produce of the island is bread-fruit, plantains, cocoa-nuts, a fruit like a nectarine, yams, tarra (a sort of potato), sugar-cane, wild figs, and some other fruits and nuts.

"Hogs did not seem to be scarce, but we saw not many fowls. These are the only domestic animals they have.

"I believe these people live chiefly on the produce of the land, and that the sea contributes but little to their subsistence. Whether this arises from the coast not abounding with fish, or from their being bad fishermen, I know not; both causes, perhaps, concur."—"Cook's Second Voyage," vol. ii., p. 77.

New Caledonia.—The inhabitants "subsist chiefly on roots and fish and the bark of a tree, which, I am told, grows also in the West Indies. This they roast and are almost continually chewing. It has a sweetish, insipid taste, and was liked by some of our people. Water is their only liquor—at least I never saw any other made use of."—Ibid., vol. ii., p. 123.

Island of Savu (between Australia and Java).—"The food of these people consists of every tame animal in the country, of which the hog holds the first place in their estimation, and the horse the second; next to the horse is the buffalo, next to the buffalo their poultry, and they prefer dogs and cats to sheep and goats. They are not fond of fish."

The fan-palm is at certain times a succedaneum for all other food, both to man and beast. A kind of wine called toddy is procured from this tree.—"Cook's First Voyage" (Hawkesworth, vol. iii., pp. 688, 689.)

Sandwich Islands.—"The food of the lower class of people consists principally of fish and vegetables, such as yams, sweet potatoes, tarrow, plantains, sugar-canes, and bread-fruit. To these the people of a higher rank add the flesh of hogs and dogs, dressed in the same manner as at the Society Islands. They also eat fowls of the same domestic kind with ours; but they are neither plentiful nor much esteemed by them."— "Cook's Third Voyage," vol. iii. (by Capt. King), p. 141.

"The principal food of the lower class of the population, and, in fact, the favorite food of all classes, is *poi.*" This "is a sort of paste made from the root of the kalo (*Arum esculentum*), a water plant, cultivated to a great extent throughout all the islands." "The kalo is much used by the foreign residents as a substitute for potatoes, or rather for bread, being for this purpose either boiled or fried."

"These (their fish) the natives prefer in a raw state, on the ground that they lose their flavor in cooking, considering it as the richest possible treat, when on their aquatic excursions, to haul a fish from the water and literally eat it to death."—"Sir George Simpson's Journey Round the World," vol. ii., pp. 31–41. 1847.

CHINA.—"The Chinese, again, have no prejudice whatever as regards food; they eat anything and everything from which they can derive nutrition. Dogs, rats, mice, monkeys, snakes, sea-slugs, rotten eggs, putrefied fish, unhatched ducks and chickens." "Both in eating and drinking the Chinese are temperate, and are satisfied with two daily meals; the morning rice about 10 A.M., and the evening rice at 5 P.M. The only repugnance I have observed in China is to the use of milk." "I never saw or heard of butter, cream, milk, or whey, being introduced at any Chinese table."—Bowring: *Statistical Society Journal*, vol. xx., p. 47.

"Their famous gin-sing, a name signifying the life of a man (the *Panax quinquefolium* of Linnæus), on account of its supposed invigorating and aphrodisiac qualities, was for a length of time weighed against gold. The sinewy parts of stags and other animals, with the fins of sharks, as productive of the same effects, are purchased by the wealthy at enormous prices; and the nests that are constructed by small swallows on the coasts of Cochin China, Cambodia, and other parts of the East, are dearer even than some kinds of gin-sing. Most of the plants that grow on the sea-shore are supposed to possess an invigorating quality, and are, therefore, in constant use as pickles or preserves, or simply dried and cut into soups in the place of other vegetables. The leaves of one of these, apparently a species of that genus called by botanists *fucus*, after being gathered, are steeped in fresh water and hung up to dry. A small quantity of this weed boiled in water gives to it the consistence of a jelly, and when mixed with a little sugar, the juice of an orange, or other fruit, and set by to cool, I know of no jelly more agreeable or refreshing."

"The great officers of state make use of these and various other gelatinous viands for the purpose of acquiring, as they suppose, a proper degree of corpulency."—"Barrow's Travels in China," pp. 551, 552. 1806.

"The food of these people [Chinese laborers] is of the simplest kind, namely, rice, vegetables, and a small portion of animal food, such as fish or pork. But the poorest classes in China seem to understand the art of preparing their food much better than the same classes at home. With the simple substances I have named, the Chinese laborer contrives to make a number of very savory dishes, upon which he breakfasts or dines most sumptuously."—"Fortune's Residence among the Chinese," p. 42.

JAPAN.—Japan surpasses most other countries hitherto known to us in the multiplicity of the articles of food to be met with in its islands and the surrounding ocean.

"Rice, which is here exceedingly white and well-tasted, supplies with the Japanese, the place of bread; they eat it boiled with every kind of provisions.

"Miso soup, boiled with fish and onions, is eaten by the common people, frequently three times a days, at each of their customary meals.

Misos are not unlike lentils, and are small beans gathered from the *Dolichos soja.*
" Fish is likewise a very common dish with the Japanese, both boiled and fried in oil. Fowls, of which they have a great variety, both wild and tame, are eaten in great abundance; and the flesh of whales, though coarse, is in several places, at least among the poorer sort, a very common food."
" In preparing their victuals they make use of expressed oils of several different sorts." " In their victuals they make a very plentiful use of mushrooms, and the fruit of the *Solanum melongena* (egg-apple), as well as the roots of the *Solanum esculentum* (batatas), carrots and several kinds of bulbous roots and of beans."
" Of oysters and other shell-fish several different sorts are eaten, but always boiled or stewed, as likewise shrimps and crabs."—" Thunberg's Travels," vol. iv., pp. 35-39. 1795

INDIA.—From the earliest period the most general food in India has been rice, which is still the most common food of nearly all the hottest countries of Asia. It is not, however, so much used in the south of Hindostan as formerly, and has been replaced by another grain, called ragi. —" Buckle's History of Civilization," vol. i., pp. 64, 65.

" The principal food of the people of Hindostan is wheat, and in the Deccan, jowár and bájra; rice, as a general article of subsistence, is confined to Bengal and part of Behár, with the low country along the sea all round the coast of the peninsula. In most parts of India it is only used as a luxury. In the southern part of the table-land of the Deccan the body of the people live on a small and poor grain, called ragi (*Cynosurus corocanus*). Though these grains each afford the principal supply to particular divisions, they are not confined to their own tracts." Pulse, roots, and fruits are largely eaten.—" Elphinstone's History of India," vol. i., pp. 12, 13.

CEYLON.—" The ordinary diet of the people is very meagre, consisting of rice seasoned with salt, the chief condiment of the East, and a few vegetables, flavored with lemon-juice and pepper, from which they will make at any time a hearty meal. Beef is forbidden, being an abomination. Flesh is scarce, and fish not always plentiful, but when it is they prefer selling it to Europeans to keeping it for themselves. It is considered anything but a reproach to be sparing in diet, but rather a credit to live on hard fare and suffer hunger.

" The hondrew class are rather more luxurious, eating from five or six sorts of food, one or two of which consists of meat or fish, and the remainder of vegetable dishes. Their chief food, however, is rice, the other dishes being used principally for a relish."—" Pridham's Ceylon," vol. i., p. 263. 1849.
Almost endless cocoa-nut forests in Ceylon provide the native with the most important necessary for supporting existence.—" Voyage of the Novara," vol. i., p. 366.

EGYPT.—Beef and goose constituted the principal part of the animal food throughout Egypt.
" The advantages of a leguminous diet are still acknowledged by the inhabitants of modern Egypt. This, in a hot climate, is far more conducive to health than the constant introduction of meat, which is principally used to flavor the vegetables cooked with it."
Vegetables form the principal food of the lower orders, and lentils are a chief article of diet.—" Wilkinson's Ancient Egyptians," vol. ii., pp. 368-388.

"The usual season for sowing the doura, which constitutes almost the whole subsistence of the peasantry, is soon after the commencement of the inundation."—" Hamilton's Ægyptiaca," p. 419. 1809.

SAHARA.—" Dates are not only the principal growth of the Fezzan oases, but the main subsistence of their inhabitants. All live on dates—men, women, and children, horses, asses, and camels, and sheep, fowls, and dogs."—" Richardson's Travels in the Great Desert," vol. ii., p. 323. 1848.

NUBIA.—" We have another example of a race subsisting entirely on animal food, in the Arabs who inhabit the Nubian desert—a district which consists principally of hills varying from 1,000 to 1,800 feet high, and is destitute of all vegetable products suitable for human food. Their camels subsist on the thorny shrubs growing among the rocks; and the milk and flesh of these animals (with salt) constitute their sole ordinary food. On their occasional journeys into Egypt, to sell camels, they usually bring home a small quantity of wheat, which is never ground, but boiled into a kind of frumenty, and eaten as a luxury, but it must not be reckoned as an ordinary element in their diet."—" Odontological Society Transactions," vol. ii., new series, p. 45.

ABYSSINIA.—" An instinctive feeling, dependent upon the pleasures of a state of warmth, has taught the Abyssinians that flesh of animals eaten raw is a source of great physical enjoyment by the cordial and warming effects upon the system produced by its digestion, and to which I am convinced *bons vivants* more civilized than the Abyssinians would resort if placed in their situation. Travellers who have witnessed their "brunde" feasts can attest to the intoxicating effects of this kind of food, and they must have been astonished at the immense quantities that can be eaten in the raw state compared to that when the meat is cooked, and at the insensibility which it sometimes produces." This raw meat, however, is considered a luxury, and is only indulged in at festivals.—" Johnston's Travels in Southern Abyssinia," vol. ii., p. 226. 1844.

"The Abyssinians suffer considerably in their health from the difficulty of obtaining salt."—Ibid., vol. ii., p. 175.

DAHOMEY.—" The diet is simple, consisting chiefly of messes of meat and vegetable, mixed with palm oil and pepper, with which is eaten a corn-cake, called kankee, or dab-a-dab. There is very little variety. A mixture of beans, peppers, and palm oil, is made into a cake and sold to travellers; yams and cassada form the staples of food. Foreign liquors are scarce and expensive; and as palm wine is forbidden by the king, the chief drinks are a very palatable malt called pitto, and a sort of burgoo called ah-kah-sar."—" Forbes' Dahomey and the Dahomans," vol. i., pp. 29, 30. 1851.

"THE WABORI are small and shrivelled black savages. Their diminutive size is, doubtless, the effect of scanty food, continued through many generations." "The principal articles of diet are milk, meat, and especially fattened dogs' flesh, of which the chiefs are inordinately fond, maize, holcus, and millet. Rice is not grown in these arid districts." "Burton's Lake Regions of Central Africa," vol. ii., p. 273.

WAMRIMA OR COAST CLANS.—" Their food is mostly ugali, the thick porridge of boiled millet or maize flour, which represents the 'staff of life' in East Africa. They usually feed twice a day, in the morning and at nightfall. They employ the cocoa-nut extensively; like the Arabs of Zanzibar, they boil their rice in the thick juice of the rasped albumen kneaded with water, and they make cakes of the pulp mixed with the flour of various grains. This immoderate use of the fruit, which, according to the people, is highly refrigerant, causes, it is said, rheumatic and other diseases. A respectable man seen eating a bit of raw or undressed cocoa-nut would be derided by his fellows."—Ibid., vol. i., p. 35. 1860.

EAST AFRICANS.—" With the savage and the barbarian, food is the all-in-all of life; food is his thought by day—food is his dream by night."

" The principal articles of diet are fish and flesh, grain and vegetables; the luxuries are, milk and butter, honey, and a few fruits, as bananas and Guinea-palm dates; and the inebriants are pombe or millet-beer, toddy, and mawa or plantain wine."

" The Arabs assert that in these latitudes vegetables cause heartburn and acidity, and that animal food is the most digestible. The Africans seem to have made the same discovery. A man who can afford it almost confines himself to flesh, and considers fat the essential element of good living."—Ibid., vol. ii., pp. 280–287.

CABANGO (a village situated on the banks of the Chihombo).—"The chief vegetable food is the manioc and lotsa meal. These contain a very large proportion of starch, and when eaten alone for any length of time produce most distressing heartburn. As we ourselves experienced in coming north, they also cause a weakness of vision, which occurs in the case of animals fed on pure gluten or amylaceous matter only. I now discovered that when these starchy substances are eaten along with a proportion of ground-nuts, which contain a quantity of oil, no injurious effects follow."—"Livingstone's Missionary Travels and Researches in South Africa," p. 455. 1857.

KAFFIRS.—" The principal diet of the Kaffir is milk, which he eats rather than drinks, in a sour and curdled state. One good meal a day, taken in the evening, consisting of the curdled milk and a little millet, is almost all that he requires, and with this he is strong, vigorous, and robust, proving that large quantities of animal food are by no means necessary for the sustenance of the human frame."

A Kaffir will never touch pork. Fish is likewise abstained from by him. He will eat the flesh of an ox, cooked or raw.—"Simmonds' Curiosities of Food," p. 39.

BOSJESMANS.—"The African Bushmen, who have few or no cattle, live upon what they can get. Hunger compels them to eat everything—roots, bulbs, wild garlic, the core of aloes, the gum of acacias, berries, the larvæ of ants, lizards, locusts, and grasshoppers—all are devoured by these poor wanderers of the desert. Nothing comes amiss to them."—Ibid., p. 38.

HOTTENTOTS.—"The victuals of the Hottentots are the flesh and entrails of cattle, and of certain wild beasts, with fruits and roots of several kinds."

They "rarely kill cattle for their own eating but when they are at a loss for other sustenance. The cattle they devour between the Andersmakens are for the most part such as die naturally, and they reckon 'em, as I have said, very delicious eating."

" The entrails of cattle, and of such wild beasts as they kill for food, they look upon as most exquisite eating. They boil 'em in beast-blood, if they have any, to which they sometimes add milk. This they look upon as a glorious dish. If they have not blood to boil 'em in, they broil 'em. And this they do on the bare fire, for they have no such thing as a gridiron."

" They eat everything in such a hurry, and with so much indecency, that they look extremely wild and ravenous at meals, particularly when they eat flesh, which being always serv'd up to 'em half raw or more, they make a very furious use of their hands (where they have no knives) and of their teeth to tear and devour it."

"Many are the sorts of fruits and roots the Hottentots eat, and the fields up and down for the most part abound with 'em. These, as I have said, are gather'd wholly by the women. In the choice of roots and fruits for food they follow the hedgehog and the bavian, a sort of ape, and will not taste of any sort which those creatures do not feed upon " (for fear of poison).

"The Hottentots have no set times for their meals. They have no notion of dividing them, as we do, into breakfast, dinner, and supper, but take 'em at random, as humor or appetite calls, without any regard to the hour of the day or the night."

They "have traditionary laws, forbidding the eating of certain meats, which they accordingly abstain from very carefully. Swine's flesh and fishes that have no scales are forbidden to both sexes. The eating of hares and rabbits is forbidden to the men, but not to the women. The pure blood of beasts and flesh of the mole are forbidden to the women, but not to the men."

"The Hottentots, when they are in great strait for food, will devour the rings of leather which the women wear upon their legs. They will likewise, in the same strait, eat old cast-off shoes " [which they lay up against a time of want].

"Their manner of dressing 'em is this : They singe off the hair, then having soak'd 'em a little in water, broil 'em upon the bare fire till they begin to wrinkle and run up, and then they devour 'em."

The Hottentots never eat salt among themselves, but " they are not a little delighted with the salt and otherwise high-seasoned victuals of the Europeans." [Such food, however, disagrees with them, and those who eat with the Europeans are subject to many maladies, and don't attain a great age.]

"The ordinary drink of the Hottentots is milk and water."

"Men and women are doatingly fond of tobacco."—"Kolben's State of the Cape of Good Hope," pp. 200–208. 1731.

Thus it is seen that a great diversity exists as regards the food consumed by the human race in different parts of the globe. Instances are to be found where life is sustained upon a wholly vegetable, a wholly animal, and a mixed diet. The mixed diet, however, may be regarded as that which, in the plan of nature, is designed for man's subsistence. It is upon this that he appears to attain the highest state of physical development and intellectual vigor. It is this which, certainly in temperate climates, he is led to consume by general inclination, when circumstances allow the inclination to guide him; and, lastly, it is this which stands in conformity with the construction of his teeth and the anatomy of his digestive apparatus in general.

Notwithstanding these considerations there are those—but few in number, it is true—who contend that vegetable food alone is best adapted to meet our requirements. Under the style of vegetarians,* they act

---

* Payen (Substances Alimentaires, 4me éd.. p. 561. Paris, 1865), after expressing himself in condemnation of restriction to vegetable products. says: " Cependant en Angleterre, ce pays des excentricités, où l'on voit une belle et progressive civilisation marcher dans presque toutes les directions avec quelque accompagnement de barbarie, une secte nombreuse tend à exclure la chair des animaux du régime alimentaire de la population ; elle prêche d'exemple et fait quelques prosélytes."

upon the principle they profess. It is true that vegetable food, with its large proportion of non-nitrogenous matter, yields, in a simple and direct manner, according to the views now entertained and fully discussed in an earlier part of this work, the requisites for force- as well as heat-production; and, in order to show that vegetable food is better adapted than animal for contributing to the performance of muscular work, reference has been made to our beasts of burden, which, as is well known, belong almost exclusively to the herbivorous tribe. That carnivorous animals, however, are not unsuited for such purpose is proved in the case of dogs, which, in some northern and other countries, are very extensively employed for the performance of work. To regard man's maintenance too closely in association with the mere performance of mechanical work —to look upon him, in other words, as though he were solely designed for the conversion of food into mechanical power, is not, it may be also said, taking a high view of his position.

Vegetarians, however, as has been remarked, are by no means numerous. Indeed, the prevailing tendency, certainly in the England of the present day, is to give an undue weight to the value of animal food, and this has been encouraged by the teachings of Liebig regarding the origin of muscular power—teachings which, during the last few years, have been shown to be untenable.

Many people seem to look upon meat almost as though it formed the only food that really nourished and supplied what is wanted for work. The physician is constantly coming across an expression of this view. Undoubtedly a greater feeling of satiety is produced by meat than by other food. It forms a greater stay to the stomach, but this arises from · the stomach constituting the seat of its digestion, and a longer time being occupied before it passes on and leaves the organ in an empty condition.

Against those who think that a large consumption of meat is a *sine quâ non* for the maintenance of health and strength, the experience of vegetarians may be adduced. In the effects of the Scotch prison dietaries corroborative testimony is afforded. Dr. J. B. Thomson, for instance, resident surgeon to the General Prison for Scotland, writing in the *Medical Times and Gazette*, vol. i., 1868, speaks in favor, from ten years' experience, of a diet into which meat entered very sparingly, and which contained instead a moderate amount of milk. He says since the employment of the improved dietaries sanctioned by the Secretary of State in 1854, the dietary in the General Prison for Scotland for all adult male prisoners, under sentence of nine, and not exceeding twenty-four months, had consisted of bread, oatmeal, barley, 1 oz. of meat per diem, made into soup, with succulent vegetables, and 20 oz. of skimmed or butter milk. One day in the week fish had been substituted for the soup. The health of the prisoners had been uniformly good. Weighing on admission and liberation had been carried out, and 88 per cent. were found to have gained or maintained their weight. Again, as shown by one of Dr. E. Smith's reports, it is not uncommon to find, amongst the agricultural laborers of Scotland, that no meat is consumed, oatmeal and milk forming the staple articles of diet. Further, Dr. Guy,* from his observations in the case of English prisons, gives as one of his deductions, "that we possess conclusive evidence of the sufficiency of a diet from which meat is wholly excluded, and even of a diet consisting wholly of vegetable matter."

---

* On Sufficient and Insufficient Dietaries, with especial reference to the Dietaries of Prisoners: Journal of the Statistical Society, vol. xxvi , p. 280. 1863.

I have introduced these particulars, not for the purpose of showing that a diet without meat is to be considered desirable, but for strengthening the argument that the consumption of meat to the extent that many persons believe necessary for the maintenance of health and strength is not in reality so. It has been before stated that physiological considerations point to a mixed diet as being most in harmony with our nature, and it may probably be considered that the most suitable admixture contains about one-fourth, or rather more, of animal food. With more animal food than this, the excretory organs are unnecessarily taxed, and the system exposed to contamination with impurities, for the nitrogen of the superfluous nitrogenous matter has to be eliminated, and is found to escape, in combination with other elements, under the form of certain excretory products, without having contributed to any useful purpose. A defective transformative and eliminative action will lead to a retention of the products of metamorphosis of this superfluous nitrogenous matter in the system, and there is reason to believe that gouty affections, and other morbid states, are sometimes induced in this way.

It has been pointed out, under the head of "Principles of Dietetics" (*vide* p. 303), how an admixture of animal and vegetable food is better fitted to yield what is wanted than either consumed alone. It is assumed that, for a man of medium stature and in moderate work, about 300 grains of nitrogen and 4,800 grains of carbon are daily required to be introduced into the system with the food. Now, this is yielded, as nearly as possible, in the case of both elements, by 2 pounds of bread and ¾ pound of meat—that is, 44 ounces of solid food, of which about one-fourth consists of animal matter. If the lean of meat only were consumed (for the proper adjustment could equally be made with meat and fat), rather over 6 pounds would be needed to furnish the requisite amount of carbon, and there would be a very large surplus of nitrogen; whilst if bread only were taken, the amount necessary to supply the requisite quantity of nitrogen would be rather more than 4 pounds, and this contains nearly double the amount of carbon demanded.

Whilst speaking of the proper food for man it may be stated that, for the perfect and prolonged maintenance of health, it is necessary that a portion of what is consumed should be in the fresh state. This applies to both animal and vegetable kinds of food. Neither one nor the other in a salted, cured, or dried state will serve to keep the body in health. Former experience has but too painfully shown that disease and death are induced by withholding all fresh articles of food. There may be no lack of quantity, and yet the body shall fail to be maintained in a proper state. Affections of the scorbutic class are produced, which are only to be checked and removed by the supply of some kind of fresh food, or, what has been found to equally answer the purpose, the juice of some kind of succulent vegetable or fruit. The efficacy of lemon and lime juice, for instance, is well known in the cure and prevention of scurvy.

DIETETIC RELATIONS AND EFFECTS OF ANIMAL AND VEGETABLE FOOD COMPARED.

Animal food, being identical in composition with the structures to be built up and maintained, contains neither more nor less than what is required for the growth and renovation of the body. It might be assumed from this relation that nutrition upon a supply of animal food would be carried on in a more simple way than nutrition upon vegetable food, where no such identity is observable, and which contains various principles, such as lignine, cellulose, starch, etc., which have no existence in the animal body. Nutrition, however, is not effected in this simple manner. With animal as well as with vegetable food, a transformation has to take place before absorption can occur.

It was shown by Mulder, and confirmed by Liebig, that the nitrogenous alimentary principles of the vegetable agree in composition with those of the animal kingdom, and it has been ascertained by physiologists that all alike undergo metamorphosis under the influence of the digestive process into a certain product, which is characterized by the possession of properties, viz., those of great solubility and diffusibility, that specially adapt it for transmission by absorption from the alimentary canal into the blood-vessels, by which it is conveyed to organs that elaborate and convert it into the nitrogenous principles existing in and applied to the purposes of the system. Thus, we elaborate for ourselves the constituent nitrogenous principles of our bodies out of a certain product of digestion, instead of deriving them directly from our food, and this brings alimentation, as far as these principles are concerned, to the same position, whether upon animal or vegetable products. There is only this difference to be noted—that animal nitrogenous substances appear to be more easily digested than vegetable.

With fats the same process occurs, whether they are of animal or vegetable origin; but, as with nitrogenous substances, it is believed that animal fats are more easy of digestion or preparation for absorption than vegetable.

Nitrogenous substances and fats may be said to comprise the organic portion of animal food. In vegetable food we encounter, besides, such principles as starch, sugar, gum, lignine, and cellulose, which belong to the group of carbohydrates. The two latter of these are scarcely, if at all, susceptible of any digestion, certainly by the human digestive organs, and, therefore, simply traverse the alimentary canal, and add to the bulk of the alvine dejections. The others are susceptible of utilization, and what digestion is required is, as in the case also of fat, carried on in the intestine, and not in the stomach. The physiological application of these principles, which are peculiar to vegetable food, has previously received attention, and need not be adverted to here.

Although animal food certainly taxes the *stomach* more than the ordinary forms of vegetable food that we consume, as is well known by those who have weak digestive power, yet, taking digestion and assimilation as a whole, a more complex process has to be gone through where vegetable food has to be dealt with. Accordingly we notice that the digestive apparatus of the herbivora is developed upon a more extended scale than in the carnivora. The difference, for instance, in the length of the intestinal canal is exceedingly marked, and, as already mentioned, it is especially here where the digestion of the principles that preponderate in vegetable products occurs. A portion of the large intestine, also, known as the crecum, which is not developed in the carnivora to any particular extent, attains, in many of the herbivora, enormous dimensions, and it can scarcely be doubted that this is designed for affording some kind of extra assistance in the digestive process.

Looked at now in relation to their effects upon the system, there are several points that call for consideration.

It is asserted by Lehmann that animal food increases the amount of fibrine in the blood, and also raises the amount of the phosphates and of the salts generally. A diet abounding in animal food appears also to render the blood richer in red corpuscles.

Animal food, with its preponderance of nitrogenous matter, tends to produce firmness of muscle with an absence of superfluous fat. Vegetable food, on the other hand, tends to increase the deposition of fat. Messrs. Lawes and Gilbert found in their experiments that animals consuming food containing an excessive quantity of nitrogenous matter showed a greater disposition to increase in frame and flesh. If we direct our attention to the animals around us, it is open to common observation to notice that vegetable feeders show a greater proneness to become fat than animal feeders. The animals we fatten all belong to the herbivora, and even dogs and cats become fatter on vegetable food—a proof that it is more the nature of the food than the kind of animal that makes the difference. Mr. Banting found that limiting his supply of vegetable food enabled him to reduce his corpulence, and it is upon the application of this principle that the system of " Bantingism " rests.

It appears from the experiments of Pettenkofer and Voit that increasing the proportion of nitrogenous matter in the food determines an increased absorption of oxygen by the lungs. Nitrogenous matter it is which starts the changes occurring in the system, and the suggestion presents itself that upon the amount of nitrogenous matter may to some extent depend the application of oxygen to the oxidation of fatty matter. Under this view the success of Mr. Banting's system may be due, not exclusively to a restriction of the principles that tend to produce fat, but in part, also, to an increased oxidizing action promoted by the large amount of nitrogenous matter consumed.

It has been observed that the amount of urine secreted is notably influenced by the nature of the food. Bischoff and Voit noticed, in the case of the dog, that, upon giving a liberal supply of meat after the animal had been previously subsisting upon vegetable food, the urine was greatly increased in quantity. A striking example is also afforded by a series of experiments by Mr. Savory upon rats.* Three pairs of rats that had been fed upon wheat were placed, one pair upon non-nitrogenous food, a second pair upon lean meat, and the third pair upon mixed food. The urine was collected for the twenty-four hours upon three occasions, at intervals of a week, and each time the urine associated with the meat diet was in very large excess of what it had been previously, and of that derived from the other animals. The amount of nitrogenous matter passed, in accordance with what might have been expected from the results that have been referred to in a previous part of this work, bore a corresponding relation, and it may be that the two stand in the position of cause and effect. The effete nitrogenous matter, in escaping, may carry with it a flow of water. The extra quantity of water eliminated was met by an extra quantity of fluid consumed.

Besides the influence just referred to on the amount of urine, the solid matter is likewise, to a marked extent, influenced by the nature of the food. There is a well-known augmentation in urea, etc., produced by the ingestion of animal food, and, at the same time, an increase in the sulphates and phosphates. The reaction of the urine is also modified. Under an animal diet it is strongly acid, whilst a vegetable diet disposes to alkalinity. During fasting, it is true, the urine of the herbivora is acid, but after food its reaction is alkaline. Bernard* has dilated upon this point, which must be regarded as being of considerable importance with reference to the therapeutic employment of food. He mentions an experiment upon himself, in which, from previously presenting a strongly acid reaction, his urine was rendered alkaline in the course of twenty-four hours by restriction to a vegetable diet. In the sucking calf, as in the carnivora, the urine is acid, whilst it afterward assumes the character belonging to the herbivora.

Animal food appeases hunger more thoroughly than vegetable, and satisfies longer. In other words, it gives, as general experience will confirm, greater stay to the stomach. It also exerts a greater stimulating effect upon the system generally. Accounts are related of the stimulant properties of animal food having sufficed, in certain instances, as after starvation and in those accustomed only to a vegetable diet, to produce a state resembling intoxication. Dr. Dundas Thompson † quotes a narrative of the effects of a repast of meat on some native Indians, whose customary fare, as is usual amongst the tribe, had consisted only of vegetable food. "They dined most luxuriously, stuffing themselves as if they were never to eat again. After an hour or two, to his [the traveller's] great surprise and amusement, the expression of their countenances, their jabbering and gesticulations, showed clearly that the feast had produced the same effect as any intoxicating spirit or drug. The second treat was attended with the same result."

Dr. Druitt, in describing the properties of a liquid essence of beef,‡ which had been prepared according to his instructions, speaks of it as exerting a rapid and remarkable stimulating power over the brain, and introduced it to notice as an auxiliary to, and partial substitute for, brandy, in all cases of great exhaustion or weakness, attended with cerebral depression or despondency. Correspondingly stimulating properties have also been recognized as an effect of the copious employment of Liebig's Extractum Carnis.

The general character of an animal is related to its food. Liebig says § it is essentially their food which makes carnivorous animals in general bolder and more combative than the herbivora which are their prey. "A bear kept at the Anatomical Museum of Giessen showed a quiet, gentle nature, as long as he was fed exclusively on bread, but a few days' feeding on meat made him vicious and even quite dangerous. That swine grow irascible by having flesh food given them is well known—so much so, indeed, that they will then attack men."

It must be considered as a part of the plan of Nature that this relation should exist. It need not be that the animal food gives origin to the ferocity, but that the ferocity exists to enable the animal to obtain its food. In the case where a bloodhound is rendered dangerous by being fed upon flesh, and also in Liebig's citation, the result need not be attributable to the food otherwise than by the taste of it arousing the natural instinct of the animal.

* Physiologie Expérimentale, tome ii., p. 459. Paris, 1856.
† Experimental Researches on the Food of Animals, p. 24. London, 1846.
‡ Trans. of the Obstetrical Society, vol. iii., p. 143, 1861.
§ Lancet, vol. i., p. 186, 1869.

PROPER AMOUNT OF FOOD.

The amount of food required depends upon the existing circumstances. No fixed quantity can be given as suited to all cases. Variation in external temperature, the amount of work performed, and individual peculiarities, occasion a variation in the amount of material consumed in the body; and in a properly arranged diet the food should be adjusted accordingly. For this adjustment Nature has provided by the instinct or sensation with which we are endowed. Appetite, or, in its more exalted character, hunger, apprises us that food is required, and produces an irresistible desire to seek and obtain its supply. By attending to its dictates a knowledge is also afforded of the proper amount to be consumed. We may ascertain by observation the precise amount by weight that is necessary to keep the body in a properly nourished condition, but Nature's guide was in operation before weights and scales were invented. Speaking of the natural state, it is only where the strict margin, on the score of economy, as in the feeding of large bodies of men, has to be regarded, that a process of weighing need be employed.

In taking appetite as a guide in regulating the supply of food, it must not be confounded with a desire to gratify the palate. When food is not eaten too quickly and the diet is simple, a timely warning is afforded by the sense of satisfaction experienced as soon as enough has been taken; and not only does a disinclination arise, but the stomach even refuses to allow this point to be far exceeded. With a variety of food, however, and especially food of an agreeable character to the taste, the case is different. Satiated with one article, the stomach is still ready for another, and thus, for the gratification of taste, and not the appeasement of appetite, men are tempted to consume far more than is required, and also, it must be said, often far more than is advantageous to health.

Whatever the precise immediate cause of the sensation constituting appetite, the source of it is a want of solid matter in the system. Now, this want will vary with the consumption going on, which is greater under exposure to cold and during the performance of work than under opposite conditions; and in harmony therewith it is noticeable that the appetite is sharpened and diminished accordingly. The dictates thus afforded should be obeyed. They are not likely to be disregarded when the appetite is increased, and they should likewise be complied with when it is diminished. Concern is sometimes experienced at the falling off of the appetite that occurs during the heat of summer in our own climate, and that is noticed by Europeans on visiting the tropics, and attempts are sometimes made to counteract it by the employment of condiments of a stimulating nature to the stomach. This, however, is clearly an error, and one which is calculated to lead to baneful results, as in other instances where Nature's indications are set aside in favor of artificial devices.

Thirst is an expression of the want of liquid in the system as hunger is of that of solids. It leads us to adjust the supply to the demand arising from the loss that has been sustained.

Under the head of Principles of Dietetics reference has been made (*vide* p. 291 *et seq.*) to the amount of food found by observation to be consumed by various classes of persons. As already mentioned, no fixed amount can be given as suited to all individuals and conditions. In . Moleschott's representation of a model diet (*vide* p. 288) the daily quantity of food, estimated in a water-free or anhydrous state, amounts to about

23 ounces. To represent the amount of food in the ordinary state to which this corresponds, we must allow for the water present. According to the table at p. 291 bread contains 37 per cent. of water, cooked meat 54 per cent., and vegetables upward of 70 per cent. Say the food consumed contained 45 per cent. of water—probably a low estimate—the 23 ounces of water-free material would correspond to 45 ounces of ordinary food. For people engaged in laborious occupations, judging from Playfair's tables of the food actually consumed, this is evidently none too much, and is even under the amount actually consumed by many. For people, however, who lead a sedentary and in-door mode of life considerably less will suffice. I find from observation of my own diet, my height being rather over 5 feet 9 inches, and weight rather more than 10 stone, that 30 ounces fully cover what I ordinarily consume, the food consisting of the usual admixture of animal and vegetable articles, and being weighed in the state in which it is placed on the table; 8 ounces for breakfast, 6 for luncheon, and 16 for dinner, give me the outside of what I feel I require.

The middle diet at Guy's Hospital—the diet on which the majority of the patients are placed—gives a mean daily allowance of 29¼ ounces of solid food, apart from the liquids supplied. Taking solids and liquids together, and calculating from the composition of the articles according to the table at p. 291, the water-free material amounts to 16¾ ounces. The food actually supplied consists of 4 ounces of meat in the cooked state, 12 ounces of bread, 8 ounces of potatoes, 1 ounce of butter, ¾ ounce of sugar, ¼ ounce of tea, and—say 3½ ounces (8 ounces three times a week is the exact quantity) of rice pudding made of rice, sugar, and milk. Besides this solid food there is a daily allowance of half a pint of porter and 2½ ounces of milk, with half a pint of mutton broth when boiled meat is given, which is four times a week. Experience shows this diet to be sufficient for bodily maintenance under a condition of freedom from labor. A conclusion may be drawn, as the subsistence on it often extends over a considerable period, and amongst the inmates there are many in an ordinary state so far as their constitutional condition is concerned, some local complaint, unaffecting their general health, having led to their admission.

Besides treating of the gross amount of food, attention must be given to the relative proportion of the constituent alimentary principles. Unless these are so related as to be adjusted to the demands of the system, more food is required to be taken than would otherwise be the case, and waste is the result. As a deduction from a review of the dietaries referred to in a preceding part of this work (*vide* p. 292 *et seq.*), the following summary account may be given of the respective amounts of the alimentary principles required. The table furnished at p. 291 will supply the means for determining the constitution of a given diet in respect of alimentary principles.

The nitrogenous matter should constitute about one-fifth of the water-free food, and, under medium conditions, from 4 to 5 oz. may be looked upon as the quantity that should be supplied daily. With an inactive life much less will suffice, viz. 3 or 3½ oz. In Playfair's subsistence-diet (p. 292) the quantity is rather under 2½ oz. Exposure to hard work leads, judging from observation, to the instinctive consumption of food yielding a full supply of nitrogenous matter. In some of the collected dietaries the nitrogenous matter amounts to from 5 to 6 oz.

It has been mentioned that about one-fifth of the water-freed food should consist of nitrogenous matter, and this, in the case of bread and meat, is afforded by an admixture of about one part of animal with three

21

parts of vegetable material. Now, such an admixture, as before shown (p. 302), is also that which is adjusted to replace without waste the carbon and nitrogen passing out of the system. It was pointed out that if bread alone, or meat alone, were consumed, in order to supply the requisite quantity of both elements, a considerable waste of either one or the other would in each case ensue, because in the articles of food taken separately they are not in the proper proportion to balance the loss occurring. For example, 2 pounds of bread and ¾ pound of lean uncooked beef contain, as nearly as possible, the amounts of carbon and nitrogen represented as escaping from the body under average circumstances. In this admixture, amounting to 44 oz., the meat (12 oz.) forms, with only a slight excess, a fourth of the whole; and if we look to the composition of it, we find that in a water-free state about one-fifth consists of nitrogenous matter. The following representation of the amounts of the alimentary principles contained in it, calculated from the table furnished at p. 291, will be seen to bear out this statement.

	Bread 2 lbs.	Lean beef ¾ lb. uncooked.	Total.
	Oz.	Oz.	Oz.
Nitrogenous matter,	2.592	2.316	4.908
Fat, ...	0.512	0.432	0.944
Carbohydrates, . .	16.320	—	16.320
Mineral matter, . .	0.736	0.612	1.348
			23.520

It may be noticed, further, that the composition of these 2 pounds of bread and ¾ pound of meat agrees pretty closely with that of the model diet of Moleschott (p. 287), framed upon grounds of quite a different nature. The whole difference of any account is in the respective amounts of fats and carbohydrates; but what is deficient in the one is balanced by a surplus in the other, and, in an alimentary point of view, the two are capable, to a certain extent, of replacing each other.

Fat appears to influence favorably the assimilation of the other principles, and to be intimately concerned in tissue formation and nutrition, besides contributing to force production; and it is believed that a deficiency of it in the food is sometimes the source of the development of the scrofulous and strumous states. The supply, it may be considered, ought not to be less, even with inactivity, than one ounce daily, and the composition of dietaries usually shows considerably more. About 2¼ oz. appears to form the average amount in the diets of various working classes.

The carbohydrates may be looked upon as forming a supplementary group of principles. They have no existence in an animal diet, and in a mixed diet should be in such quantity as to fill up what is defective for force-production—heat and mechanical work—in the other principles. Looking at the various dietaries of mixed food to which the attention of the reader has been already directed, and leaving out of consideration the lowest or subsistence diet, the supply of carbohydrates is seen to range in amount from between 14 and 15 to 22 oz. per diem.

The amount of mineral matter required may be set down at from ¾ oz. to 1 oz. daily.

Water is needed beyond that contained in our food. It may be reckoned that we receive from about 15 to 25 oz. of fluid into the system mixed with the solid food that is consumed; and besides this, it is advisable that about 60 to 70 oz., or even in some cases more, should be taken. The average amount of urine passed daily may be said to be about 50 oz., and there is a considerable loss of fluid from the skin and the lungs. To meet these sources of elimination, compensation must be effected by a corresponding ingestion, and, as long as the fluid taken is devoid of noxious properties, a free supply must be regarded as beneficial, forming, as it does, a means of carrying off impurities from the system. Perhaps the benefit derivable from a course of water-treatment is often, in a great measure, due to this cause. I am strongly inclined to think so.

Having spoken of the proper amount of food, let me next direct attention to the effects produced by a deficiency and excess in its supply. I may commence by saying that there is far more evil to be encountered attributable to too much food being taken than to too little. It is only in exceptional cases that the latter kind is met with; whilst the amount of disorder, disease, and likewise even curtailment of life, attributable to excess in eating and drinking is immeasurably great. Where the living is plain and simple, and the dictates of Nature are followed, there is no need for weights and scales; but how many are there who would not be in an infinitely better state if they lived upon a weighed and measured allowance of food and drink! Seeking for what is pleasurable instead of natural, the promptings of instinct are overruled, and it is the inclination instead of appetite that regulates what is consumed. Were it not for the temptation to exceed, induced by the refinements of the culinary art, the physician's aid would be much more rarely required.

Amongst the effects arising from excess in feeding may be mentioned an oppressed stomach, deranged digestion, a loaded tongue, vitiated secretions, with disordered action of the bowels, a gorged liver, obesity, plethora and its consequences, a sluggish brain and troubled sleep, surcharged urine, leading to deposits, perverted nutrition from the preternatural accumulation of products of disintegration in the system, and, as a concomitant, gouty and rheumatic affections. Such, and others too, are the ills arising from over-feeding. Excess in animal food is worse than excess in vegetable food, especially when combined with sedentary habits. It is true, vegetable food especially leads to the production of obesity, and this may amount to such as to constitute a serious evil, but, being less charged with nitrogenous matter, there is less of the nitrogenous products of disintegration for elimination—products which unless oxidized and metamorphosed to a full extent by free exercise, and so placed in a favorable position for discharge, are apt to accumulate in the system, and thence impair the performance of the functional operations of life. Some of the phenomena of gout, for example, are due to this defective metamorphosis and retention of nitrogenous products within the system.

The effects of privation and insufficiency of food constitute the well-known phenomena comprised under the terms inanition and starvation. As we can have no manifestation of vital properties without chemical change, a consumption of material must be constantly going on, and, unless a supply equal to the loss is provided, a progressive wasting of the body and failure of its powers must ensue. These, therefore, form the necessary concomitants of starvation, and it is only a question of time for the exhaustion of material to proceed to a point sufficient to render the continuance of life impossible.

From the elaborate series of experiments performed by Chossat,[*] it has been shown that the immediate cause of death from starvation is a decline of the animal temperature. He found during the first portion of the period a gradual, but not very extensive, fall. Then it diminished more rapidly, and when it reached about 29° or 30° (Fahr.) below the normal point the animal died. A state of torpor preceded death, and it was noticed by Chossat that when this stage was reached a restoration of consciousness and muscular power could be effected by exposing the subject of experiment to artificial warmth, and thereby raising its temperature. Some of his animals were thus rescued from impending death, and afterward completely restored by supplying them with food. In fact, the operations of life can only be carried on—that is, in the case of ourselves and other warm-blooded animals—within a certain range of temperature, and if from any cause, either external or internal, this range is passed, no matter whether on the side of excess or deficiency, death is the inevitable consequence.

The usual length of time that life continues under complete abstinence from food and drink may be put down at from eight to ten days. Longer periods, however, in exceptional instances, have been noticed, and the duration, indeed, is liable to be influenced by the surrounding circumstances, such as the amount of available material accumulated in the system at the commencement of starvation, the surrounding temperature, and the state of the atmosphere as regards the amount of moisture present.

It will be readily understood that, other circumstances being equal, the greater the amount of combustible material to draw upon, the longer will the capacity exist for maintaining the heat of the body, and with it life. An instructive instance bearing upon this point is afforded by the fat pig referred to at p. 58. In Chossat's experiments the animals provided with most fat lived the longest, and it was, moreover, found that they lived until the fat was nearly exhausted. It seemed, indeed, as though the approach of death was coincident with the consumption of nearly all the disposable combustible material. The animals lost, on an average, about 40 per cent. in weight—in other words, about two-fifths of their original weight disappearing—before the occurrence of death. In the case of the fat of the body, taken alone, the loss amounted to upward of 90 per cent. The waste of this material, it was found, far exceeded that of any other.

As regards the surrounding temperature, it is a well-known fact that exposure to cold in conjunction with starvation very much accelerates death.

The presence of moisture in the atmosphere to some extent favors the prolongation of life, and evidently by diminishing the exhalation of water from the body. Persons, for instance, have been excavated alive after confinement in a mine, or have continued alive whilst placed under such-like circumstances, for periods considerably longer than the usual time.

In the absence of both food and drink, the distress from thirst is far greater than that from hunger. With access to water and a very small supply of food, life may be prolonged for an extensive period.

The Welsh fasting girl, about whom so much excitement prevailed in 1869, lived exactly eight days from the time that she was placed under systematic inspection. The supply of food under which, it may be assumed, she had for some time previously subsisted had, doubtless, been very irregular and scanty, but then she lay in bed and passed her time in

---

* Recherches Expérimentales sur l'Inanition.   Paris, 1843.

a perfectly quiescent state—conditions that would diminish, to the fullest extent, the waste or consumption of material. The deception was so successfully carried out, and it was so stoutly affirmed by the parents of the girl that she had existed for many weeks without touching food, that many believed it as a fact, and she was daily visited by numbers of persons from far and near. So much wonder and excitement did the case create, that it was ultimately arranged to place the girl under such supervision as would secure that no access to food existed. The problem, in reality, that was thus systematically arranged to solve was tantamount to whether a fire could continue to burn without being replenished with fuel. The watching commenced at 4 P.M. on Thursday, December the 9th, and the girl died at 3 P.M. on Friday, the 17th. She was cheerful, and nothing extraordinary presented itself during the first part of the period. As time advanced, it was found that she could not be kept warm. She then sank into a state of torpor from which she could not be roused. This occurred only a short time before death.

The most prominent symptoms of starvation, says Dr. Carpenter,* as they have been noted in the human subject, are as follows: In the first place, severe pain in the epigastrium, which is relieved on pressure; this subsides after a day or two, but is succeeded by a feeling of weakness and sinking in the same region; and an insatiable thirst supervenes, which, if water be withheld, thenceforth becomes the most distressing symptom. The countenance becomes pale and cadaverous; the eyes acquire a peculiar wild and glistening stare; a general emaciation soon manifests itself. The body then exhales a peculiar fetor, and the skin is covered with a brownish, dirty-looking, and offensive secretion. The bodily strength rapidly declines; the sufferer totters in walking; his voice becomes weak, and he is incapable of the least exertion. The mental powers exhibit a similar prostration; at first there is usually a state of stupidity, which gradually increases to imbecility, so that it is difficult to induce the sufferer to make any effort for his own benefit; and on this a state of maniacal delirium frequently supervenes. Life terminates, either calmly, by gradually increasing torpidity, or as occasionally happens, suddenly, in a convulsive paroxysm.

In many respects the effects on the brain have a close resemblance to those produced by exposure to cold. In consequence of the torpor of the brain and intellectual faculties, it is often difficult to obtain from the sufferer information regarding his state. Instead of showing any anxiety to communicate the particulars about himself, or to relate the privations he has undergone, he generally shows an unwillingness to be questioned, lies in a listless or lethargic state, taking but little notice of what is going on, and seeming desirous only of not being disturbed. It is of the deepest importance that such symptoms should be recognized by the medical practitioner in their proper light, and that they should not be mistaken for the effects of narcotism produced by drinking.

Sudden transitions are always prejudicial, and where abstinence has prevailed for some days the return to a supply of food should be practised with caution. At first the supply should be very limited, and then gradually increased. There is reason to believe that death, which might otherwise have been averted, has been, in some instances, occasioned by the too free ingestion of food and fluid when succor has been obtained. The system should have time to accommodate itself to the new condition.

---

* Principles of Human Physiology, 4th ed., p. 396.

No matter whether a change be from the natural to the unnatural or from the unnatural to the natural state, it is always a sudden change that is especially difficult to be borne.

TIMES OF EATING.

Next to the quality and quantity of food, attention must be given to the mode of taking it. That the food should be taken with regularity, and at proper periods is almost as necessary for the maintenance of health and a vigorous state of the energies as that it should be of a proper nature and in proper quantity. Frequently recurring instances present themselves to the medical practitioner of evils arising from the non-observance of the precepts that should be followed in reference to this point.

We know that a certain amount of food is required to be consumed daily in order that the body may be properly maintained. Discarding for the moment the practices of mankind, let us look at the evidence that can be adduced to enable us to arrive at a rational determination of the manner in which it is best that our food should be taken.

Carnivorous animals appear to thrive best upon food taken at long intervals. It is the custom in zoological menageries to feed the wild animals once a day only, and it is stated that they have been found, by observation, to do better when fed in this way than upon the same allowance of food given to them twice daily. Now, if we look to the habits of these animals, we notice that their mode of existence entails the occurrence of more or less protracted intervals between the times of feeding. Their supply is precarious and irregular, having to be captured as the opportunity presents itself, by the exercise of stealth and cunning. The food obtained is voraciously devoured to repletion, and then, from the heavy tax imposed upon the powers by the loaded state of the stomach, the animal remains for some time in a sluggish or inactive and drowsy condition.

Such is the result where long intervals elapse between the periods of consumption of food. From the nature of the circumstances, it is a matter of necessity with these animals that this should be their mode of feeding. There are those amongst mankind, however, who have been satisfied with one meal a day. But is it in conformity with our nature that our food should be taken in this way? In proportion to the length of the interval, so must be the amount of food consumed at one time, and in proportion to this so will be the degree and duration of the inaptitude for the performance of any bodily or mental work. The feast of the glutton places him for awhile in the position of the brute, that is by nature compelled to fill his stomach to repletion when the opportunity occurs. The monks of the monastery of La Trappe, near Nantes, says Dr. Combe, make it a part of their religion to eat only once a day. While travelling upon a French diligence journey, Dr. Combe was thrown in contact for three days with one of the order, and was surprised at the store of food consumed at each daily meal—a store appearing "sufficient to last a week instead of a day." But, as in the case of the boa constrictor, under similar circumstances, remarks Dr. Combe, "a deep lethargy immediately succeeded, and it was not till four or five hours afterward that his almost apoplectic features became again animated and expressive."

Now, looking to our relation to the supply of food, which involves no necessity for protracted intervals between the times of eating, and to the fact that our mental capacity constitutes our characteristic attribute, and that this is notably blunted after repletion of the stomach to the extent incurred where only one meal a day is taken, we have physiological grounds for dismissing from consideration such a mode of life as unsuited to our position.

With the vegetable feeders, we pass to an illustration of the other extreme. These animals, constantly within reach of their food as they are, pass a considerable portion of their time in feeding. We do not find that they gorge themselves at a repast so as to become placed in the same inactive condition as the carnivorous animal, but that they, instead, leisurely and frequently partake of the food within their reach.

Is this, it may next be asked, the mode of taking food that is adapted for mankind? To consume what is eaten in small quantities and at frequently repeated intervals would, doubtless, serve our purpose so far as alimentation is concerned, but experience shows that it is not necessary, and much of our usefulness would be lost by the time devoted to the consumption of food. Indeed, as we are designed by Nature for a mixed diet, so it may be considered that the most appropriate mode of taking food is something between that adopted by the animal and the vegetable feeder; and this happens to accord with the general practice of the majority of nations. The prevailing custom—and, doubtless, this has arisen from instinct and from what has been found by experience to be best suited to our requirements—is for three meals of a substantial nature to be taken during the day, at intervals of about five or six hours' duration. Observation has shown that an ordinary meal is digested and has passed on from the stomach in about four hours' time, and thus, according to the precept laid down, the stomach is allowed to remain for a short period in a state of quiescence before it is filled with food again.

It is important that we should break our fast, or, as the term goes, "breakfast," without much delay after rising. The length of time that has elapsed since the last meal of the previous day leads to a demand for food for the ordinary purposes of life. The system, moreover, at a period of fasting—as experience has but too plainly, and it may be said, on some occasions, painfully testified—is more prone to be perniciously influenced by infection, miasmata, exposure to cold, and other morbid conditions, and less adapted for sustaining fatigue than at any other time. In any case, therefore, where exposure to influences of this kind has to be undergone, it becomes of the deepest importance that food should be previously taken.

The size of the meal should be regulated by collateral circumstances. If food has been taken late in the previous evening, the appetite is not great for food in the morning. Where considerable exertion has to be afterward sustained, a substantial meal may be looked upon as advisable. Otherwise, however, a light meal will be found most conducive to health and activity. A maid of honor, it is stated, in the court of Elizabeth, breakfasted upon beef and drank ale after it. Such may be compatible with plenty of out-door exercise to carry off the meal, but not so with the in-door life which is led by so many of the present generation.

Supposing breakfast to be taken at 8 or 9 A.M., the next meal, no matter by what name it is called, should follow about 1 or 2. A fairly substantial meal should be taken at this time, and it does not signify whether it goes under the name of luncheon or dinner. Some dine in the

middle of the day, and make this their heaviest repast. To many, however, it is inconvenient to give up the amount of time that is usually devoted to the principal meal of the day at such a period, and, moreover,
the more or less marked disposition to inactivity that follows a heavy meal
may interfere with the subsequent engagements. Under these circumstances, the less ceremonious and lighter repast, designated luncheon, will
best fall in with the daily arrangements. The *déjeuner à la fourchette*
in France represents our luncheon, but is usually more substantial and
taken rather earlier, and the amount of food that has been consumed previously having been but slight.

The error is often made of omitting to take food in the middle of the
day, or of only taking biscuit or something of equal insignificance. There
are many business or professional men who, after leaving home for their
office or chambers in the morning, do not taste food, or, if they do, take
only a minute quantity, until they return in the evening. Actively engaged all day, the system becomes exhausted, and they arrive home in a
thoroughly jaded or worn-out condition. They expect that their dinner
is to revive them. It may do so for a while, but it is only a question of
time how long this system can be carried on before evil consequences
arise. They begin to feel heavy, drowsy, and uncomfortable after dinner, and no wonder from the amount of food that it has been necessary
to introduce at one time into the stomach to supply the requisite material for meeting the wants of the system, and also from the exhaustion of
power produced by the work performed and the long abstinence from
food. Vigor is required for digestion equally as much as for muscular
or any other action, and it is not to be expected that it can properly proceed under the state that has been described. Added to these indications that the digestive power is not equal to the amount of work thrown
upon it, evidences of disordered action begin to show themselves. The
sufferer becomes dyspeptic, and the heart and brain may sympathize with
the derangement. The physician is frequently encountering instances of
the description I have depicted; and when advice is given that food in
proper quantity should be consumed in the middle of the day, the usual
answer met with is that if a luncheon were taken it would have the effect
of rendering the person unfit for his employment afterward. It is a *sine
qua non*, however, that the interval should be broken by a repast between
an early breakfast and a late dinner, and no medical treatment will suffice
to afford relief unless attention is given to this point. When once the
alteration has been made and persevered in a short time, as much reluc-
tance will be felt in omitting the luncheon upon any single occasion as
was experienced in taking it to begin with. Often, in cases where indigestion forms the chief complaint, will it be found to have arisen from
some unwitting breach of the principles of dietetics, and thence it frequently happens that instruction on the dietetic precepts requiring to be
obeyed for the maintenance of health will be all that is needed to set
matters right.

When the middle of the day is allotted to dinner, the evening meal is
designated supper, and as this is not usually taken till an advanced hour
of the evening an intermediate light repast is generally introduced under
the name of tea. A heavy supper, especially if taken only a short time
before going to bed, is unquestionably bad. During sleep there is a diminished activity of all the bodily functions, and the condition is not favorable for the due performance of digestion. He who retires to rest with
a full stomach is fortunate if he escape passing a restless night, being

troubled with dreams, and rising in the morning with a foul mouth. The supper, when supper at all is taken, should be, as far as practicable, made to approach to the early part of the evening—that is, supposing the usual hour for retiring to rest be observed; and where the engagements of life render such a course inconvenient, the meal should be light and a heavier tea consumed.

The best arrangement for health is that the third substantial meal should be taken about six or seven in the evening—in other words, that breakfast, luncheon, and dinner should form the order observed. The opportunity is thus given for digestion to have approached completion before the night's sleep is begun. In fashionable society it is now common to find the dinner postponed till a later hour, bringing it, in fact, nearly to the old-fashioned period for supper. If the time of retiring to rest is proportionally late, as is usually the case, there is nothing seriously objectionable in the course adopted, but if early, the remark applies with equal force that has been made under the head of supper. A dinner at eight or half-past eight, however, calls for an intermediate light repast, under the form of tea, to break the length of interval that would otherwise occur. But, besides being customary under these circumstances for tea to be taken about five, fashion has led to its being also taken when the dinner hour is earlier, and against a simple cup of tea at this time nothing can be said. It serves to refresh, although it cannot be considered as needed. Temptation, however, is also offered to partake of food, and when this is done to any extent, it must be looked upon as pernicious, by impairing the appetite for one of the principal meals.

After a late dinner, and with the observance of ordinary hours, no further food is required. The tea, therefore, which is generally taken afterward, should be confined to liquid, and a cup of warm tea, coffee, or cocoa, has the effect of arousing the energies, and apparently also of favorably influencing digestion.

The error of going to bed upon a full stomach has been alluded to. It is also equally unadvisable that the stomach should be in a perfectly empty condition. Fasting excites restlessness and watchfulness, and many a person has needlessly passed sleepless hours through retiring to rest after too long an interval since the last meal. The literary man, for example, who carries his labors far into the night, goes to bed with an empty stomach and finds that he cannot sleep. Let a little food, however, be taken, and it will be found to exert a tranquillizing and comforting effect, and so will dispose to sleep.

I have been speaking of the meals adapted for a state of health. Three substantial meals—morning, mid-day, and evening—should be taken, and, unless the interval between one or the other be considerably prolonged, no intermediate repast of solid food is required. Indeed, it is not beneficial for a person to be constantly eating through the day. Some are in the habit of taking food at odd times between the meals, but such a practice is not to be upheld. Eating should be confined to the meals, otherwise a constant state of repletion is kept up, and the stomach has no opportunity of resting. In sickness, it is true, advantage is gained by the frequent administration of food, but then only a small quantity at a time can be taken. The stomach will not bear, or the invalid cannot take, more than a very limited amount at once; and to compensate for this, and enable a sufficiency to be ingested, more frequent administration is required. In proportion to the limited amount that can be taken at a time, so, it may be said, should be the frequency of administration.

Infants and young children require food more frequently than grown-up persons. They dispose of what is taken more rapidly, and do not bear fasting well. Less lengthy intervals should therefore be allowed to elapse between the periods of eating. The best arrangement of meals for children that are a little older is—breakfast, dinner, tea, and supper: the supper consisting of light but nutritious food. A late dinner is to be strongly condemned. There are many children whose delicate health and feeble constitution is owing to the error of their parents in making them join in a late dinner. Instead of dining, say at seven or after, it would be better for them to be going to bed, and the evils of going to bed upon a heavy meal have already been adverted to.

In connection with these remarks upon the times of taking food, I may refer to the following collateral points.

A hearty meal should neither immediately follow nor precede violent exercise. In each case the stomach is rendered unfit for the vigorous discharge of its office.

A hearty dinner taken in the evening after an unusual day's exertion is sure to be followed by more or less indigestion, and, it may be, vomiting. Sportsmen and pedestrians are acquainted by experience with this fact. The depression of general bodily power occasioned by the fatigue endured is incompatible with the possession of full energy by the stomach. By a little repose, however, time is given for the production of fresh power to raise the system from its previous state of exhaustion, and render the stomach equal to the easy digestion of a moderate meal.

The sensation experienced on undertaking any violent bodily exertion immediately after a hearty meal is sufficient to show that the task imposed is greater than the system is adapted for. With a loaded stomach, the fullest amount of energy that can be given is required to enable it to get through its work. We notice, indeed, under such circumstances, that the energies are so concentrated upon what the stomach is doing that an indisposition, and even incapacity, for vigorous and sustained mental or bodily exertion is induced. Whilst after a light meal, muscular or mental work can with ease and comfort be performed, after a heavy meal an effort to accomplish it so diverts from the stomach the energy required of it as to occasion manifest signs of incapacity for the function to be discharged. The process of digestion fails to be carried on as it ought to be. The food remains longer than it should within the stomach, and ultimately, it may be, is rejected by vomiting.

If sharp exercise after a hearty meal is to be avoided, is it desirable, it may be asked, to encourage the inclination for repose, and allow indulgence in a *siesta?* A short and light nap after dinner will not be sufficient to do any harm, but if the nap is permitted to pass into a profound and a prolonged sleep, unquestionably a retarding influence is exercised upon digestion, and a prejudicial influence upon the stomach. However agreeable, therefore, it may be to gratify the desire for a nap, if there is danger of its passing into a lengthy and heavy sleep, it is well to have recourse to some light mental or bodily employment, whether under the shape of one of the various games of amusement, as billiards, bagatelle, cards, chess, etc., or otherwise to obviate its occurrence. But, with a natural state of things, there ought to be no strong desire for sleep after a meal. If there be such, it may be concluded that some fault exists: either the meal has been excessive, in consequence of yielding to the gratification of the palate, or of eating largely to make up for a too prolonged fast, or else the digestive power is below the healthy standard.

A cheerful state of mind is conducive to the easy digestion of a meal. The influence exerted by states of the mind upon the appetite and digestion, as well as the nutrition of the body generally, is a matter of common observation. A person receiving a piece of unwelcome intelligence just before the commencement of a repast may be unable to eat a mouthful, no matter what might have been the appetite previously. Henry VIII. frowning upon Wolsey, and handing him papers notifying his disgrace, is made by Shakespeare to say—

> ———" Read o'er this ;
> And after this ; and then to breakfast *with*
> *What appetite* you have."

" Experience," says Dr. Combe,* " must have taught every one with what zest we sit down to enjoy the pleasures of the table, and how largely we incline to eat, when the mind is free, unburdened, and joyous, compared with the little attention we bestow on our meals when we are overwhelmed with anxiety, or have the whole energies of the mind concentrated on some important scheme." " Laughter," also says Hufeland, of Berlin,† " is one of the greatest helps to digestion with which I am acquainted; and the custom prevalent among our forefathers, of exciting it at table by jesters and buffoons, was founded on true medical principles. In a word, endeavor to have cheerful and merry companions at your meals; what nourishment one receives amidst mirth and jollity will certainly produce good and light blood."

CULINARY PREPARATION OF FOOD.

Several important purposes are fulfilled by the process of cooking. By it our food is rendered more pleasing to the eye, agreeable to the palate, and digestible by the stomach. We all know, for example, the influence exerted by the appearance presented by food—how, if pleasing to the eye, it becomes tempting to the palate, and, if revolting to the sight, the stomach may turn against it. Again, food which is savory— and cooking has the effect of developing flavor—excites the inclination in a manner peculiar to itself. Lastly, by the alterations it induces of a physical and chemical nature, cooking renders our food more easy of digestion, and may remove an obnoxious property by killing parasites or their germs, where such exist.

Cooking lessens cohesion and alters the texture in such a manner as to render a substance more easy of mastication and subsequent reduction to a fluid state by the stomach.

The effect upon meat is to coagulate albumen and coloring matter; to solidify fibrine, and gelatinize tendinous, fibrous, and connective tissues. A piece of meat, for instance, which before cooking is tough, tenacious, and stringy, so as to be insusceptible of proper mastication, has firmness or solidity given to the muscular fibres, whilst the connective tissue is transformed into a soft gelatinous material. The connective tissue being softened, the muscular fibres are loosened. Thus, the whole substance becomes less coherent, and is easily broken down by the application of pressure. It is thereby more digestible, for the digestibility of meat may

---

* Physiology of Digestion, 2d ed., p. 300. Edinburgh, 1836.
† Art of Prolonging Human Life, English ed., p. 282. London, 1829.

be regarded as standing in proportion to its tenderness or want of cohesion. Tenderness and digestibility are influenced by the circumstances antecedent to cooking. If flesh, whether of fish, fowl, or any other animal, be cooked before *rigor mortis* has set in, its texture is looser, and the article is thereby more easy of digestion than when cooked after this state has passed off. It is rare, however—seldom practicable indeed—for cooking to be performed at so early a period after death, and when the flesh has set, its tenderness and digestibility are increased by its being kept for a time. The flesh of an animal, also, which has been driven or hunted just prior to death is more tender and digestible than where it has been previously quiescent. Bruising loosens the texture of meat, and makes it more tender when cooked: hence the advantage of the process of beating to which steaks and chops are, in many households, subjected.

The effect of cooking upon vegetables is to soften their consistence, and so allow them to be more readily masticated or broken up in the mouth. It also loosens their intercellular structure, and thereby facilitates the penetration of digestive juices into their substance. It further aids, in an important manner, digestibility, by its physical action on the starch granule—an ingredient which enters more largely than any other into the constitution of vegetable aliment. It causes this granule to swell up, and its outer envelope to burst. The digestive fluids are thus permitted to come in contact with the central part. In the absence of this change, the starch granule is much less easily attacked, its outer covering being hard and offering considerable resistance to digestive action. Albuminous and fibrinous matters, as with those in meat, are coagulated; and, in the case of boiling, some of the gummy, saccharine, coloring, and saline matters are extracted. This occurs to a less extent when vegetables are boiled in hard water, or water impregnated with salt, than when boiled in soft water, but the article is, at the same time, less tender and digestible. The effect of a little salt added to the water in which vegetables are boiled in preserving their color, is well known to those versed in the economy of the kitchen, but the eye is pleased at the sacrifice of tenderness.

The warmth imparted to food by the process of cooking aids the digestive action of the stomach, and, where fatigue or exposure to cold has been sustained, exerts a reviving effect upon the system.

With these observations of a general nature, I will now offer some remarks on the various modes of cooking in common use, which may be enumerated as follows: Boiling, roasting, broiling, baking, frying, stewing.

Boiling.—There is an art in cooking food in such a manner as to cause as little loss as possible of its nutritive principles.

If the object to be attained should be the extraction of the goodness of meat into the surrounding liquid, as in making *soups*, *broths*, etc., the article should be minced or cut up finely, and placed in cold water. After soaking for a short time, heat should be applied, and the temperature gradually raised. For broths, no actual boiling is needed—it is desirable, indeed, that it should be avoided, so as not to consolidate and lose more than possible of the albumen. For soups, however, prolonged boiling is necessary, in order fully to extract the gelatine. It is this, in fact, which forms the basis of soup, for the floating albumen is hardened or condensed and got rid of by straining.

Thus treated, the principles of the meat, so far as circumstances will allow, pass out into the surrounding liquid, and as this gains in flavor and nutritive properties, so the meat becomes impoverished, a hard, fibrous, and insipid residue being produced.

Where, however, it is desired that the flavor and nutritive properties should be retained in the meat, an opposite process must be adopted. The piece of meat should be large, and it should be plunged suddenly into boiling water, and the process of boiling briskly maintained for about five minutes. This coagulates the albuminous matter upon the surface, and leads to the formation of a more or less impermeable external layer, which precludes the escape of the juices from the substance of the meat. After this object has been fulfilled, instead of boiling being continued, a temperature of between 160° and 170° Fahr. constitutes what is wanted, and this degree should be maintained until the process of cooking is completed. Cooked in this way, the central part of the meat remains juicy and tender, and possesses, in the highest degree, the properties of nutritiveness and digestibility. Unless exposed throughout to the temperature named, the albuminous and coloring matters are not properly coagulated, and the meat presents a raw or underdressed appearance. If exposed to a temperature much above 170°, the muscular substance shrinks and becomes proportionately hard and indigestible. The usual fault committed in cooking meat is keeping the water in which it is being boiled at too high a temperature after the first exposure to brisk ebullition is over.

Fish is rendered firm in proportion to the hardness of the water in which it is boiled. Hence, fish boiled in sea-water or in water to which salt has been added, is firmer, and, at the same time, more highly flavored, than when boiled in soft water, on account of the less solvent action exerted.

Upon the principle of endeavoring to retain, so far as practicable, the soluble constituents of an article of food, potatoes should be boiled in their skins, and the object aimed at is still further secured by the addition of a little salt to the water. By steaming, instead of boiling, the result is still more completely attained.

Boiled food is more insipid than food cooked in other ways. From the lower temperature employed, no empyreumatic products are developed. Being more devoid of flavor, it is less tempting to the palate, but sits more easily on a delicate stomach.

In cooking, meat loses about one-fourth or more of its weight. The loss varies with the quality of the meat and the process of cooking employed. According to Dr. Letheby, the ordinary percentage of loss is about as follows:

	Boiling.	Baking.	Roasting.
Beef generally,	20	29	31
Mutton generally,	20	31	35
Legs of mutton,	20	32	33
Shoulders of mutton,	24	32	34
Loins of mutton,	30	33	36
Necks of mutton,	25	32	34
Average of all,	23	31	34

Thus, the loss by baking is greater than by boiling, and by roasting greater than all. The loss arises chiefly from the evaporation of water and the melting down and escape of fat, although some is due to the destructive action of the heat and the exudation of nutritive juice under the form of gravy.

Roasting should be conducted upon the same principle as boiling. In order, as far as possible, to retain the nutritive juices, meat should first be subjected to a sharp heat. This leads to the formation of a coagulated layer upon the surface, which subsequently offers an impediment to the escape of the fluid matter within. After a short exposure to a sharp heat, the meat should be removed to a greater distance from the fire, so as to allow a lower heat gradually to penetrate to the centre. In this way the albumen and coloring matters are coagulated without the fibrine being corrugated and hardened.

As has been already stated, on account of the great heat employed, roasted meat is more savory than boiled. The surface also is more or less scorched, and a portion of the fat is melted, and drops away under the form of dripping. Some of the fat likewise, under a prolonged exposure to a strong heat, undergoes decomposition, attended with a production of fatty acids, and an acrid volatile product known as acroleine, which may cause derangement of a weak stomach. In boiling, the temperature is not sufficient to incur the risk of rendering the fat in a similar way obnoxious.

When properly roasted, the meat is juicy enough within to lead to the escape of a quantity of red gravy when the first cut is made into it.

Broiling produces the same effect as roasting, but the proportion of scorched material is greater, on account of the relatively larger amount of surface exposed. The principle of cooking should be the same, in order to retain the central portion juicy.

Baking renders meat more impregnated with empyreumatic products, and therefore richer or stronger for the stomach than any other process of cooking. The operations being carried on in a confined space the volatile fatty acids generated are prevented from escaping, and thus permeate the cooked articles. Meat cooked in this way is ill adapted for consumption where a delicate state of system exists.

Frying is also an objectionable process of cooking for persons of weak digestive power. The heat is applied through the medium of boiling fat or oil. The article of food thus becomes more or less penetrated with fatty matter, which renders it, to a greater extent than would otherwise be the case, resistent to the solvent action of the watery digestive liquid secreted by the stomach. It is apt also to be impregnated with fatty-acid products arising from the decomposition of the fat used in the process. These are badly tolerated by the stomach, and, whether generated in this way or when the food is in the act of undergoing digestion, appears to form the source of the gastric trouble known as heartburn.

Stewing places food in a highly favorable state for digestion. The articles to be cooked are just covered with water, and should be exposed to a heat sufficient only to allow of gentle simmering. A considerable portion of the nutritive matter passes into the surrounding liquid, which is consumed as well as the solid material. Properly cooked in this way, meat should be rendered sufficiently tender to break down under moderate pressure. If boiling be allowed to occur, the meat becomes, instead, tough and hard.

Hashing is the same process applied to previously cooked instead of fresh meat.

By surrounding the vessel in which the article of food is contained with water, so as to secure that no burning shall occur, meat may be stewed in its own vapor. For example, a chop or other piece of meat taken upon a small scale, may be placed in an ordinary preserve-jar, and this tied over at the top, and partially immersed in water contained in a saucepan. The water in the saucepan is made to simmer or gently boil, and when the proper time has elapsed, the meat is found perfectly soft and tender, and surrounded by a liquor derived from the juice which has escaped during the process. Meat thus prepared is in an exceedingly suitable state for the convalescent and invalid.

It is upon this principle that the action of Captain Warren's "cooking-pot" depends. This consists of a kind of double saucepan, the inner vessel containing the joint or other article to be cooked, and the outer some water, through the medium of which the cooking is effected, but without its coming into actual contact with the food. The utensil constitutes, in fact, a *bain-marie*, or water-bath. There need be no loss whatever of any of the solid matter of the meat, and the loss of weight that occurs in a joint is considerably less than when cooked by roasting. If it be desired to increase the flavor, the joint may be first roasted for a short time before being stewed.

I may here refer to the "*Norwegian nest*," or "self-acting cooking apparatus" which was introduced to notice in this country a few years back. Messrs. Silver & Co., of Cornhill and Bishopsgate street, are now the patentees and manufacturers. It consists of a box constructed upon the principle of a refrigerator, the only difference in action being that it keeps the heat in instead of keeping it out. The box, indeed, may be made use of either as a refrigerator or for the purpose of cooking. It is padded inside with a non-conducting material, arranged so as to leave a space in the centre for receiving the movable tin vessel in which the process of cooking is carried on. The vessel is lifted out from its "nest" and filled with water and the article to be cooked. Heat is applied, so as to bring the water to the boiling point, and afterward maintain it at this for a short time. The vessel is then replaced in the box and shut in by the closure of the lid. The heat being prevented from escaping, the process of cooking goes on away from the fire, and no matter in what situation the box may be placed. The contrivance recommends itself on the score of economy for household use, and the box being easily carried about, it affords the means of furnishing, without a fire being needed, hot food out of doors, as in campaigning, travelling, pleasure-making, etc. It is also susceptible of being turned to useful account as an appurtenance to the sick-room.

Soups and Broths.—The process of preparation is here directed to extracting the goodness from the article employed—the reverse of that in the case of boiling. To accomplish what is aimed at in the most complete manner, the article should be chopped or broken into fine pieces, and placed in cold water. After being allowed to macerate for a short time, for the soluble constituents to become dissolved out, it is gradually heated to a point which should vary according to the product required. In the case of broths and beef-tea, which properly contain only the flavoring principle of meat—*osmazome*—and the soluble constituents with finely coagulated albuminous matter, all that is required is to produce gentle simmering, and this should be kept up for about half an hour. In the case of soups a prolonged gentle boiling is required, in order that the gelatine may be extracted, this being the principle which gives to good soup its property of solidifying on cooling. Bones require boiling a longer time than meat. The chief principle they yield is gelatine, and its extraction is greatly facilitated by the bones being broken into fine fragments previous to being used.

Salting, pickling, and smoking are processes to which articles of food are sometimes subjected for the purpose of enabling them to be preserved previous to cooking. These processes have been already referred to under the head of "Preservation of Food" (p. 270), but may be alluded to here for the sake of stating that by their hardening action they give an article of difficult digestibility, which cannot be overcome by cooking. Food, therefore, which has been submitted to these processes should be avoided by the dyspeptic, except, it may be said, in the case of bacon, which happens, as a rule, to sit easily on the stomach. Indeed, according to general experience, the cured article (particularly the fat belonging to it) is here more digestible than the fresh—that is, than either pork or pig-meat.

DIET OF INFANTS.

The importance of this branch of dietetics can scarcely be overrated. At no period of life is discreet management throughout so much called for as during the helpless condition of early infancy, and nothing constitutes so fruitful a source of infantile sickness and mortality as injudicious feeding.

The *proper* food during the first period of infancy is that, and that only, which has been provided by Nature for the young of mammals, viz., milk General observation and carefully collected statistics agree in conclusively showing that nothing can adequately replace this natural food. "The infant," says Dr. West,[*] "whose mother refuses to perform toward it a mother's part, or who, by accident, disease, or death, is deprived of the food that Nature destined for it, too often languishes and dies. Such children you may see with no fat to give plumpness to their limbs—no red particles in their blood to impart a healthy hue to their skin—their face wearing in infancy the lineaments of age—their voice a constant wail—their whole aspect an embodiment of woe. But give to such children the food that Nature destined for them, and if the remedy do not come too late to save them, the mournful cry will cease, the face will assume a look of content, by degrees the features of infancy will disclose themselves, the limbs will grow round, the skin pure red and white, and when, at length, we hear the merry laugh of babyhood, it seems almost as if the little sufferer of some weeks before must have been a changeling, and this the real child brought back from fairy-land."

Formed for the special purpose of constituting the sole nourishment during the first period of infantile life, milk not only contains the principles required for the growth and maintenance of the body, but contains them under such a form as to be especially adapted to the state of the digestive powers then existing. It must be remembered that the exercise of the digestive organs only comes into operation after birth. At the time of birth these organs are in a comparatively immature state of development, and it is only gradually that their full power becomes evolved. For the first few months it appears that no saliva at all is secreted; and it is true, under natural circumstances, from the character of the food and the absence of masticatory organs, that it is not required. The alimentary canal is short, and that portion of it called the cæcum very

---

[*] Lectures on the Diseases of Infancy and Childhood, fifth edition, p. 532. 1865.

small. The teeth, as is well known, do not appear until after the lapse of several months. Besides these evidences of immature development, experience shows that the alimentary canal is in an exceedingly susceptible state, and most easily deranged by slight deviations in the character of the food. So strikingly, indeed, is this the case, that the mother, whilst suckling, knows that for the sake of her infant's comfort it is necessary to exercise care over what she herself eats. All this points to feeble digestive capacity, and suggests a want of power of adaptiveness to alien articles of food. It may be considered .that, up to about the eighth month, the infant is designed to be sustained solely by its parent's milk. The teeth, which about this time begin to show themselves, indicate that preparation is now being made for the consumption of food of a solid nature, and the most suitable to begin with will be one of the farinaceous products. Bread, baked flour, biscuit-powder, oatmeal, or one of the numerous kinds of nursery biscuits that are made, may be employed for a time as a supplement to the previous food. Then, at about the tenth month, the maternal supply, which should have been already lessened, should be altogether stopped, and the child started upon the life of inde-, pendence that is to follow. For a while, milk and the farinaceous products referred to above still form the most suitable food; but as the child advances in its second year and the teeth become more developed, meat may be added.

Such forms the natural course to be pursued, but it often happens, either as the result of choice or of necessity—either because she *will not* or *cannot*—that the mother's part fails to be fulfilled. Under these circumstances, the question of the nature of the supply to be provided as a substitute has to be decided upon.

Undoubtedly the nearest approach to the actual food which has been designed to be given is the milk furnished by another woman, and amongst the more wealthy classes this is often had recourse to. Now, in the selection of a wet-nurse there are certain points which, in the interest of the infant to be reared, require to be attended to. It is scarcely necessary to say that the woman should be free from constitutional taint and in a healthy condition. The most suitable age is from twenty to thirty. The milk should be sufficient in quantity and good in quality, and as its composition alters to some extent as time advances from the date of confinement, it is desirable that the infant should be nourished by a person who has given birth about the same time as its own mother. A *brunette* is considered to make a better nurse than a *blonde.* Upon the authority of the analyses of L'Héritier, the milk of the former is said to be richer in solid constituents than the latter; but, besides this, the difference in temperament exerts its influence in maintaining a more steady condition in the one case than in the other. For example, the sanguine temperament, with its associated susceptible organization, belonging to the *blonde,* disposes to a greater liability of sudden alterations from mental causes than the phlegmatic temperament, with its less impressionable organization, of the *brunette.*

Next in appropriateness to the food supplied by a wet-nurse comes the milk derived from one of the lower animals; and this may be employed either to make up for a deficient supply from the mother, or as the sole article of nourishment. It is obvious that the milk to be selected should be that which is readily obtainable, and which presents the closest approximation to the infant's natural food. The cow, goat, and ass are the animals which best answer the conditions required; and reference to the

22

analytical table at p. 117 will show which of the three furnishes the most appropriate kind of milk.   In the first place, the milk of the ass, although it has had its advocates as a food for infants, presents considerable disparity in composition from that of the human subject.   Whilst being richer in sugar and soluble salts, it shows a marked deficiency in both nitrogenous matter and fat.   It may be adapted for the delicate stomach of a person reduced by illness to a great state of debility, but it can hardly be looked upon as representing what is most suitable for a growing child. The milk of the cow gives the nearest approach to what is wanted, and it happens, also, that this in general is more easily procurable than that of any other animal.   In Payen's table (*vide* p. 117), cow's milk is represented as richer in all its solid constituent principles than woman's, and slight dilution with water will be all that is required to bring it to a sufficiently close approximation for serving as a substitute.   The analyses given by other authorities, however, render it presumable that the sugar of woman's milk is under-estimated in the table in question; and that, whilst the caseine and butter are in less quantity than in cow's milk, the lactine, on the other hand, is in excess.   The practical management of infants shows that in employing cow's milk, it is desirable to sweeten as well as dilute it.   Instead of simply adding water, a solution of sugar, or, what is more in conformity with the natural state, sugar of milk, in the proportion of an ounce to three-fourths of a pint, may be used, and at first mixed to the extent of about one-third with two-thirds of milk. Later on, the quantity of the diluent may be somewhat diminished.   The milk of the goat is even richer in solid constituents than that of the cow, and, therefore, stands somewhat further removed from that of the human subject.   Goat's milk also possesses a strong and peculiar odor of its own, but, in the case of infants, this does not seem to form any serious obstacle to its use, for, if repugnant at first, custom soon overcomes the difficulty.

The importance of securing, as far as practicable, that the milk is derived from an animal in a healthy state, and surrounded by wholesome conditions, will be readily understood.   The alimentary canal of infants, and particularly of some, is exceedingly impressionable to unwholesome food, and the milk of cows kept, as cows in large cities and towns not unfrequently are, in an unnatural state, may prove the source of violent irritation of the stomach and bowels, and lead, if persevered in, to serious impairment of the health, terminating ultimately, it may be, in a fatal result.

There can be little doubt of the desirability of always obtaining the supply from the same animal, instead of indiscriminately from any cow, and arrangements for this are generally made in dairies.   In the case of the goat, the animal is often kept solely for the purpose under consideration, and has before now been domesticated, and tutored to discharge its office in the manner of a wet-nurse.

Respecting the use of condensed milk as food for infants, the reader's attention is directed to the foot note at p. 122.   The milk, as sold, is already in a highly sweetened condition.

Articles of a farinaceous nature, such, for instance, as bread, biscuit-powder, baked flour, rusks, and a variety of biscuits and preparations sold at different establishments, which enter so extensively into general nursery use, must be looked upon as foreign to the diet of infants of tender age. Constituted in great part, as these articles are, of a principle—starch—which has no existence in milk, and which requires to undergo a special kind of digestion to fit it for absorption, it is presumable that the digestive organs are not adapted at this stage properly to meet the demand that is made when these substances are consumed. From the fact that they are light and nourishing for older children, there is a popular tendency to regard them as forming suitable food for early infancy; but all authorities concur in condemning them as improper for use at such a period. It is true, later on they represent the most appropriate solid material to begin with; but this is when the digestive organs have reached a more advanced stage of development. Liebig, in his pamphlet * on the "Food for Infants" devised by himself, goes so far as to assert that the usual farinaceous foods are the cause of most of the diseases and of half of the deaths of infants.

Looking at its composition, the sweet almond has properties which furnish a food more analogous to milk than the farinaceous products. Pounded and made into an emulsion, a liquid is obtained which, as regards the chemical nature of its constituents and the physical condition in which the fatty matter exists, presents a close alliance to milk.

Liebig has introduced a food for infants, devised upon chemical principles, to form a substitute for the mother's milk. It is derived from malt-flour, wheat-flour, cow's milk, bicarbonate of potash, and water. For further particulars regarding its precise mode of preparation, *vide* p. 122. It appears to be extensively used in Germany, and has been brought prominently into notice in England. To avoid the uncertainty arising from not properly attending to the directions given, it is manufactured and sold in a dried state, the preparation thus supplied keeping for an indefinite time, and requiring only to be dissolved in a certain quantity of warm water to be rendered fit for use. Infants, as a rule, take it readily, and seem to thrive satisfactorily upon it.

The amount of milk consumed by a child fed naturally at the breast, has been determined by weighing immediately before and immediately after suckling. Dr. West, upon the authority of M. Guillot's results, obtained at the Foundling Hospital in Paris, says that the increase in weight has been found to vary from 2 to 5 ounces in infants under a month old, and that 2¼ pounds avoirdupois has been concluded to form the smallest quantity that will suffice for the daily nourishment of a healthy infant during the first month of its existence. It is suggested, however, that the observations made were not numerous enough to furnish more than a rough approximation to the truth.

DIET FOR TRAINING.

The object of training is the preparation of the system for some unusual feat of exertion, and the results which the art aims at producing are (1) increased muscular strength, (2) increased power of endurance, and (3) "improvement of the wind." It is principally by attention to diet and exercise that these results are attained, and about six weeks is the time usually devoted to the process when fully carried out. Under a successful progress the muscles increase in bulk, grow firmer, and become more subordinate to the influence of the will, thereby leading to the production of a feeling of freedom and lightness, or "corkiness," as it has

* Food for Infants. Walton, Gower street, 1867.

been termed, of the limbs. The muscular tissue, in fact, increases in quantity and improves in quality. There is a removal of superfluous fat and water, and by "over-training" the body may become so completely deprived of fat, or the muscles so finely drawn, as to lead to a loss, instead of gain, of the power of enduring prolonged exertion. The skin becomes clear, smooth, fresh-colored, and elastic. There is no part of the body, it is said, on which training produces a more conspicuous effect than on the skin, and by its state a criterion is afforded which enables an experienced person to judge of the fitness of the individual for the task in view.

The rule as regards exercise is to begin with a moderate amount, and gradually increase it, and the muscles which are to be specially called into play require to be systematically trained in excess of the others. Running is the kind of exercise which most "improves the wind," and, whatever the feat to be performed, it is usual to enforce a certain amount of running daily, for the special object of making the person "longer winded."

There is a general agreement regarding exercise, but respecting diet and other measures most fanciful notions have been held. Emetics, purgatives, and sometimes diaphoretics, were formerly recognized as forming an essential part of the process of training. Sir John Sinclair,* in his article on "Training," says, "With a view of clearing the stomach, and getting rid of all superfluities, either of blood or anything else, and also to promote good digestion afterward, medicines are given when the training is commenced. They begin with an emetic, and in about two days afterward give a dose of Glauber's salts, from one to two ounces; and, missing about two days, another dose, and then a third. It is supposed that one emetic and three doses of physic will clear any man of all the noxious matter he may have had in his stomach and intestines." It is scarcely necessary to state that no such heroic measures are now deemed advisable, and, if our present ideas are correct, considerable harm must have frequently resulted from their employment.

The tendency of the present day is not to attach so much importance to strictness of diet as formerly, and perhaps the latitude given is sometimes beyond what is desirable. There can be no doubt that, to begin with, there should be no sudden deviation of a marked nature from the accustomed diet, and afterward that the restriction should not be so severe as to excite any repugnance. Sudden changes always incur the risk of a disturbance of health, and, unless the food subsequently allowed proves grateful to the palate, the dietetic scheme may fail to secure the fully nourished condition that is needed.

Lean meat has always entered largely into the diet for training, and experience shows that it contributes in a higher degree than other food to the development of strength and energy. If we look to the lower animals, and compare the carnivora with the herbivora, we notice a striking contrast in their muscular vigor and activity. It has been ascertained physiologically that animal food disposes to the removal of superfluous water (*vide* the effect in increasing the flow of urine, p. 318) and fat, and makes the muscles firm and rich in solid constituents. The accounts that are furnished by travellers point to the aptitude of a meat diet for increasing the power of performing muscular exertion. Dr. Livingstone† says: "When

---

* The Code of Health and Longevity, 4th ed., p. 32. 1818.
† Livingstone's Zambesi, p. 272.

the Makololo go on a foray, as they sometimes do, a month distant, many of the subject tribes who accompany them, being grain-eaters, perish from sheer fatigue, while the beef-eaters scorn the idea of ever being tired." Sir Francis Head,* when crossing the Pampas, got tired at first with the constant galloping, and was obliged to ride in a carriage after passing five or six hours on horseback; but after, he says: "I had been riding for three or four months, and had lived on beef and water, I found myself in a condition which I can only describe by saying that I felt no exertion could kill me. . . . This will explain the immense distances which people in South America are said to ride, which," adds Sir Francis Head, "I am confident could only be done on beef and water." The Guachos, belonging to South America, are a race of people well known for the extraordinary number of hours they pass in active exercise on horseback, and they are observed to subsist almost entirely on animal food. It will thus be seen that evidence is not wanting to substantiate the position accorded to meat in the trainer's regimen.

Roasting and broiling are considered to be the best modes of cooking. All are agreed that the meat should not be over-cooked, but some have advocated that it should be eaten very much underdone. Perhaps in the latter state it possesses higher stimulating properties, but reason calls for its being cooked sufficiently to be palatable and susceptible of mastication. There can be no doubt that, by over-cooking, its digestibility and virtue are lessened.

Beef and mutton are the meats to be preferred, and it is not necessary that all the fat should be excluded. Stale bread or dry toast, potatoes, and some kind of green vegetable in moderation, are the appropriate articles to be taken in conjunction. Water-cresses are considered good. Pastry, flour-pudding, sweets, and made dishes, should find no place in the dietary of the man in training. The farinaceous articles, as rice, sago, etc., are allowable, but should only be taken to a moderate extent. To avoid too great sameness is an important point, especially with those who have been previously accustomed to a liberal diet; at the same time it is not desirable that the person should be tempted to eat to satiety. A full stomach, as is well known, disposes to inactivity. Condiments, as pickles, sauces, etc., are objectionable, on account of their effect being to force the appetite, which should be simply allowed to have its natural play.

In former times it was the practice to rigorously restrain the consumption of liquids to the lowest point that could be borne. Sir John Sinclair † states: "There is no circumstance which seems to be more essential in training up persons to the acquisition of athletic strength, than to permit them to take only a small quantity of liquid food. . . . The ancient *athletæ* were allowed but a very small quantity of fluid. This *dry diet*, as it is termed, seems to have formed an essential and important part of their regimen." Such a course of procedure must evidently be wrong in principle. The exercise undertaken involves an extensive loss of fluid, and it is only natural that this should be replaced in proportion as thirst indicates its requirement. In proof of the actual amount of loss occurring during active exercise, Maclaren ‡ says: "In one hour's energetic fencing, I found the loss by perspiration and respiration, taking the average of six consecutive days, to be about 3 lbs., or, accurately, 40 oz., with a varying range of 8 oz." The sensation of thirst may be taken as af-

---

* Journeys Across the Pampas, p. 51. 1828.   † Op. cit., p. 33.
‡ Training in Theory and Practice, by A. Maclaren, p. 89. 1866.

fording a correct guide upon the point of the amount of liquid to be consumed, but instead of drinking freely at a draught to satiety, the liquid should be sipped in small quantities, to give time for absorption, and thus satisfy thirst, without incurring the risk of introducing a surplus amount into the stomach. In this way the error is not likely to be committed of drinking too much. The liquids consumed must be of a simple and unexciting nature, Beer and the light wines are allowable, but spirits should be scrupulously avoided. Tea, coffee, and cocoa may be taken according to inclination, and, as a simple diluent, nothing is better than toast and water, or barley water.

The proper number of meals to be taken during the day consists of three—viz., one about 9 A.M., the second between 1 and 2 P.M., and the third in the early part of the evening.

It has been mentioned that, at the commencement of training, instead of plunging suddenly into a severe system of diet and exercise, a gradual advance should be made. The same equally applies to the cessation of training, and there is reason to believe that the seeds of more or less serious mischief are often sown by the sudden retreat that is customarily made from the life of discipline that has been practised.

Subjoined are the training tactics employed for rowing at Oxford and Cambridge, according to the tables contained in the appendix to the work of Maclaren already referred to.

THE OXFORD SYSTEM.

A day's training for the summer races.—Rise about 7 A.M. A short walk or run. Breakfast at 8.30 of meat (beef or mutton, underdone), bread (the crust only recommended), or dry toast, and tea (as little as possible recommended). Dinner at 2 P.M., of meat (much the same as for breakfast), bread, and no vegetables (a rule, however, not always adhered to), with one pint of beer. About 5 P.M. a row twice over the course on the river, the speed being increased with the strength of the crew. Supper at 8.30 or 9, of cold meat and bread, with perhaps jelly or water-cresses, and one pint of beer. Retire to bed about 10.

A day's training for the winter races.—Rise about 7.30 A.M. A short walk or run. Breakfast at 9, as for the summer races. Luncheon about 1, of bread or a sandwich, and half a pint of beer. About 2 a row twice over the course. Dinner at 5, of meat, as for the summer races; bread; vegetables, the same rule as for the summer races; pudding (rice) or jelly, and half a pint of beer.

It is particularly impressed on men in training that as little liquid as possible is to be drunk, water being strictly forbidden.

THE CAMBRIDGE SYSTEM.

A day's training for the summer races.—Rise at 7 A.M. A run of 100 or 200 yards as fast as possible. Breakfast at 8.30 of meat—beef or mutton—underdone; dry toast; tea—two cups, or toward the end of training a cup and a half only; and water-cresses occasionally. Dinner about 2 of meat—beef or mutton; bread; vegetables—potatoes, greens; and one pint of beer. (Some colleges have baked apples, or jellies, or rice puddings). Dessert—oranges, or biscuits, or figs, with two glasses of wine. About 5.30 a row to the starting-post and back. Supper about 8.30 or 9 of cold meat; bread; vegetables—lettuce or watercresses, and one pint of beer. Retire to bed at 10.

A day's training for the winter races.—Rise about 7 A.M. Exercise as for the summer races. Breakfast at 8.30, as for the summer races. Luncheon about 1 of a little cold meat, bread, and half a pint of beer; or biscuit with a glass of sherry—perhaps the yolk of an egg in the sherry. At 2 a row over the course and back. Dinner about 5 or 6, as for summer races. Retire to bed about 10.

THERAPEUTIC DIETETICS.

HOLDING the position that food does in relation to the operations of life, the art of dietetics not only bears on the maintenance of health, but is capable of being turned to advantageous account in the treatment of disease.

Under natural circumstances, instinct guides us in the selection and consumption of food and drink. Whilst keeping to simple articles of diet, it may be left to the sensations of hunger and thirst to regulate the amount of solids and liquids taken. In many disordered conditions, however, there is such a perverted state existing that the promptings of nature fail to be evoked, and it devolves upon reason to assume the initiative and dictate the supply to be furnished. Under these circumstances the nature and amount of food administered will often exert a most potent influence for good or evil, and the art of dietetics thus comes into great importance. Skill and attention are called into requisition— indeed, it is not too much to say that success in the treatment of disease is largely dependent upon a display of judicious management with regard to food.

It frequently happens that the difficulty encountered in the sick-room is to get what may be considered a proper amount of food taken. The inclination to eat depends upon the state both of the body and the mind. The food must be rendered pleasing to the eye and agreeable to the palate; and in order to rouse and keep in action a flagging appetite, a suitable variety in what is provided must be secured. Herein lies a great point in catering for sick people, and but too often the error is committed of allowing an excess of sameness to prevail.

It must be borne in mind that the demand for food is dependent upon its proper application, and failure of the appetite is often due to the defective manner in which nutrition is performed. It is not what we eat, but what we digest, assimilate, and apply, that concerns us as regards nutrition. Food introduced into the stomach, but not digested, assimilated, and employed, is calculated to prove a source of irritation and to do harm. It is not, therefore, to be thought that because it is got down it must needs prove of service. Judicious persuasion should be exercised, but I believe that much needless worry is often inflicted by the incessant solicitation, however well meant, that is frequently made by those around a patient to get food taken. The disinclination, indeed, for taking food is sometimes such that the thought of it is sufficient to excite a feeling of repulsion, which, more powerful over the muscles concerned than the will, overcomes any effort that may be made to swallow it.

The quantity of food administered at a time should be in proportion to the power of digesting it, and to properly compensate for a diminished quantity there should be a corresponding increase in the frequency of administration. " Little and often " is the maxim upon many occasions to be followed, and much will sometimes depend upon the strictness with which it is carried out; for, apart from complying with what is wanted upon the principle that has been just referred to, it meets the defective aptitude that exists in sickness for sustaining any lengthened duration of absence of food.

As a natural result of the administration of food at short intervals, no appetite is at any time experienced, even although the circumstances may be such as would otherwise allow it to become developed. The fact must not be lost sight of, that the return of a feeling of desire for food may be kept back in this way; and the expediency must always be held in view of conforming as soon and as far as is allowable with what is natural. Under all circumstances, it may be said, the rule should be to follow, alike as to quality, quantity, and periods of taking food, as closely as the conditions to be dealt with will permit, the course that is natural in health.

It devolves upon the physician, in the dietetic management of his case, to point out the suitable kinds and quantities of food to be taken, but it depends upon the system of his patient whether his recommendation can be carried out. It is no good to lay down and attempt to enforce, as may be done in health, rigid dietetic regulations, founded upon the number of grains of carbon and nitrogen required for carrying on the operations of life. The difficulty with which the practitioner is more often than not assailed is as to what *can*, and not as to what *should*, be taken.

As the principles of dietetics have become better understood, we do not hear of those disastrous consequences of improper dieting, affecting large numbers of people, that were formerly from time to time recorded. There is still, however, a large amount of scattered evil to be met with, in many instances directly dependent on the food that is taken, and in others, if not directly occasioned by the food, at all events removable by an altered system of dieting. It may happen that this evil arises out of poverty or ignorance, but more frequently it is the fruits of indiscretion. Much of the deranged health which the physician is called upon to treat, stands as the offspring of some kind of error in eating or drinking, and his first concern should be to find out what is wrong, in order that he may know how to shape his advice advantageously.

In speaking of the appropriate diets to be employed in various morbid conditions, attention will require to be directed to the particular diatheses or states of the body which different kinds of food tend to induce, for it may be considered that the information thus supplied often directs us to a rational mode of procedure in therapeutic dietetics.

It may be premised, to start with, that our natural diet consists of an admixture of animal and vegetable food; that different combinations of alimentary principles are best suited for particular modes of life; and that, if the combination supplied be wrongly adjusted, a tendency to the development of an unhealthy state will exist.

The effect of a highly nitrogenized diet—and it is animal food which is characterized by richness in nitrogenous matter—is to throw upon the system a large amount of eliminative work. The nitrogenous matter in excess of that which is directly applied to the growth and renovation of the structures of the body undergoes a process of retrograde metamorphosis, and is resolved in part into certain useless nitrogenous products which have to be cast out by the agency of the glandular organs with which we are provided. Now, as long as free exercise is taken and the circulation is kept in an active state, favorable circumstances exist for the absorption of oxygen and the proper occurrence of metamorphosis and elimination. Thus circumstanced, a diet into which animal food enters largely—a diet that is rich in nitrogenous matter—is borne with ease, and indeed may be said to conduce to increase tissue-formation and the development of a high state of bodily health and strength. Conjoined with sedentary habits, however, a different result is observed. The sluggish circulation which such habits tend to occasion naturally entails defective oxygenation. This, in its turn, leads to imperfect metamorphosis, and the two together conspire to induce deficient eliminative action. Thus the system becomes more or less clogged with effete products, which act perniciously in various ways upon the body. For instance, there is reason to believe that they may sometimes in a direct manner constitute the source of gouty deposits in the joints. They undoubtedly give rise to the presence of a preternatural amount of solid matter in the urine, manifesting a proneness to become deposited under the form of sand, gravel, or stone. They likewise disturb the action of the liver, producing a disposition to the occurrence of bilious derangement. Besides these effects, evidence is not wanting to show that through their influence the other functions of life are to a greater or less extent interfered with. To obviate, therefore, the production of these disordered actions, those who lead an inactive life should not allow their diet to contain a preponderance of nitrogenous food—that is, they should abstain from partaking largely of animal products.

Gout has been enumerated above amongst the evils that may arise from the consumption of a highly nitrogenized diet, and the present opportunity may be taken for referring to the appropriate dietetic course to be pursued by those who are suffering from, and those who desire to avert the invasion of, the disorder. Cullen remarked that gout seldom attacks persons employed in constant bodily labor, or those who live principally upon vegetable diet, and general observation confirms the truth of this statement. If not completely proved, it is nevertheless highly probable, that gout is the offspring of an undue accumulation of imperfectly metamorphosed nitrogenous products within the body, and that either an excess of nitrogenous matter in the food, a deficiency on the part of the metamorphosing capacity of the system (such as may be produced by an inactive life), or the ingestion of certain alcoholic drinks which appear to contain extractive matter prone to undergo imperfect metamorphosis (vide p. 240), and perhaps to impede the metamorphosis of other substances, may be the source of this condition. Whether or not the above reasoning is correct, it is known as the result of experience that a highly animalized diet, sedentary habits, and indulgence in the use of the richer varieties of wine and beer, individually and conjointly tend to encourage the development of gout. It has been previously stated that a diet rich in animal food may be consumed with advantage where much muscular work is performed. It seems, under these circumstances, to be both promotive of health and bodily vigor. Not so, however, where sedentary habits prevail, and particularly is this the case where a gouty disposition exists. With those who have already experienced symptoms of gout, and those also who have grounds for apprehending its invasion, it is important that an excess of nitrogenous food should be avoided. The diet should be simple, in order that the temptation may be avoided of eating too much, and should at the same time be adjusted to the mode of life, the principle to observe being, that the higher the degree of inactivity the greater ought to be the preponderance of food derived from the vegetable kingdom.

Even of more importance than what is eaten is what is drunk, where the question of gout is concerned, and observation shows that it is not distilled spirits, but the stronger wines and malt liquors which favor the production of the disorder. Nothing is more potent than port wine in leading to the production of gout, and a few years' liberal indulgence in it has often been known to be instrumental in bringing it on where no family predisposition had existed. Dry sherry and the light wines, as claret, burgundy, hock, champagne, etc., may be drunk, certainly in moderation, with comparatively little or no fear of inducing the disease, although any kind of wine appears capable of sometimes acting as the exciting cause of a paroxysm where the gouty disposition is already established. Stout, porter, and the stronger ales, especially those which have become hard from age, rank next to port wine in their power of predisposing to gout. As regards the light bitter beers, which are so extensively used at the present time, the same must be said of them as of the light wines— viz., that with little, if any, disposition to induce the disease, they nevertheless appear capable of sometimes exciting its manifestation in a gouty subject. A pure spirit, as whiskey, hollands, or brandy, diluted with water, often forms the only kind of alcoholic drink that is found to agree with those who are suffering from gout.

The effect of a deficiency of nitrogenous matter is to tell prejudicially upon nutrition and vigor. Forming, as it does, the essential basis of living structures, a definite quantity is indispensable for the proper development and maintenance of the body. However freely the other elements of food may be supplied, an ill-nourished and feeble condition, such as was formerly noticeable amongst the potato-eating Irish, must necessarily follow a scanty allowance of nitrogenous matter. As the instrument of living action, power will be proportionate, other circumstances being equal, to the amount of nitrogenous matter existing in operation.

Fatty matter occupies a position of considerable importance as an alimentary agent. Apart from its high capacity as a force-producing agent, its presence seems to be essential to tissue-formation, and, rightly or wrongly, the belief is entertained that the existence of a deficiency for application in this way furnishes a source of diseased action in the direction of scrofula and tubercle. Experience shows the beneficial effect that is often derivable from the administration of cod-liver oil in the scrofulous and tubercular diatheses. Now, it is probably to the increased systematic employment of fatty matter that this effect is to a large extent due, and it is only reasonable to infer that a measure which proves of efficacy in removing an unhealthy condition would also tend to prevent its development.

Taken in excess, fatty matter is apt to derange the alimentary canal. It is always more or less trying to the stomach, and particularly so when it has undergone change from keeping or from prolonged exposure to heat. Entering the bowels beyond the capacity that exists for effecting its digestion and absorption, it is liable to set up diarrhœa.

Starchy and saccharine matters form advantageous constituents of our food, and serve to take the place that would otherwise require to be filled by any extra amount of fat. Consumed in moderate amount they are utilized by application to the operations of life; but taken to a large extent, and in association with a proper proportion of albuminous and fatty matter, they lead to an advancing deposit of fat, which may proceed to such a point as to prove a source of serious evil. They possess the convenient quality of taxing lightly the digestive organs, and thereby usefully contribute to afford appropriate food for sick and delicate persons. Used in excess and too exclusively, however, they are liable to give rise to acidity of stomach and flatulence.

The present may be looked upon as forming the most fitting opportunity for referring to the kind of food best suited for increasing and diminishing stoutness. The condition of the body is to a large extent dependent on the quality and quantity of food consumed. It is not, however, wholly the question of food that is concerned, but also the temperament or nervous organization belonging to the individual. It is well known that, whatever and however much some people may eat, they always remain thin, whilst others grow stout although eating comparatively little. The same holds good in the case of the lower animals, and fatteners of animals for the table are practically made aware that a restless disposition is unfavorable to successful fattening. "A restless pig," states Liebig,[*] upon the strength of practical information furnished to him, " is not adapted for fattening, and, however great the supply of food, it will not grow fat. Pigs which are fit for fattening must be of a quiet nature; after eating they must sleep, and after sleeping must be ready to eat again."

From what is contained in the foregoing pages, we learn that the increase of muscle is most promoted by a diet which is rich in nitrogenous matter conjoined with exercise. It is simply, however, a growth of muscular tissue which occurs under these conditions. The fat undergoes no increase. Indeed, the effect of such a regimen is to lead to a reduction of fat if a superfluity has existed at the commencement. These are facts which have long been known, and are constantly being attested by the results obtained by training. It has been equally well known that the conditions most conducive to the accumulation of fat are a diet which is rich in either fat or carbohydrates (provided the requisite amount of nitrogenous matter be present for affording what is wanted for the operations of life), exposure to a warm atmosphere, and inactive habits. The food used for the fattening of domestic animals by those who have acquired the knowledge by experience of what is best, is of the nature described. The efficacy of sugar in promoting fatness is displayed by the change that occurs in the condition of the negro during the sugar-making season in the West Indies. The ordinary food of these people, I was informed by a plantation proprietor belonging to Barbadoes, consists of Indian corn-meal, rice, butter, and salt, with, during a portion of the year, the sweet potato, which is grown as a succession-crop for the sugar-cane. I learnt from the same source, in confirmation of what has been mentioned by others, that during the season for gathering the sugar-cane, which extends through March, April, and May, the work-people are noticed to grow conspicuously stouter, and that this change is attributed (and doubtless correctly so) to their habit of constantly chewing pieces of the succulent cane whilst they are working amongst it.

That a supply of fat should tend to augment the accumulation of fat in the body is simple and intelligible enough. Digestion, absorption, and accumulation when in excess of the immediate requirements of the body, follow its ingestion as natural sequences. With the carbohydrates, however, an elaborating process has to be carried out—they necessarily require, in

---

* Animal Chemistry, 2d ed., p. 312.

the first place, to become converted by assimilative action into fat before they can lead to the accumulation of this principle. Although the point was at one time disputed, precise experimental evidence is now adducible (*vide* p. 76 *et seq.*) showing that this assimilative power is enjoyed by the animal system, and common observation affords confirmatory testimony. For the conversion to take place, the food must contain a due proportion of nitrogenous matter. Without this nutrition suffers, and the carbohydrates fail to produce an increase of fat. The presence of a certain proportion of fatty matter seems also to promote the conversion of the carbohydrates into fat. I have found, for example, in experimenting upon the subject, that the addition of a moderate amount of fat to a fixed daily allowance of barley-meal and potatoes, which had previously maintained a dog without any material variation in weight, caused an increase in weight beyond the amount of fat administered. The food employed, also, for fattening the goose and obtaining the *foie gras*, consists of Indian corn, which is characterized amongst farinaceous seeds by the large proportion of fatty matter it contains.

Guided, then, by the information we possess, the dietary to be prescribed, where the aim is to produce increased stoutness, should comprise such articles as fat meats, butter, cream, milk, cocoa, chocolate, bread, potatoes, peas, parsnips, carrots, beet-root, farinaceous and flour puddings, pastry, almond puddings and biscuits, custard, frumenty, oatmeal porridge, sugar and sweets, sweet wines, porter, stout, sweet ales, and liqueurs. Women in the Bey's seraglio at Tripoli we are told (Mrs. Walker's " Female Beauty ") " are fattened against a certain day by means of repose and baths, assisted by a diet of Turkish flour mixed with honey."

For reducing stoutness, just the converse mode of dieting is naturally dictated; and that there is nothing new in applying dietetics to this purpose is shown by the subjoined extract from the writings of Sir John Sinclair. Amongst the remedies for corpulency, the following dietary rules are given: "*Liquid food*—Acid wines, like hock, ought to be preferred to sweet wines, and cider to malt liquors; for when the former is the usual beverage the people are leaner than when the latter is usually drunk. Plain water, or mixed with a small proportion of the best vinegar, may be taken. Vinegar is better than the juice of lemons, having passed through the process of fermentation. Tea and coffee should be taken by corpulent people without cream. *Solid food*—The bread should have the bran in it, so as to be more digestible. Vegetable diet to be preferred; hard dumplings excellent. If any animal food is taken, let it be fish or lean and dry meat. No eggs or butter, and the less sugar the better." * We cannot now, it is true, subscribe in their entirety to the recommendations here furnished, for, in some respects, owing to the imperfect knowledge of physiology which prevailed in Sir John Sinclair's time, they stand at variance with the precepts founded on the teachings of modern science.

A few years ago a great stir was made about the treatment of corpulency by the publicity given by Mr. Banting to his own case, in which, after unsuccessfully trying other means, he reduced himself from cumbersome to comely dimensions by dietetic measures. His original dietary table, Mr. Banting tells us, consisted of "bread and milk for breakfast, or a pint of tea with plenty of milk, sugar, and buttered toast; meat, beer, much bread, and pastry for dinner; the meal of tea similar to that of

* The Code of Health and Longevity, 4th ed., p. 530. 1818.

breakfast; and generally a fruit tart or bread and milk for supper." For this he substituted—*Breakfast* at 9 A.M.: five or six ounces of either beef, mutton, kidneys, broiled fish, bacon, or cold meat of any kind except pork or veal; a large cup of tea or coffee (without milk or sugar), a little biscuit or one ounce of dry toast: making together six ounces of solids and nine of liquids. *Dinner* at 2 P.M.: five or six ounces of any fish except salmon, herrings, or eels; any meat except pork or veal; any vegetable except potato, parsnip, beet-root, turnip, or carrot; one ounce of dry toast; fruit out of a pudding not sweetened; any kind of poultry or game, and two or three glasses of good claret, sherry, or madeira—champagne, port, and beer forbidden: making together ten to twelve ounces of solids and ten of liquids. *Tea* at 6 P.M.: two or three ounces of cooked fruit, a rusk or two, and a cup of tea without milk or sugar: making two to four ounces of solids and nine of liquids. *Supper* at 9 P.M.: three or four ounces of meat or fish, similar to dinner, with a glass or two of claret or sherry and water: making four ounces of solids and seven of liquids.

With this change of diet Mr. Banting states that he fell in weight from 14 stone 6 pounds to 11 stone 2 pounds in about a year. Such is nothing more than, without the aid of experience afforded by his case, would have been physiologically looked for. If he had been trying before the change to increase his corpulence he could scarcely have selected a more appropriate diet. The transition, having in view the object to be obtained, and speaking upon the strength of previously acquired physiological knowledge, was from an erroneously to a properly constructed dietary.

No new principle of action was brought to light, but there is this to be said, that before the introduction of "Bantingism" it was not sufficiently realized that dietetics might be turned to such practical account as it is really susceptible of for the reduction of corpulency.

It must not be lost sight of that the *quantity* of food in Mr. Banting's dietary is such as would be calculated to contribute its share of influence toward reducing the weight of the body; and it certainly must not be looked upon as safe to be indiscriminately followed—indeed, there is reason to believe that, when the popular rage for "Bantingism" prevailed, many persons incurred a serious impairment of health by keeping too strictly to the letter of the recommendation given. The dietary provides twenty-two to twenty-six ounces of solid food, with thirty-five ounces of liquids, *per diem*. The twenty-two to twenty-six ounces of solid food may be taken as representing about eleven to thirteen ounces of water-free material, and if reference be made to Playfair's dietaries (*vide ante*, p. 202), it will be seen that this fails to come up to what is classed as only a "subsistence diet." The middle diet of Guy's Hospital, which forms the general diet upon which the inmates of the institution are placed, and which experience shows can scarcely be regarded as furnishing much, if anything, beyond what is really required for the support of life under a quiescent state, furnishes 29¼ ounces of solid food, and represents 16¾ ounces of water-free material (*vide* p. 321). With these comparisons the reader is supplied with data for forming his own judgment upon the point in question.

Dr. Parkes, after remarking that an excess of albuminates causes a more rapid oxidation of fat, says,[*] "It is now generally admitted that the success of Mr. Banting's treatment of obesity is owing to two actions: the increased oxidizing effect of fat consequent on the increase of meat

---

(especially if exercise be combined), and the lessened interference with the oxidization of fat consequent on the deprivation of starches." Whether or not an increase of meat produces the alleged effect of promoting the oxidation of fat, it is practically evident that enough to account for what occurs is to be found in the spare allowance of food and the restraint imposed in the use of fat and fat-forming principles.

As a *résumé* for the guidance of the corpulent, it may be said that the fat of meat, butter, cream, sugar and sweets, pastry, puddings, farinaceous articles, as rice, sago, tapioca, etc., potatoes, carrots, parsnips, beet-root, sweet ales, porter, stout, port wine, and all sweet wines, should be avoided or only very sparingly consumed. The articles allowable, and they may be taken to the extent of satisfying a natural appetite, are lean meat, poultry, game, eggs, milk (moderately), green vegetables, turnips, succulent fruits, light wines (as claret, burgundy, hock, etc.), dry sherry, bitter ale (in moderation), and spirits. Wheaten bread should be consumed sparingly, and brown bread is to some extent better than white. The gluten biscuits which are prepared for the diabetic may, on account of their comparative freedom from starch, be advantageously used as a substitute for bread in the treatment of obesity.

In *diabetes mellitus* a morbid condition exists, attended with a want of assimilative power over the starchy and saccharine principles of food, and in order to keep down the symptoms of the disease, the dietary requires to be framed so as to secure as far as practicable an exclusion of these principles. The following is the dietary plan for this complaint, introduced into my work "On the Nature and Treatment of Diabetes."

DIETARY FOR THE DIABETIC.

MAY EAT.—Butcher's meat of all kinds, except liver; ham, bacon, or other smoked, salted, dried, or cured meats; poultry, game, shell-fish and fish of all kinds, fresh, salted, or cured; animal soups, not thickened, beef-tea, and broths; the almond, bran, or gluten substitute for ordinary bread,* eggs dressed in any way, cheese, cream-cheese, butter, cream, greens, spinach, turnip-tops, † turnips, † French beans, † Brussels sprouts, † cauliflower, † broccoli, † cabbage, † asparagus, † seak-ale, † vegetable marrow, mushrooms, water-cress, mustard and cress, cucumber, lettuce, endive, radishes, celery, vinegar, oil, pickles, jelly (flavored, but not sweetened), savory jelly, blanc-mange (made with cream, and not milk), custard (made without sugar), nuts of any description (except chestnuts), olives.

MUST AVOID EATING.—Sugar in any form, wheaten-bread and ordinary biscuits of all kinds, rice, arrow-root, sago, tapioca, macaroni, vermicelli, potatoes, carrots, parsnips, beet-root, peas, Spanish onions, pastry and puddings of all kinds, fruits of all kinds, fresh and preserved.

MAY DRINK.—Tea, coffee, cocoa from nibs, dry sherry, claret, dry Sauterne, Burgundy, Chablis, hock, brandy, and spirits that have not been sweetened, soda-water, Burton bitter ale in moderate quantity.

MUST AVOID DRINKING.—Milk (except sparingly), sweet ales (mild

---

* These substitutes may be obtained at Mr. Blatchley's, 362 Oxford street; Mr. Van Abbot's, 5 Prince's street, Cavendish square; and Mr. Bonthron's, 106 Regent street.

† Those marked with a dagger may only be eaten in moderate quantity, and should be boiled in a large quantity of water.

and old), porter and stout, cider, all sweet wines, sparkling wines, port wine (unless sparingly), liqueurs.

Experience has shown that, for the proper maintenance of health, a certain proportion of the food must be consumed in the fresh state. The ill effects that are producible by a too exclusive restriction to salted and dried provisions are now recognized in their true light; and with the knowledge that has been obtained, means have been placed at our command for averting those calamitous results due to scorbutic affections, which were formerly so common, particularly amongst the maritime classes. Without being able to give the precise reason for what occurs, it is evident that there is something absent from dried and salted food which the system requires, for under restriction to its use for a lengthened period, a state of poverty of the blood is induced which leads to the various manifestations of defective nutrition that accompany scurvy; and, moreover, by the employment of a certain amount of fresh or succulent vegetable food, and even of vegetable juices (lemon-juice and lime-juice are specially used for the purpose), not only may the evils of scurvy be averted, but the diseased condition when established may be cured. It is generally considered that the anti-scorbutic virtue of the articles named is owing to the vegetable acids which they contain; but it must be remarked that the pure acids cannot be efficaciously used as a substitute.

A beneficial influence may be exerted in certain states of the system by regulating the amount of fluid taken.

The supply of a certain amount of fluid is as indispensable as that of solid matter for the performance of the operations of life. One use of the fluids taken is to furnish the requisite liquid material for carrying the effete products from the body. With increased water-drinking there is an increased discharge of urine, and with it an increased removal of solid matter; and there can be no doubt that, in certain states, a powerful influence for good may be exerted by putting this principle of action into force. With those, for instance, who lead a sedentary mode of life, and are accustomed to full living, the effect of the free consumption of a watery fluid may be to rid the system of impurities which might otherwise lead to evils, such as liver disorder, gout, gravel, etc. Probably much of the benefit in many instances derived from undergoing the course of treatment pursued at a watering-resort is in great part due to the eliminative effect of the water drunk.

The *restriction* of fluids is also sometimes capable of effecting good. It constitutes a recognized therapeutic agency that is occasionally employed in certain cases under the denomination of the "dry treatment." It has been recommended for cutting short a common head-cold, and when so employed must be put in force at the very commencement of the attack. No liquid of any kind is to be drunk until the disorder is gone, the object being to avoid supplying fluid for discharge from the inflamed mucous membrane of the nose. The treatment is affirmed to be less distressing to bear than might be thought, and to be capable of effecting a cure in forty-eight hours. In pleurisy, with serous effusion, feeding the patient upon the driest possible diet, and withholding liquids as far as practicable, has, in some cases, proved successful in leading to an absorption of the fluid. The restriction of fluids likewise forms a part of Mr. Tufnell's plan of treatment of internal aneurisms by "position and diet." The treatment is specially advocated for aneurisms of the thoracic and abdominal aorta, which cannot be otherwise treated, and several examples of successful issue have been placed on record. The points aimed at are to diminish the volume of blood and reduce the activity of the circulation, so that coagulation of fibrine within the sao may be favored. Conjoined with a strict maintenance of rest in the recumbent position for eight or ten weeks, the daily diet recommended for use consists of two ounces of white bread with butter, and two ounces of cocoa or milk, for breakfast; three ounces of broiled or boiled meat, with three ounces of potatoes or bread, and four ounces of water or light claret, for dinner; and two ounces of bread and butter, with two ounces of milk or tea, for supper; making, altogether, *ten ounces of solid and eight ounces of fluid food in the twenty-four hours.*

The nature of the food exerts a marked influence on the urine, and the effect may be turned to useful account therapeutically.

Physiology teaches us that the kidneys perform an eliminative office. The water which they remove in regulating the amount of fluid in the system is made the vehicle for carrying off solid matter, consisting of useless products of metamorphosis of the food and effete materials resulting from the disintegration of the tissues, which poison and produce death if allowed to accumulate in the blood. As long as the kidneys are acting healthily, these matters are discharged as fast as they are formed, and no danger of their undue retention within the body is incurred. The kidneys, however, are liable to become the seat of disease of a character to lead to their eliminative capacity being interfered with. Bright's disease is of this nature, and one mode of fatal termination in this affection is by uræmic poisoning—in other words, by coma attributable to the imperfect removal of urinary products.

Now, the amount of urinary matter to be discharged is largely dependent upon the nature of the food. The fats and carbohydrates throw no work upon the kidneys. The products of their utilization—carbonic acid and water—pass off through another channel. The nitrogenous ingesta, on the other hand, as explained in a previous section of this work (*vide* p. 42), in great part undergo metamorphosis, and yield their nitrogen to be carried off in combination with a portion of their other elements, under the form of urinary products. In this way the kidneys become taxed by the food. Under an ordinary mixed diet, indeed, the chief part of the solid matter of the urine consists of nitrogenous products, and observation has shown that it is to the nitrogenous matter ingested that these stand related. Upon the principle, therefore, of endeavoring to lighten the work of an affected organ, it is reasonable to infer that good may be done in Bright's disease by arranging the diet so as not to lead to the introduction of more nitrogenous matter into the system than is absolutely needed, and this may be effected by allowing vegetable food to preponderate.

It must not be lost sight of that the escape of albumen might be brought forward as affording an argument in favor of an extra amount of nitrogenous matter being required in order to compensate for the waste occurring. In the form of Bright's disease, however, where the greatest impairment of functional capacity of the kidney is encountered—viz., in the contracted kidney—the amount of albumen escaping is frequently insignificant, and sometimes, even, there may be none. It may be presumably considered, in fact, that the effect of the mere loss of albumen is not so much to be dreaded as the danger of uræmia, which is constantly impending, and which is the most likely to be staved off for a time by the

23

dietetic measures that are calculated to lead to a limited production of urinary matter for discharge.

The reaction of the urine is also susceptible of being influenced by the character of the food, and this likewise may be turned to account therapeutically. The effect of animal food is to increase the acidity, whilst that of vegetable food is to diminish it, and even to produce alkalinity. The urine of the dog, like that of the carnivora generally, is strongly acid, but it may be rendered alkaline by a diet of potatoes. The urine of the herbivora, although acid during fasting or during the intervals of digestion, tends to become alkaline and to remain so for a certain period after feeding. The ordinary reaction of the urine of man—a mixed feeder—is acid, but after fruits and other vegetable articles, partaken of largely, it has been observed to present an alkaline behavior. Bernard conducted an observation upon himself bearing on this point, and obtained a strongly marked attestation. His urine, to start with, was examined, and found to possess its ordinary acid character; and, moreover, was sufficiently loaded with lithates to throw down a deposit on cooling. He began in the morning, and confined himself throughout the day to vegetables, fruit, and butter. The urine remained acid till night, but on the following morning it was decidedly alkaline, and no longer threw down the lithate deposit that had been noticed before. He partook at 8 A.M. of coffee and milk and bread, and at noon of meat, eggs, cheese, and wine. At 2 P.M. the urine was still alkaline, but at 4 P.M. it had become neutral, and at 6 P.M. acid, in which state it afterward remained, and again threw down the lithate deposit.

Dr. Bence Jones pointed out that the effect of the ingestion of food, without reference to any special kind, is to diminish for a time the acidity of the urine. He found, as the result of an examination conducted at short intervals, that a notable falling off in its acidity was discoverable after a meal; and that in numbers of healthy persons it became neutral or alkaline for two or three hours after breakfast and dinner. Dr. Bence Jones regarded this result as dependent on the withdrawal of acid from the blood into the stomach for the purpose of digestion, the blood being thereby left for the time less capable of yielding acid to the urine. Dr. Roberts [*] has discussed the subject, and refers the phenomenon to the effect of the entrance of the newly digested food into the blood. He says, "If, as is believed, the normal alkalescence of the blood is due to the preponderance of alkaline bases in all our ordinary articles of food, a meal is *pro tanto* a dose of alkali, and must necessarily, for a time, add to the alkalescence of the blood; and as the kidneys have delegated to them the function of regulating the reaction of the blood, the urine immediately reflects any undue addition to or subtraction from the blood's proper alkalescence." Without detracting from the validity of the explanation suggested by Dr. Bence Jones—for the abstraction of acid from the blood by the stomach may help to produce the result—Dr. Roberts' view is in harmony with the circumstance that the effect of food in the way mentioned is most strikingly apparent in the vegetable feeder, where the saline matter ingested has the greatest capacity for giving alkalescence. In the rabbit, for instance, the urine, which is acid and clear during fasting, becomes, as an everyday occurrence, opaque and milky after the ingestion of food, in consequence of the deposition of earthy phosphates resulting from the marked degree of alkalescence acquired.

---

[*] On Urinary and Renal Diseases, 2d ed., p. 50.

From what has preceded, it is seen that an excess of acidity and of solid matter may be reduced by means of a preponderance of vegetable food in the diet. With those suffering from the lithic acid diathesis— those in whom the urine may throw down red sand, or simply be unduly loaded and acid—a most beneficial effect may be produced by arranging the diet so that a limited allowance only of animal food is consumed, and that succulent vegetables and fruits, with the light wines, as claret, hock, etc., obtain a conspicuous place. On the other hand, where there is a tendency to alkalinity and the deposition of the earthy phosphates, exactly the opposite course should be adopted; but it must be remarked that the same degree of success is not always in this case to be obtained; and, where the urine is alkaline from the presence of ammonia, no decided effect must be looked for.

I have hitherto been speaking of the therapeutic application of dietetics through influences exerted upon the system, and have shown that various morbid conditions are capable of being beneficially affected by appropriately regulating the nature of the food consumed. I will now pass to the consideration of the application of dietetics to the treatment of diseased and disordered conditions of the digestive organs, and, here dealing with the immediate reciprocity that is observed to exist, the character of the food forms an all-important matter in the management of the case; indeed, it is not too much to say, that there is usually more to be done by proper dieting than by the agency of drugs; and, without some attention to dietetics, drugs will rarely be found to prove efficacious in affording relief.

It is as organs in the exercise of their functional capacity that the digestive organs are brought into relation with food; and it may be remarked, as a preliminary point of consideration, that, besides the absolute character of the food, there are conditions of a collateral nature connected with its ingestion which exert their influence for good or evil, and demand attention. In the first place, much depends upon the state in which the food reaches the stomach. Thorough mastication affords great assistance to the performance of digestion, and derangement of the digestive system is not unfrequently attributable to the food being swallowed in an imperfectly masticated state. The dental art may here prove of incalculable service, and sometimes it may be found advisable to recommend that the food should be finely minced before being eaten—an operation which may be most effectually achieved by having recourse to the aid of a mincing apparatus, and small mincing machines have been specially constructed for the purpose. Taking the food at regular periods also tends to promote the orderly working of the digestive organs, and, where derangement has to be rectified, should be carefully attended to. The amount of food that can be taken at a time should form the guide for regulating the frequency of taking it. The smaller the amount tolerated at once, the more frequent should be its administration. An interval of more than four or five hours' duration between the meals is to be avoided. It acts perniciously in more ways than one. By inducing an exhausted state of the system, it diminishes the energy of the digestive organs, and, whilst having this effect, it at the same time calls for the exercise of increased energy, on account of the larger amount of food which requires to be taken at each meal, as a compensation for the duration of the interval that has elapsed. It is with digestion as with other kinds of work: the effect of allowing it to be leisurely accomplished, as by taking moderate-sized meals at intervals of moderate duration, instead of crowding it into limited periods, as by taking larger meals with intervals of longer duration, is to render it more easily performed.

In giving attention now to the kind of food best adapted for employment in different disordered states of the alimentary canal, the rational course will be to take the influence exerted by the various groups of alimentary articles as affording a guiding principle of action.

The office of the stomach is to dissolve nitrogenous matter, and as animal food is characterized by a preponderating amount of such matter, it specially taxes the powers of the organ in question. Peas, beans, and other leguminous seeds are, amongst vegetable articles, the richest in nitrogenous matter, and hence, as common experience testifies, prove more trying than other vegetable products to gastric digestion.

In febrile, acute inflammatory, and other conditions where an absence of digestive power prevails, it is not only useless to introduce food of the nature above referred to into the stomach, but absolutely pernicious, as, from its remaining undigested, it can only prove a source of irritation and disturbance. Whatever is given should be susceptible of passing on without requiring the exercise of functional activity on the part of the stomach. Hence the food in such cases should be confined to such articles as beef-tea, mutton-, veal-, or chicken-broth, whey, calf's foot and other kinds of jelly, arrow-root and such like farinaceous articles, barley-water, rice-mucilage, gum-water, fruit-jelly, and the juice of fruits, as lemons, oranges, etc., made into drinks. Besides its objectionable nature as concerns the stomach, it may be presumed that, if nitrogenous food were digested and absorbed, it would be calculated afterward to prove obnoxious to the system, on account of the products it gives rise to creating the demand they do for the performance of glandular eliminative work. With articles of the carbohydrate group, on the other hand, no such glandular work is called into requisition. Where a little latitude is allowable, the employment of milk, and of eggs in a fluid form, may be sanctioned. Bread-jelly, which is made by steeping bread in boiling water and passing through a sieve whilst still hot, is also an article that may be used under similar circumstances, either alone or boiled with milk. From this, as the circumstances permit, an advance may be made to solid substances which do not throw much work on the stomach, such as rice, sago, tapioca, bread and custard puddings, and stale bread or toast sopped. Next may be allowed fish; and the varieties to select are whiting, sole, flounder, or plaice, which should be boiled or broiled, and not fried. Whiting, of all fish, is that which proves the lightest to the stomach. As power becomes restored, calves' feet, chicken, game, and butcher's meat—mutton to begin with—may be permitted to follow. The exciting action of animal food upon the system of the invalid is exemplified by its liability to occasion a relapse in cases of rheumatic fever when administered at too early a period in convalescence.

I have been referring to the appropriate food to be made use of where defective digestive power depends upon the general state; but cases are frequently presenting themselves where the source of defect primarily belongs to the stomach, and equal care is required in adapting the food to the amount of power that exists.

It may be advisable, in some cases, to refrain altogether for a time from introducing any kind of food into the stomach, and here recourse should be had to the employment of enemata, consisting of articles fitted to undergo absorption into the blood-vessels. Amongst these, in the foremost rank as a desirable agent for use in such cases, is a preparation that has been made at my suggestion by Messrs. Darby & Gosden, of 140 Leadenhall street, London, and called "Fluid Meat." It constitutes meat that has been reduced to a fluid state by artificial digestion; and, representing, as it does, a product of digestion, it furnishes a material in identically the same favorable state for absorption as that which naturally passes on from the stomach. It may be mixed with sugar and thickened with mucilage of starch or arrow-root, and, if necessary, a little brandy may be added. In the absence of this, the usual agents employed as nutritive enemata are concentrated beef-tea, eggs, and milk.

In cases of ulcer of the stomach, acute gastric catarrh, and vomiting, whether from these or from some other cause, the food must be selected from that which is nutritious, and which, at the same time, taxes least the digestive powers. Milk—and this is often better borne after being boiled—milk and lime-water, or milk and soda-water, will frequently be found to be tolerated when other articles excite irritation and are returned. Sometimes the milk may be advantageously mixed with isinglass, arrow-root, ground rice, or biscuit-powder. The addition of agents like the three last-named articles increases the consistence and improves the alimentary value of the food. They at the same time, by virtue of their presence, lessen the cohesiveness of the mass which is formed by the process of curdling which the milk undergoes on arriving in the stomach.

Where chronic impairment of power exists, as in ordinary dyspepsia, the patient must be guided by what it is found from experience will agree. Whilst avoiding that which is known to be of an indigestible nature, and whatever, through idiosyncrasy, may happen in particular instances to upset the stomach, the maxim of management should be to keep the diet as closely to what is natural as the circumstances of the case will permit. Frequently, because a person is suffering from dyspepsia, he is recommended to leave off this and that article of food, and may, perhaps, in the course of time be reduced to taking exclusively, or almost exclusively, liquid nourishment. Such in itself is sufficient to lower the already enfeebled power of the stomach. The organ, getting no employment, becomes weaker and weaker, and is also prejudicially influenced by the defectively nourished state of the system. The aim of the physician in these cases should be rather to raise by appropriate treatment the digestive capacity to the level of digesting light but ordinary food, than to reduce the food to an adjustment with a low standard of digestive power. The food for the dyspeptic cannot be too simple or too plainly dressed. Of meats, mutton is almost invariably found to be the most suitable, and will often sit lightly on the stomach when even beef lies heavily. Chicken and game are allowable, also white fish (boiled or broiled), as whiting, sole, etc. (but not cod). Stale bread and dry toast, floury potatoes, rice, and the various farinaceous articles, form the kind of food derived from the vegetable kingdom to be selected.

The fatty constituents of food pass through the stomach to undergo emulsification or preparation for absorption in the small intestine. When fats are in a perfectly fresh state, and are not taken in excess, they pass on without giving signs of producing any effect upon the stomach. If taken in excess, however, they are apt to excite nausea and sickness, and also subsequently, from their influence in the bowels, diarrhœa. From their proneness to undergo change, and to give rise to the production of volatile fatty acids, they are likewise liable, under certain circumstances, to excite derangement. When delayed, for instance, for a long time in the stomach, this change becomes induced, and acrid eructations, with a burning sensation in the stomach and throat—phenomena constituting heartburn—are apt to follow. If the fat has been exposed to a strong heat before being consumed, it is already partially decomposed, and now with great facility leads to the gastric trouble that has been referred to. It is for this reason that anything containing fatty matter which has been baked, as pastry, etc., and fried articles, prove obnoxious to the stomach unless the digestive power is strong. Dishes consisting of meats, etc., cooked a second time, are similarly unsuited for the dyspeptic, on account of the effect of the prolonged exposure to heat that has occurred. Apart from exposure to heat, butter, or any other fatty article that has undergone change—turned rancid, as it is termed—by keeping, is also particularly prone to upset the stomach and occasion heartburn. It is unnecessary, therefore, to say, that fatty matter in the least degree rancid should be scrupulously avoided by the dyspeptic.

As with fatty matter, the principles of the carbohydrate group are not digested in the stomach. Similarly, also, they are liable to undergo change, during their sojourn in the organ, that may prove the source of discomfort. Starchy and saccharine matters, in certain states of the stomach, seem to be transformed into lactic acid to such an extent as to give a highly preternatural acidity to its contents. Acid eructations that may set the teeth on edge are apt to occur; and, as though the acid diffused itself along the mucous tract, a constantly sour taste is often experienced in the mouth. Sweet things are more likely than starchy to give rise to acidity. Amongst the latter, oatmeal and potatoes seem the most, and rice the least, disposed to prove obnoxious.

A result not unfrequently arising from impaired digestion is the production of an inordinate quantity of gas and its accumulation, so as to give rise to an inconvenient distention of the stomach and bowel. Vegetable food, it is found, is more apt to create flatulence than animal, and articles belonging to the cabbage tribe are particularly to be regarded as objectionable by those who have a tendency to this form of derangement.

Common observation suffices to show that the bowels are susceptible of being in a marked manner influenced by different kinds of food: diarrhœa, constipation, flatulence, and colic, constituting the effects by which the influence is betrayed.

In the healthy state no particular effect is observed to be produced by ordinary animal food; but, as previously stated, the ingestion of a large quantity of fat is apt, not only to derange the stomach, but likewise the bowels, and thus to produce diarrhœa.

The tendency of eggs is well known to very decidedly favor costiveness.

The alimentary products derived from the farinaceous seeds, and also other dried farinaceous articles, are more easily borne by the bowels than any other kind of food. They pass with ease through the whole digestive tract, but, whilst their freedom from exciting action renders their employment advantageous in irritable states of the canal, they fail to supply the stimulus that is needed to keep the bowels adequately moved where a sluggish disposition exists.

Succulent vegetable food, on the other hand, whether consisting of fruit or vegetables, has the effect of encouraging alvine evacuations, and thereby of promoting a free state of the intestinal canal. A liberal employment of food of this kind is thus indicated where a costive habit prevails; and it is not unfrequently found that, by partaking to a special extent of fruit, particularly in the early part of the day, persons otherwise troubled with constipation may succeed in procuring a proper activity of the bowels. Carried too far, an actual state of looseness may be established; and, from the excited muscular action brought about, griping or colicky pains may also be induced. As an extensive use of succulent vegetable food is indicated in cases of costiveness, so it is contraindicated where a tendency to looseness prevails. With some persons it very easily occasions colic and diarrhœa; and it is well known how readily, even without such a tendency, fruit in an unripe or overripe state gives rise to these phenomena.

The leguminous seeds, peas and beans, etc., and the products derived from the cabbage tribe, seem to be the most prone of all alimentary articles to give rise to intestinal flatulence.

A dietetic measure that has long met with extensive employment for rendering assistance in overcoming habitual constipation is the use of brown instead of white bread. The particles of bran contained in it, being of an indigestible nature, produce a certain amount of mechanical irritation, which is often found to supply the requisite stimulus to glandular and muscular action to correct the effects of a sluggish intestine where the want of activity is not very great.

In dysentery, and other forms of ulcerative disease of the intestine, scrupulous attention requires to be paid to diet. The object to be held in view is to keep the intestine in as tranquil a state as practicable. The food should consist of articles which are known to exert the least stimulant and irritant action on the mucous membrane and muscular fibres, and those which best meet the demand in question are such as milk, isinglass, and the various farinaceous products, amongst which rice is pre-eminently valuable. Next to these come eggs, white fish (particularly whiting and sole); white-fleshed poultry, fresh game, and fresh meat—mutton in preference to all other kinds. Salted and dried meats are highly objectionable. Their pernicious effect is quickly felt, and apparently arises from their difficult digestibility in the stomach, leading to an undue excitement of the circulation throughout the alimentary canal. Fruits and succulent vegetables, with the exception of a floury potato, which is often easily borne, should be strictly shunned.

DIETETIC PREPARATIONS FOR THE INVALID.

PANADA.—Take the white part of the breast and wings, freed from skin, of either roasted or boiled chicken; or the under side of cold sirloin of roasted beef; or cold roasted leg of mutton, and pound in a mortar with an equal quantity of stale bread. Add either the water in which the chicken has been boiled, or beef-tea, until the whole forms a fluid paste, and then boil for ten minutes, stirring all the time.

BEEF-TEA.—Mince finely one pound of lean beef and pour upon it, in a preserve-jar or other suitable vessel, one pint of cold water. Stir, and allow the two to stand for about an hour, that the goodness of the meat may be dissolved out. Next, stand the preserve-jar or other vessel in a saucepan of water, and place the saucepan over the fire or a gas-stove, and allow the water in it to boil gently for an hour. Remove the jar and pour its contents on to a strainer. The beef-tea which runs through contains a quantity of fine sediment, which is to be drunk with the liquid, after being flavored with salt at discretion. The jar or other vessel in which the beef-tea is made may be introduced into an ordinary oven for an hour, instead of being surrounded by the water in the saucepan.

Beef-tea, thus prepared, represents a highly nutritive and restorative liquid, with an agreeable, rich, meaty flavor. It is a common practice, however, amongst cooks, to make it by putting it into a saucepan, and subjecting it to prolonged boiling or simmering over the fire; but the product then yielded constitutes in reality a soup or broth instead of a tea. The prolonged boiling leads to the extraction of gelatine, and the liquid gelatinizes on cooling (which is not the case when prepared as above directed), but, at the same time, the albuminous matter becomes condensed and agglomerated in such a manner as to subsequently form a part of the solid rejected residue. The liquid also loses in flavor and invigorating power. All that is wanted is that the cold infusion should be heated to about 170° Fahr. This just suffices to coagulate the albumen and coloring matter, and thus deprive the product of its character of rawness.

The difficulty is often experienced of getting beef-tea made in the kitchen in a careful and proper manner; and to render the patient, as far as this is concerned, independent of the cook, Messrs. Darby & Gosden, of 140 Leadenhall street, London, have arranged, at my suggestion, a contrivance for conducting the process without the aid of fire or lamp in the sick chamber or anywhere that may be desired. The contrivance consists of the Norwegian box or "nest" referred to at page 335, and a double tin case provided with a suitable sized central space for receiving the vessel containing the article to be cooked. The tin appliance is removed from the box and sent into the kitchen for the outside chamber to be filled with water, which is then to be made to boil over a gas-stove or fire. The boiling water thus provided furnishes the heat which is subsequently required. The apparatus, with its store of heat, is carried back and deposited in the non-conducting box, and the vessel containing the article to be cooked is placed in the central chamber. The lid of the box being closed, the heat is retained and communicated to the · contents of the central chamber. About an hour suffices for cooking a pint of beef-tea, but the beef-tea may be retained in the apparatus as long as may be desired—for several hours or all night if necessary—and will keep hot all the while. Other articles, as a chop, pigeon, etc., may be likewise cooked by the store of heat contained in the boiling water; and there is this advantage in the use of the apparatus, that, after sufficient time has been allowed for the process of cooking, it does not signify whether the food is eaten at once or not for several hours: it is always hot and ready whenever it may happen to be required.

The apparatus is also susceptible of being turned to account for preserving a moderate store of ice in the apartment of a sick person.

SAVORY BEEF-TEA.—Take three pounds of lean beef chopped up finely, three leeks, one onion with six cloves stuck into it, one small carrot, a little celery-seed, a small bunch of herbs, consisting of thyme, marjoram, and parsley, one teaspoonful of salt, half a teacupful of mushroom-ketchup, and three pints of water. Prepare according to the directions already furnished.

LIEBIG'S BEEF-TEA.—Take half a pound of raw lean beef (chicken or any other meat may be similarly used) and mince it finely. Pour on to it, in a glass or any kind of earthenware vessel, three-quarters of a pint of water to which has been added four drops of muriatic acid and about half a saltspoonful of salt. Stir well together, and allow it to stand for an hour. Strain through a hair sieve and rinse the residue with a quarter of a pint of water. The liquid thus obtained contains the juice of the meat with the albumen in an uncoagulated state, and syntonine, or muscle fibrine, which has been dissolved by the agency of the acid. It is to be taken cold, or, if warmed, must not be heated beyond 120° Fahr. It will be observed that no cooking is here employed, and, although much richer in nutritive material and more invigorating than ordinary beef-tea, the raw-meat color, smell, and taste that it possesses sometimes cause it to be objected to.

CHICKEN-, VEAL-, OR MUTTON-TEA.—To be prepared like beef-tea, substituting either of the meats referred to.

If *broths* instead of a tea are required, boil the article in a saucepan for two hours and strain.

Pearl barley, rice, vermicelli, or semolina may sometimes be advantageously added to give increased nourishing power.

The fleshy part of the knuckle of veal is the best for veal-broth.

For chicken-broth, the bones should be used as well as the flesh, and all chopped up. The feet strongly add to the characteristic flavor.

LIEBIG'S EXTRACTUM CARNIS.—This article is largely sold, and, from the prestige afforded by its inventor's name, has obtained a world-wide notoriety. Its true position, as I pointed out in my work on "Digestion, its Disorders and their Treatment," in 1867, is scarcely that of an article of nutrition, and this is now beginning to be generally recognized. The fact that from thirty-four pounds of meat only one pound of extract, as stated by Liebig, is obtained, shows how completely the substance of the meat, which constitutes its real nutritive portion, must be excluded. The article, indeed, is free from albumen, gelatine, and fat, and may be said to comprise the salines of the meat, with various extractive principles, a considerable portion of which, doubtless, consists of products in a state of retrograde metamorphosis and of no use as nutritive agents. If not truly of alimentary value, the preparation nevertheless appears to possess stimulant and restorative properties which render it useful in exhausted states of the system. It may be given in extreme cases, in combination with wine. Being rich in the flavoring matter (termed osmazone) of meat, it is often used for imparting additional flavor to soups.

FLUID MEAT.—This article forms a complete representative of lean meat. Acting upon my suggestion, Messrs. Darby & Gosden, of 140 Leadenhall street, undertook its preparation, and since 1867, when it was first introduced, it has steadily advanced into public favor. It consists of meat which has been liquefied by artificial digestion, and, therefore, not only includes all the elements of the meat, but contains them in the same state as they are naturally placed by the stomach—that is, in a fit state for absorption, without requiring any further aid from digestion. It resembles in character a fluid extract, and is used in various ways, either alone or in combination with other articles of food.

From the properties it possesses as a product of artificial digestion, it may be spoken of as forming exactly what is wanted where recourse requires to be had to the employment of nutrient enemata. Used for this purpose, two tablespoonfuls, which about correspond with a quarter of a pound of meat, may be mixed with two ounces of white sugar, and dissolved in six ounces of mucilage of starch or arrow-root.

ESSENCES AND SOLID EXTRACTS OF MEAT, AND MEAT LOZENGES.—These are sold at various establishments. They may be obtained, as well as a number of other articles for the sick room, at Mr. Van Abbott's special dietary depôt for the invalid, No. 5 Princes street, Cavendish square, London; and of Messrs. Brand & Co., at No. 11 Little Stanhope street, Hertford street, Mayfair. Brand's " Essence of Beef " has obtained a high reputation, and is very extensively employed.

MILK AND SUET.—Boil one ounce of finely chopped suet with a quarter of a pint of water for ten minutes, and press through linen or flannel. Then add one drachm of bruised cinnamon, one ounce of sugar, and three-quarters of a pint of milk. Boil again for ten minutes, and strain. A wineglassful to a quarter of a pint forms the quantity to be taken at a time. It constitutes a highly nutritive and fattening article, but if given in excess is apt to derange the alimentary canal and occasion diarrhœa.

FLOUR AND MILK.—Fill a small basin with flour and tie it over with a cloth, or, if preferred, simply tie the flour up tightly in a cloth. Immerse it in a saucepan of water and boil slowly for ten or twelve hours. The flour becomes agglomerated into a hard mass, and is only wetted on the surface. After drying, add one grated tablespoonful to a pint of milk, and boil. A nourishing and useful article of food for irritable states of the stomach and bowels, and particularly suitable in dysentery and diarrhœa.

Plain biscuit-powder may be substituted, if thought proper, for the cooked flour.

EGG AND BRANDY (BRANDY MIXTURE).—Take four ounces of brandy, the same quantity of cinnamon-water, the yolks of two eggs, and half an ounce of loaf sugar. Rub the yolks of the eggs and sugar together, and add the cinnamon-water and brandy. Given in two to four teaspoonful doses as a restorative and stimulant.

BREAD-JELLY.—Steep stale bread in boiling water, and pass through a fine sieve while still hot. A light nourishing article for a weak stomach, which may be taken alone or after being mixed and boiled with milk.

OATMEAL PORRIDGE.—Mix a large tablespoonful of oatmeal with two tablespoonfuls of cold water. Stir well, to bring to a state of uniformity, and pour into a pint of boiling water in a saucepan. Boil and stir well for ten minutes. Flavor either with salt or sugar, as preferred. Milk may be used instead of water, or the boiling may be continued for half an hour and the porridge turned out into a soup-plate and cold milk poured over it: thus prepared, the porridge sets and acquires a solid consistence; the milk and porridge are mixed together little by little as they are eaten with a spoon.

If the coarse Scotch oatmeal is used—and this is generally considered the best—two tablespoonfuls may be sprinkled into a pint of boiling water and stirred and boiled for half an hour. At the end of this time the oatmeal is sufficiently cooked, but many allow the porridge to continue simmering for two or three hours. It may be turned out into a soup-plate and eaten with milk, after the manner mentioned above.

Porridge is a nourishing article of food, but is sometimes apt to give rise to water-brash and acidity, and from its slightly irritant properties, whilst advantageous for constipation, must be looked upon as objectionable where diarrhœa, or a tendency to it, exists.

OATMEAL GRUEL.—Mix thoroughly one tablespoonful of groats with two of cold water, and pour over them one pint of boiling water, stirring all the while. Boil for ten minutes, and still continue to stir. Sweeten with sugar, and add, if desired, a little sherry or brandy. A soothing and nutritive food, holding a totally different position, on account of the nitrogenous matter present, from the farinaceous preparations, as arrow-root, etc. Milk may be used, if required, instead of water.

ARROW-ROOT.—Mix thoroughly two teaspoonfuls of arrow-root with three tablespoonfuls of cold water, and pour on them half a pint of *boiling* water, stirring well during the time. If the water is quite boiling, the arrow-root thickens as it is poured on, and nothing more is necessary. If only warm water is used, the arrow-root must be afterward boiled until it thickens. Sweeten with loaf-sugar, and flavor with lemon-peel or nutmeg, or add sherry or brandy, if required. Milk may be employed instead of water, but when this is done no wine must be added, as it would be otherwise curdled.

Tous-les-mois, another farinaceous preparation, may be substituted for arrow-root.

BARLEY-WATER.—Take two ounces of pearl barley, and wash well with cold water, rejecting the washings. Afterward boil with a pint and a half of water for twenty minutes, in a covered vessel, and strain. The product may be sweetened and flavored with lemon-peel, or lemon-peel may be introduced whilst boiling is carried on. Lemon-juice is also sometimes added to flavor. A bland, demulcent, and mildly nutritive beverage.

ORGEAT.—Blanch two ounces of sweet almonds and four bitter almond-seeds. Pound with a little orange-flower water into a paste, and rub this with a pint of milk diluted with a pint of water until it forms an emulsion. Strain and sweeten with sugar. A demulcent and nutritive liquid.

RICE-WATER, OR MUCILAGE OF RICE.—Thoroughly wash one ounce of Carolina rice with cold water. Then macerate for three hours in a quart of water kept at a tepid heat, and afterward boil slowly for an hour, and strain. A useful drink in dysentery, diarrhœa, and irritable states of the alimentary canal. When circumstances permit, it may be sweetened and flavored in the same way as barley-water.

GUM-WATER.—Take half an ounce to an ounce of gum arabic and wash with cold water. Afterward dissolve by maceration in two pints of cold water. Lemon-peel may be added to impart flavor.

LINSEED-TEA.—Place one ounce of bruised linseed and two drachms of bruised liquorice-root into a jug, and pour over them one pint of boiling water. Lightly cover, and digest for three or four hours near a fire. Strain through linen to render fit for use. A mucilaginous liquid possessing demulcent properties. Frequently used as a drink in pulmonary and urinary affections. It is rendered more palatable by the addition of sliced lemon and sugar-candy.

DECOCTION OF ICELAND MOSS.—Wash one ounce of the moss in cold water to remove impurities. Then heat with water up to nearly the boiling point, and reject the liquid, which has extracted much of the bitter principle. Next boil with a pint of water for ten minutes in a covered vessel and strain with gentle pressure while hot. A mucilaginous demulcent liquid, with mild bitter tonic properties. It may be flavored with sugar, lemon-peel, white wine, or aromatics; or milk may be used instead of the water, by which a nourishing liquid is obtained.

DECOCTION OF CARRAGEEN MOSS.—Macerate half an ounce of Carrageen moss in cold water for ten minutes. Remove and boil in three pints of water for a quarter of an hour, and strain through linen. It possesses the same kind of properties as, and may be flavored like, the decoction of Iceland moss. Milk, also, may be substituted for the water. By doubling the quantity of the moss a mucilage is obtained, and when in a highly concentrated state the product solidifies into a jelly on cooling.

WHEY.—Curdle warm milk with rennet, and strain off the opalescent liquid for use. It acts as a sudorific and diuretic, and forms a useful drink in febrile and inflammatory complaints. Holding a little nitrogenous matter in solution, and containing the lactine and saline matter of the milk, it possesses mildly nutritive properties.

WHITE WINE WHEY OR POSSET.—To half a pint of milk whilst boiling in a saucepan, add one wineglassful of sherry, and afterward strain. Sweeten with pounded sugar, according to taste. A useful drink in colds and mild febrile disorders.

TREACLE WHEY OR POSSET.—Pour two or three tablespoonfuls of treacle into a pint of *boiling* milk, and afterward let it boil up well and strain. Drunk hot, it is frequently used as a diaphoretic for a common cold.

TAMARIND WHEY.—Stir two tablespoonfuls of tamarinds into a pint of milk whilst boiling, and afterward strain. It forms a refrigerant and slightly laxative drink.

CREAM OF TARTAR WHEY.—Stir a quarter of an ounce of cream of tartar (a large teaspoonful piled up) into a pint of boiling milk, and strain. A refrigerant and diuretic drink, which is rendered more agreeable by the addition of sugar.

ALUM WHEY.—Add a quarter of an ounce of powdered alum to a pint of boiling milk and strain. An astringent drink. May be flavored with sugar and nutmeg if desired.

CREAM OF TARTAR DRINK (*Potus Imperialis—Imperial*).—Dissolve a drachm or a drachm and a half of cream of tartar in a pint of boiling water, and flavor with lemon-peel and sugar. When cold, may be taken *ad libitum*, as a refrigerant drink and diuretic.

LEMON-PEEL TEA.—Pare the rind thinly from a lemon which has been previously rubbed with half an ounce of lump-sugar. Put the peelings and the sugar into a jug and pour over them a quart of boiling water. When cold decant the liquid, and add one tablespoonful of lemon-juice.

LEMONADE.—Pare the rind from a lemon thinly and cut the lemon into slices. Put the peel and sliced lemon into a jug, with one ounce of white sugar, and pour over them one pint of boiling water. Cover the jug closely, and digest until cold. Strain or pour off the liquid.

Citron may be used instead of lemon, and likewise furnishes a grateful and refreshing refrigerant beverage.

TOAST AND WATER.—Toast thoroughly, short of burning, a slice of stale bread (or, what is better, a piece of crust) or a biscuit, and pour over it, in a jug, a quart of boiling water. Cover it over, and place aside to cool. A small piece of orange- or lemon-peel put into the jug with the toast greatly improves the beverage.

HOSPITAL DIETARIES.

GUY'S HOSPITAL.

FULL OR EXTRA DIET.

14 oz. of bread. 1 pint of porter for males; ½ pint of porter for females. 6 oz. of dressed meat, roasted and boiled alternately, with potatoes (8 oz.). ½ lb. of rice pudding * three times a week. ½ pint of mutton-broth in addition on days when boiled meat is given (which is four times a week). Or, occasionally, 1 pint of strong vegetable soup, with meat and rice pudding,* twice a week. 1 oz. of butter each day. Porridge, gruel, and barley-water, as required.

MIDDLE OR ORDINARY DIET.

12 oz. of bread. ½ pint of porter. 4 oz. of dressed meat, roasted and boiled alternately, with potatoes (8 oz.). ¼ lb. of rice pudding * three times a week. ½ pint of mutton-broth, in addition, on days when boiled meat is given (which is four times a week). Or, occasionally, 1 pint of strong vegetable soup, with meat and rice pudding,* twice a week; with the full diet allowance of bread. 1 oz. of butter each day. Porridge, gruel, and barley-water, as required.

MILK OR PUDDING DIET.

12 oz. of bread. 2 pints of milk, or 1 pint of milk, with rice, sago, or arrow-root, boiled, or made into light pudding. ½ pint of beef-tea, when ordered. 1 oz. of butter. Gruel and barley-water, as required.

LOW DIET.

10 oz. of bread. ½ pint of beef-tea, mutton-broth, rice, arrow-root, or sago, when specially ordered. ¾ oz. of butter. Gruel and barley-water, as required.

Tea, ¼ oz.; sugar, ¾ oz.; and milk, 2½ oz., daily, with all diets.

Fish, chops, steaks, chicken, and chicken soup, eggs, and other extras, are to be specially ordered by the medical attendant, and will be given with the low diet. Wines and spirits, if continued, must be mentioned each time the physician or surgeon attends.

---

* Formula for the rice pudding—Rice, 2½ lbs.; milk, 6 quarts; sugar, 12 oz.; butter, 1 oz.; spice, 1 drachm. Loss of water in cooking, say 37 oz.

ST. BARTHOLOMEW'S HOSPITAL.

FULL DIET (MEAT).

BREAKFAST.—1 pint of tea; bread and butter.
DINNER.—½ lb. of meat when dressed; ½ lb. of potatoes; bread and beer.
TEA.—1 pint of tea; bread and butter.
SUPPER.—Bread and butter; beer.

DAILY ALLOWANCES TO EACH PATIENT.—2 pints of tea; 14 oz. of bread; ½ lb. of meat when dressed; ½ lb. of potatoes; 2 pints of beer (men); 1 pint of beer (women); 1 oz. of butter.

HALF DIET (MEAT).

BREAKFAST.—1 pint of tea; bread and butter.
DINNER.—¼ lb. of meat when dressed; ½ lb. of potatoes; bread and beer.
TEA.—1 pint of tea; bread and butter.
SUPPER.—Bread and butter; beer.

DAILY ALLOWANCES TO EACH PATIENT.—2 pints of tea; 12 oz. of bread. ¼ lb. of meat when dressed; ½ lb. of potatoes; 1 pint of beer; ¾ oz. of butter.

BROTH DIET.

BREAKFAST.—1 pint of tea.
DINNER.—1½ pint of broth; 6 ounces potatoes (mashed); ¾ oz. of butter; gruel.

MILK DIET.

BREAKFAST.—1 pint of tea.
DINNER.—1½ pint of milk, or 1 pint of milk with arrow-root, rice, or sago; bread.
TEA.—1 pint of tea; bread and butter.
SUPPER.—Bread and butter. Gruel.

DAILY ALLOWANCES TO EACH PATIENT.—2 pints of tea; 12 oz. of bread; 1½ pint of milk, or 1 pint of milk with arrow-root, rice, or sago; ¾ oz. of butter; gruel.

LOW DIET.

Bread, broth, gruel, or barley-water, as may be ordered.
Children under 9 years to receive half allowances.
EXTRAS TO BE SPECIALLY ORDERED.—Mutton chops, beefsteaks, beef for beef-tea, fish, eggs, puddings, jelly, porter, ale, wine, or spirits.
Each patient, on admission, to be placed on milk diet until a diet is ordered by the physician or surgeon.

ST. THOMAS'S HOSPITAL.

DAILY ALLOWANCE—FULL DIET.

12 oz. of bread; ¾ oz. of butter; ¾ pint of tea with milk and sugar for breakfast. The same for tea. 4 oz. of beef or mutton when dressed; roast or boiled alternately; ½ lb. potatoes or fresh vegetables; ½ pint of milk in the forenoon; porter, etc., if ordered.

MIXED DIET.

12 oz. of bread; ¾ oz. of butter; ¾ pint of tea with milk and sugar for breakfast. The same for tea. 4 oz. for men and 3 oz. for women of mutton when dressed; roast or boiled alternately; ¼ lb. of potatoes or fresh vegetables; 8 oz. of rice or bread pudding alternately; ½ pint of milk. When fish is ordered, meat to be omitted.

MILK DIET.

12 oz. of bread; ¾ oz. of butter; ¾ pint of tea with milk and sugar for breakfast. The same for tea. 8 oz. of rice or bread pudding alternately; 1½ pint of milk.

FEVER DIET.

4 oz. of bread; 2 pints of barley-water or gruel; 2 pints of milk.

CHILDREN'S DIETS.

(Intended for all Children under 10 years of age.)

MIXED.—12 oz. of bread; ¾ oz. of butter; ½ pint of milk for breakfast. The same for tea. 2 oz. of mutton when dressed, roast or boiled alternately; ¼ lb. of potatoes or fresh vegetables; 6 oz. of rice or bread pudding; ½ pint of milk.

MILK.—8 oz. of bread; ¼ oz. of butter; ½ pint of milk for breakfast. The same for tea. 6 oz. of rice or bread pudding; ½ pint of milk.

Wine, brandy, gin, porter, mutton chops, fish, eggs, beef-tea, soda-water, lemonade, and other extras, to be served when specially ordered, such order being renewed at each regular visit of the physician or surgeon.

Each patient, on admission into the hospital, to be placed on milk or fever diet until the proper diet is ordered by the physician or surgeon.

LONDON HOSPITAL.

FULL DIET FOR MEN AND WOMEN.

DAILY.—12 oz. of bread; 8 oz. of potatoes; 1 pint of porter.
BREAKFAST.—Gruel.
DINNER.—Sunday and Thursday, 6 oz. of boiled mutton.*
     Monday, Wednesday, and Saturday, 6 oz. of roast mutton.*
     Tuesday and Friday, 6 oz. of roast beef.*
SUPPER.—1 pint of broth.

* Weighed when cooked and free from bone.

MIDDLE DIET FOR MEN.

The same as full diet, except 4 oz. of meat instead of 6 oz., and ½ pint of porter instead of 1 pint.

ORDINARY DIET FOR WOMEN.

The same as middle diet for men.

MILK DIET FOR MEN AND WOMEN.

DAILY.—12 oz. of bread.
BREAKFAST.—Gruel.
DINNER.—1 pint of milk.
SUPPER.—1 pint of milk.

LOW DIET FOR MEN AND WOMEN.

DAILY.—8 oz. of bread.
BREAKFAST.—Gruel.
DINNER.—Broth.
SUPPER.—Gruel or broth.

DIET FOR CHILDREN.
(Under 7 years of age).

DAILY.—12 oz. of bread; ¼ pint of milk.
2 oz. of meat and 8 oz. of potatoes five times a week, and rice pudding twice a week.

EXTRAS.
(To be discontinued unless order renewed by the physician or surgeon at each visit.)

Mutton chops, beefsteaks, beef-tea, strong broth, puddings (rice, light, and batter, alternately. *Recipe for puddings:* Rice pudding—4 oz. of rice, 2 oz. of sugar; light pudding—6 eggs, 2 oz. of sugar, 1½ oz. of flour; batter pudding—4 eggs, 2 oz. of sugar, 6 oz. of flour, milk in each case sufficient to make up 1 quart of the mixture), eggs, bread, green vegetables, water-cresses, wine, spirits, porter.

ST. GEORGE'S HOSPITAL.

BREAD.—At discretion, to be served to the nurses at the rate of 10 oz. daily for each patient, and to be cut up by them. If more is required, this will be supplied by the steward.
BUTTER.—1 oz. daily to each patient, to be served out three times a week.
TEA.—To be served weekly to the nurses at the rate of ¼ oz. daily for each patient.
SUGAR.—To be served twice a week to the nurses at the rate of 1 oz. daily for each patient.
MILK.—¼ pint daily for each patient, for both breakfast and tea, to be served to the nurses every morning.

24

EXTRA DIET.

DINNER.—6 oz. of cooked meat, and ½ lb. of potatoes. 1 pint of porter to men above 16 years of age.
SUPPER.—½ pint of milk, or 1 pint of soup if ordered.

ORDINARY DIET.

DINNER.—4 oz. of cooked meat for men; 3 oz. for women. ½ lb. of potatoes. ½ pint of porter to men above 16 years of age.
SUPPER.—½ pint of milk, or 1 pint of soup if ordered.

FISH DIET.

DINNER.—4 oz. plain boiled white fish (as whiting, plaice, flounders, or haddock). ½ lb. of potatoes.
SUPPER.—½ pint of milk.

BROTH DIET.

DINNER.—1 pint of broth and 6 oz. of light pudding (such as tapioca, sago, rice, corn-flour, or such other pudding as the superintendent of nurses shall arrange).
SUPPER.—½ pint of milk.

MILK DIET.

DINNER.—Four days—1½ pint of rice milk.
    Three days—½ lb. of bread or rice pudding.
SUPPER.—½ pint of milk.
    Beef-tea, Yorkshire pudding, arrow-root, etc., to be specially directed.
    Ordinary diet for children under 7 years of age to consist of 2 oz. of meat, 4 oz. of potatoes, and some light pudding.

MIDDLESEX HOSPITAL.

CONVALESCENT DIET.

DAILY.—10 oz. of bread.
BREAKFAST.—½ pint of milk.
DINNER.—12 oz. of undressed meat* (roast and boiled alternately) for males, 8 oz. for females, and ½ lb. of potatoes.
SUPPER.—1 pint of gruel or 1 pint of broth.

HALF CONVALESCENT DIET.

DAILY—10 oz. of bread.
BREAKFAST.—½ pint of milk.
DINNER.—4 oz. of undressed meat * (roast and boiled alternately). ½ lb. of potatoes.
SUPPER.—1 pint of gruel or 1 pint of broth.

---

* Leg and shoulder of mutton only, except on Sundays, when the same quantity of roast sirloin and best round of beef is issued.

PUDDING AND ORDINARY DIET.

DAILY.—10 oz. of bread.
BREAKFAST.—½ pint of milk.
DINNER.—6 oz. of undressed **meat*** (roast and boiled alternately); ¼ lb. of potatoes; 1 oz. of beef suet and 2 oz. of flour for pudding.
SUPPER.—1 pint of gruel or 1 pint of broth.

ORDINARY DIET.

DAILY.—10 oz. of bread.
BREAKFAST.—½ pint of milk.
DINNER.—6 oz. of undressed meat † (roast and boiled alternately) and ½ lb. of potatoes.
SUPPER.—1 pint of gruel or 1 pint of broth.

HALF ORDINARY DIET.

DAILY.—10 oz. of bread.
BREAKFAST.—½ pint of milk.
DINNER.—3 oz. of undressed meat † (roast and boiled alternately) and ½ lb. of potatoes.
SUPPER.—1 pint of gruel or 1 pint of broth.

MUTTON-BROTH DIET.

DAILY.—10 oz. of bread.
BREAKFAST.—½ pint of milk.
DINNER.—8 oz. of undressed meat (neck of mutton only), weighed with bone before it is dressed, served in 1 pint of broth with barley.
SUPPER.—1 pint of gruel.

FISH DIET.

DAILY.—10 oz. of bread.
BREAKFAST.—½ pint of milk.
DINNER.—8 oz. of fish (whiting, sole, haddock, cod, plaice, or brill). ½ lb. of potatoes.
SUPPER.—1 pint of gruel.

MILK DIET.

DAILY.—10 oz. of bread.
BREAKFAST.—½ pint of milk.
DINNER.—Alternate days—rice pudding, containing 2 oz. of rice, half an egg, ½ oz. of sugar; sago pudding, containing 1¼ oz. of sago, half an egg, and ½ oz. of sugar; and bread pudding, containing bread, with one and a half eggs, and ¾ oz. of sugar. Extra—custard, ½ oz.
SUPPER.—1½ pint of milk.

SIMPLE DIET.

DAILY.—10 oz. of bread.
BREAKFAST.—½ pint of milk.
DINNER.—1 pint of gruel.
SUPPER.—½ pint of milk.

* Leg and shoulder of mutton only, except on Sundays, when the same quantity of roast sirloin and best round of beef is issued.
† Leg and shoulder of mutton only, weighed with the bone before it is dressed.

EXTRAS.

For supper, meat when cooked, 3 oz. Chops, ½ lb. each when trimmed. Ordinary beef-tea, ¼ lb. of clod and sticking of beef, without bone, to a pint. Strong beef-tea, 1 lb. of ditto, ditto. Broth without meat: ¼ lb. of neck of mutton with bone, to a pint; this broth is made with that for the patients on mutton-broth diet. Steaks: rump-steak, ½ lb., without bone. Tripe, chicken, oysters, greens, eggs, arrow-root, sago, jellies, porter, wine, spirits.

UNIVERSITY COLLEGE HOSPITAL.

FULL DIET.

12 oz. of bread. 8 oz of potatoes. 6 oz. meat, dressed (roast or boiled leg or neck of mutton, or roast beef). ¾ pint of broth or pea soup four times a week on alternate days. 4 oz. boiled rice or rice pudding made with milk. 1 pint of milk. 1 pint of beer.*

MIDDLE DIET.

12 oz. of bread. 8 oz. of potatoes. 4 oz. of meat or 8 oz. of fish (white). 1 pint of milk. Soup with barley, 1½ oz.; or beef-tea, 1 pint. Rice pudding made with milk, instead of soup. ½ pint of beer.*

SPOON DIET.

2 pints of milk. 1 pint of beef-tea. 12 oz. of bread. 2 oz. of arrow-root and 1 oz. of sugar made into a jelly.

The resident assistants to the physicians and surgeons are empowered, during the absence of their superior officers, to order the following extras, subject to the general supervision of the resident medical officer:—Malt liquors, spirits, port, sherry, eggs, strong beef-tea, milk, fish, chops, steaks, custard puddings, vegetables, and bread. Such orders to stand good for twenty-four hours only.

KING'S COLLEGE HOSPITAL.

MEAT DIET (MEN).

Bread 12 oz. Milk, ¾ pint. Meat,† 4 oz. cooked. Potatoes, ½ lb. Porter, ale, 1 pint. Rice or other pudding, ½ lb.

MEAT DIET (WOMEN).

Bread, 8 oz. Milk, ¾ pint. Meat,† 4 oz. cooked. Potatoes, ½ lb. Porter or ale, ¼ pint. Rice or other pudding, ½ lb.

MILK DIET (MEN).

Bread, 8 oz. Milk, 1½ pint. Eggs, 2. Rice or other pudding, ½ lb.

---

* To medical cases beer is only to be supplied when ordered.
† Sunday, roast beef; Monday, Thursday, Friday, and Saturday, roast mutton; Tuesday, boiled mutton; Wednesday, soup.

MILK DIET (WOMEN).

Bread, 6 oz. Milk, 1½ pint. Eggs, 2. Rice or other pudding, ½ lb.

Children under 10 years of age same as milk diet for women.

Beef-tea (on milk diet only), wine, and spirits, may be ordered by the resident medical officers.

Fish or mince may be added to milk diet; such addition to be authorized by the signature of the visiting physician or surgeon, to be renewed once in each week at the least.

ST. MARY'S HOSPITAL.

FULL DIET.

BREAKFAST.—Tea with sugar. Bread and butter. ¼ pint of milk.
DINNER.—6 oz. of meat (cooked). ½ lb. of potatoes.
TEA.—Tea with sugar. Bread and butter. ¼ pint of milk.
SUPPER.—Gruel.

DAILY ALLOWANCE TO EACH PATIENT.—2 pints of tea with sugar, and ½ pint of milk. 15 oz. of bread. 6 oz. of meat when dressed. ½ lb. of potatoes. ¾ oz. of butter.

ORDINARY DIET.

BREAKFAST.—Tea with sugar. Bread and butter. ¼ pint of milk.
DINNER.—4 oz. of meat (cooked). ½ lb. of potatoes.
TEA.—Tea with sugar. Bread and butter. ¼ pint of milk.
SUPPER.—Gruel.

DAILY ALLOWANCE TO EACH PATIENT.—2 pints of tea with sugar, and ½ pint of milk. 12 oz. of bread. 4 oz. of meat when dressed. ½ lb. potatoes. ¾ oz. of butter.

HALF DIET.

BREAKFAST.—Tea with sugar. Bread and butter. ½ pint of milk.
DINNER.—2 oz. of meat (cooked). ½ lb. of potatoes.
TEA.—Tea with milk. Bread and butter. ½ pint of milk.
SUPPER.—Gruel.

DAILY ALLOWANCE TO EACH PATIENT.—2 pints of tea with sugar, and 1 pint of milk. 12 oz. bread. 2 oz. of meat when dressed. ½ lb. of potatoes. ¾ oz. of butter.

BROTH DIET.

BREAKFAST.—Tea with sugar. Bread and butter. ¼ pint of milk.
DINNER.—¼ lb. meat before dressed. 1 pint of broth.
TEA.—Tea with sugar. Bread and butter. ¼ pint of milk.
SUPPER.—Gruel.

DAILY ALLOWANCE TO EACH PATIENT.—2 pints of tea with sugar, and ¼ pint of milk. 12 oz. of bread. About 4 oz. of meat when dressed. 1 pint of broth. ¾ oz. of butter.

SIMPLE DIET.

2 pints of tea with sugar, and 1 pint of milk. 12 oz. of bread. ¾ oz. of butter.

SUPPER.—Gruel.

No extras, except porter, allowed on full diet.

No extras, to be ordered by the resident medical officers in the absence of the physician or surgeon, unless in cases of great urgency, a special report of which must be made to the physician or surgeon at his next visit.

WESTMINSTER HOSPITAL.

FULL DIET.

DAILY.—14 oz. of bread.

BREAKFAST.—Tea (⅛ oz.) with milk (¼ pint) and sugar (½ oz.).

DINNER.—¼ lb. of meat, roasted, boiled, or chops. ½ lb. of potatoes.

SUPPER.—Tea (⅛ oz). with milk (¼ pint) and sugar (½ oz.).

MIDDLE DIET.

DAILY.—10 oz. of bread.

BREAKFAST.—Tea (⅛ oz.) with milk (¼ pint) and sugar (½ oz.).

DINNER.—¼ lb. of meat, roasted, boiled, or chops. ½ lb. of potatoes.

SUPPER.—Tea (⅛ oz.) with milk (¼ pint) and sugar (½ oz.).

LOW DIET (FIXED).

DAILY.—½ lb. of bread.

BREAKFAST.—Tea (⅛ oz.) with sugar (½ oz.) and milk (¼ pint).

DINNER.—No fixed diet.

SUPPER.—Tea (⅛ oz.) with sugar (½ oz.) and milk (¼ pint).

LOW DIET (CASUAL).

1 pint of broth (from 2 oz. of meat), or ½ lb. of bread or rice pudding, or 1 pint of beef-tea (from 4 oz. of beef), or a chop, or fish.

Composition of bread pudding.—Bread, ¼ lb. Milk, ½ pint. Sugar, ½oz. Flour, ¼ oz. 1 egg for every 2 lbs.

Composition of rice pudding.—Rice, 1½ oz. Milk, ½ pint. Sugar, ½ oz.

SPOON OR FEVER DIET.

DAILY.—¼ lb. of bread.

BREAKFAST.—Tea (⅛ oz.) with sugar (¾ oz.) and milk (¼ pint).

DINNER.—Barley water (from 2 oz. of prepared barley).

SUPPER.—Tea (⅛ oz.) with sugar (¾ oz.) and milk (¼ pint).

EXTRAS.

Porter, or wine, or spirits. No other extras to be allowed with full or middle diet.

Every patient admitted into the hospital is to be placed upon low diet, until a diet is ordered by the physicians or surgeons.

No extras to be placed on the diet roll by the apothecary, or to be provided by the steward or matron, other than those specified as above.

NOTE.—Arrow-root, sago, vermicelli, or coffee, allowed as extras to low and spoon diet, on the written order of the medical officers, communicated to the matron.

INCURABLES' DIET.

Bread, ¾ lb. Meat, ¼ lb. Potatoes, ½ lb. Milk, ¼ pint. Porter, 1 pint. Each daily, when not otherwise ordered.

SEAMEN'S HOSPITAL.

FULL DIET.

1 lb. of bread. ¾ lb. of meat—viz., two days roast mutton, one day boiled mutton, four days boiled beef. ¾ lb. of potatoes. 1 pint of soup (on boiled meat days).

MUTTON (OR EXTRA) DIET.

1 lb. of bread. ¾ lb. of roast mutton (boiled on Tuesdays). ¾ lb. of potatoes. 1 pint of soup (on boiled meat day).

ORDINARY DIET.

1 lb. of bread. ½ lb of meat—viz., two days roast mutton, one day boiled mutton, four days boiled beef. ½ lb. of potatoes. 1 pint of soup (on boiled meat days).

LOW DIET.

¼ lb. of bread. 1 pint of beef-tea.

MILK DIET.

1 lb. of bread. 1 quart of milk. 1 pint of beef-tea. Tea with milk and sugar, morning and evening, with all diets.

LEEDS GENERAL INFIRMARY.

LOW DIET (ADULTS).

BREAKFAST.—8 oz. of buttered bread. 1 pint of tea.
DINNER.—4 oz. of bread. 1 pint of broth.
TEA.—8 oz. of buttered bread. 1 pint of tea.
SUPPER.—1 pint of rice milk.

LOW DIET (CHILDREN).

BREAKFAST.—4 oz. of buttered bread. ⅓ pint of tea.
DINNER.—2 oz. of bread. ½ pint of broth. 4 oz. of rice pudding.
TEA.—4 oz. of buttered bread. ½ pint of tea.

ORDINARY DIET (ADULTS).

BREAKFAST.—8 oz. of buttered bread. 1 pint of tea.
DINNER.—Meat, 4 oz. (Sunday, Wednesday, and Friday, boiled beef;
Monday, roast beef; Tuesday, Thursday, and Saturday, roast mutton).
8 oz. potatoes.
TEA.—8 oz. of buttered bread. 1 pint of tea.
SUPPER.—1 pint of rice milk.

ORDINARY DIET (CHILDREN).

BREAKFAST.—4 oz. of buttered bread. ½ pint of tea.
DINNER.—Meat, 2 oz. (Sunday and Friday, boiled beef; Monday and
Wednesday, roast beef; Tuesday, Thursday, and Saturday, roast
mutton). 4 oz. of potatoes.
TEA.—4 oz. of buttered bread. ½ pint of tea.

FULL DIET (ADULTS).

BREAKFAST.—8 oz. of buttered bread. 1 pint of tea.
DINNER.—Meat, 5 oz. (Sunday and Friday, boiled beef; Monday and
Wednesday, roast beef; Tuesday and Saturday, roast mutton; Thurs-
day, boiled mutton). 8 oz. of potatoes. ½ pint of broth.
TEA.—8 oz. of buttered bread. 1 pint of tea.
SUPPER.—1 pint of rice milk.

MANCHESTER ROYAL INFIRMARY AND DISPENSARY.

GENEROUS DIET.

BREAKFAST.—1 pint of tea or coffee. 6 oz. of bread. ¾ oz. of butter.
Or boiled bread and milk; or porridge with milk.
DINNER.—Sunday, Tuesday, Thursday, and Saturday—6 oz. of beef,
roasted. 4 oz. of bread. 8 oz. of potatoes.
Monday, Wednesday, and Friday—6 oz. of mutton, boiled.
4 oz. of bread. 8 oz. of potatoes.
This diet to be changed on the alternate weeks, *i.e.*, on one week, four
days the beef is to be roasted and three days the mutton boiled; on the
other week, four days the mutton is to be roasted and three days the beef
boiled, as indicated above.
SUPPER.—The same as breakfast, except that no coffee is allowed.

COMMON DIET.

BREAKFAST.—1 pint of tea or coffee. 5 oz. of bread. ½ oz. of butter.
Or boiled bread and milk; or porridge with milk.
DINNER.—Sunday, Wednesday, and Friday—6 oz. of beef roasted. 4 oz.
of bread. 8 oz. of potatoes.

DINNER.—Monday—1 pint of good soup. 2 oz. of roast meat and potatoes. 4 oz. of bread.

Tuesday, Thursday, and Saturday—Potato hash, with 4 oz. of bread; or the option of having cold meat, with 8 oz. of potatoes, and 4 oz. of bread.

SUPPER.—The same as breakfast, except that no coffee is allowed.

MILK DIET.

BREAKFAST.—1 pint of tea or coffee. 5 oz. of bread. ½ oz. of butter. Or boiled bread and milk, with porridge and milk.

DINNER.—Sunday and Wednesday—½ pint of milk. 12 oz. of semolina pudding.

Monday, Thursday, and Saturday—½ pint of milk. 12 oz. of rice pudding.

Tuesday and Friday—½ pint of milk. 12 oz. of bread pudding.

At the option of the medical and surgical officers, ¼ pint of beef-tea may be substituted for the ½ pint of milk.

SUPPER.—The same as breakfast, except that no coffee is allowed.

LOW DIET.

BREAKFAST.—1 pint of tea. 3 oz. of bread.

DINNER.—1 pint of gruel. 2 oz. of bread.

SUPPER.—Water gruel or tea. 3 oz. of bread.

BIRMINGHAM GENERAL HOSPITAL.

LOW DIET (MEN AND WOMEN).

BREAKFAST.—1 pint of milk.

DINNER.—8 oz. of rice or sago pudding. 1 pint of broth for lunch. 12 oz. of bread.

SUPPER.—1 pint of broth or gruel.

LOW DIET (CHILDREN).

BREAKFAST.—1 pint of milk.

DINNER.—8 oz. of rice or sago pudding. 6 oz. of bread.

SUPPER.—½ pint of broth or gruel.

MILK DIET (MEN AND WOMEN).

BREAKFAST.—1 pint of milk.

DINNER.—12 oz. of bread. 1½ pint of milk.

SUPPER.—1 pint of broth or gruel.

MILK DIET (CHILDREN).

BREAKFAST.—1 pint of milk.

DINNER.—6 oz. of bread. 1½ pint of milk.

SUPPER.—½ pint of broth or gruel.

HOUSE DIET (MEN AND WOMEN).

BREAKFAST.—1 pint of milk.
DINNER.—Cooked meat (4 oz. men, 3 oz. women). 8 oz. of potatoes. 12 oz. of bread.
SUPPER.—1 pint of broth or gruel.

HOUSE DIET (CHILDREN).

BREAKFAST.—1 pint of milk.
DINNER.—2 oz. of cooked meat. 6 oz. of potatoes. 6 oz. of bread.
SUPPER.—½ pint of broth or gruel.

MUTTON DIET (MEN AND WOMEN).

BREAKFAST.—1 pint of milk.
DINNER.—Cooked mutton (4 oz. men, 3 oz. women). 8 oz. of potatoes. 12 oz. of bread.
SUPPER.—1 pint of broth or gruel.

MUTTON DIET (CHILDREN).

BREAKFAST.—1 pint of milk.
DINNER.—2 oz. of cooked mutton. 6 oz. of potatoes. 6 oz. of bread.
SUPPER.—½ pint of broth or gruel.

FULL DIET (MEN AND WOMEN).

BREAKFAST.—1 pint of milk.
DINNER.—Cooked meat (6 oz. men, 4 oz. women). 8 oz. potatoes. 12 oz. of bread.
SUPPER.—1 pint of broth or gruel.

FULL DIET (CHILDREN).

BREAKFAST.—1 pint of milk.
DINNER.—2 oz. of cooked meat. 6 oz. of potatoes. 6 oz. of bread.
SUPPER.—½ pint of broth or gruel.

NEWCASTLE-UPON-TYNE INFIRMARY.

COMMON DIET.

BREAKFAST.—1 pint of porridge and 1 gill of milk, or 1 pint of tea.
LUNCHEON.—½ pint of soup.
DINNER.—6 oz. of beef or mutton (roast, Sunday, Tuesday, Thursday, and Saturday; boiled, Monday, Wednesday, and Friday), and potatoes.
TEA.—1 pint of tea.
SUPPER.—Sunday, Tuesday, Thursday, and Saturday, 1 gill of milk. Monday, Wednesday, and Friday, 1 gill of boiled rice and milk.
  Every male to have 14 oz. of bread, and every female 12 oz., daily.
Every male to have six oz. of meat, and every female 5 oz., daily.

MILK DIET.

BREAKFAST.—1 pint of porridge and 1 gill of milk, or 1 pint of tea.
DINNER.—Sunday and Thursday, rice pudding and 1 gill of milk. Monday, Wednesday, and Friday, 1 pint of broth mixed with barley. Tuesday and Saturday, 1 pint of boiled rice and milk.
TEA.—1 pint of tea.
SUPPER.—Sunday, Tuesday, Thursday, and Saturday, 1 gill of milk. Monday, Wednesday, and Friday, 1 gill of boiled rice and milk.
Every male to have 12 oz. of bread, and every female 10 oz., daily.
All extras only by order of the medical officers.

EDINBURGH ROYAL INFIRMARY.

LOW DIET.

BREAKFAST.—Bread, 3 oz. Tea, ½ pint (tea, ⅛ oz.; milk, 1 oz.; sugar, ½ oz.).
DINNER.—Panada (bread, 3 oz.; milk, 2 oz.; sugar, ¼ oz.).
SUPPER.—Bread, 3 oz. Tea, ½ pint (tea, ⅛ oz.; milk, 1 oz.; sugar, ½ oz.).

RICE DIET.

BREAKFAST.—Bread, 3 oz. Coffee, ½ pint (coffee, ½ oz.; milk, 2 oz.; sugar, ½ oz.). One egg.
DINNER.—Beef-tea (from 8 oz. of meat), ⅘ pint. Rice pudding (rice, 1½ oz.; sugar, ½ oz.; milk, 2½ oz; half an egg; essential oil of lemon, 1 drop).
SUPPER.—Bread, 3 oz. Tea, ½ pint (tea, ⅛ oz.; milk 1 oz.; sugar, ½ oz.).

STEAK DIET.

BREAKFAST.—Bread, 6 oz. Coffee, ½ pint (coffee, ½ oz.; milk, 2 oz.; sugar, ½ oz.).
DINNER.—Potatoes, 16 oz. Beefsteak,* 4 oz. Broth, 1 pint (barley, 1 oz.; vegetables, ¾ oz.; meat, 2 oz.).
SUPPER.—Bread, 6 oz. Tea, ½ pint (tea, ⅛ oz.; milk, 1 oz.; sugar, ½ oz.).

STEAK DIET WITH BREAD.

This is the same as "Steak Diet," except that 6 oz. of bread are substituted at dinner for potatoes, and ⅘ of a pint of beef-tea for broth.

COMMON DIET.

BREAKFAST.—Bread, 6 oz. Coffee, ½ pint (coffee, ½ oz.; milk, 2 oz.; sugar, ½ oz.).
DINNER.—Potatoes, 16 oz. Broth, 1 pint (barley, 1 oz.; vegetables, ¾ oz.; meat, 2 oz.).
SUPPER.—Bread, 6 oz. Tea, ½ pint (tea, ⅛ oz.; milk, 1 oz.; sugar, ½ oz.).

---

* In this and all the other diets, the weight is to be understood as applying to the food before being cooked.

COMMON DIET WITH BREAD.

The same as "Common Diet," except that 6 oz. of bread are substituted at dinner for potatoes.

FULL DIET.

BREAKFAST.—Porridge, 1½ pint—made of oatmeal, 4½ oz. Buttermilk 1 pint (20 oz.).
DINNER.—Boiled meat, 6 oz. Potatoes 16 oz. Bread 3 oz. Broth (barley, 1 oz.; vegetables, ¾ oz.; meat, 2 oz.).
SUPPER.—Potatoes, 16 oz. New milk, ½ pint (10 oz.).

FULL DIET WITH BREAD.

The same as "Full Diet," except that bread, 8 oz., is substituted for potatoes and bread at dinner; and bread, 6 oz., for potatoes at supper.

EXTRA DIET.

BREAKFAST.—Porridge, 2 pints—made of oatmeal, 6 oz.; buttermilk, 1 pint (20 oz.).
DINNER.—Boiled meat, 8 oz. Potatoes, 20 oz. Bread, 3 oz. Broth, 1 pint (barley, 1 oz.; vegetables, ¾ oz.; meat, 2 oz.).
SUPPER.—Potatoes, 20 oz. New milk, 15 oz.

GLASGOW ROYAL INFIRMARY.

ORDINARY DIET.

BREAKFAST.—Bread, 4 oz. Butter, salt (or fresh, if specially ordered), ½ oz. Tea, 4 gills.
DINNER.—Bread, 6 oz. Broth or soup, 2 pints. Beef or mutton, boiled (cooked weight, free of bone), 4 oz.; or, beefsteak (uncooked weight, trimmed and free of bone), 4 oz.; or, mutton chop (uncooked weight, bone included), 6 oz.; or, chicken, one-fifth part of a fowl; or, fresh fish (cleaned weight), 8 oz. Potatoes, when in season, instead of bread, 1 lb. Beef-tea may be specially ordered instead of broth or soup, but, as a rule, beef-tea with bread is a dinner without beef or mutton.
SUPPER.—Bread, 4 oz. Butter, ½ oz. Coffee, 4 gills.

MILK DIET.

BREAKFAST.—Bread, 4 oz. Milk, 4 gills.
DINNER.—Rice, 2½ oz. Milk, 4 gills.
SUPPER.—Bread, 4 oz. Milk, 4 gills.

ROTATION OF BROTH OR SOUPS.

Sunday, Wednesday, and Friday, broth. Monday and Thursday, rice soup. Tuesday and Saturday, pea soup.
Chicken soup. Beef-tea.

EXTRAS, WHICH CAN BE HAD TO ORDER.

Porridge and buttermilk—4 oz. meal and 4 gills of milk. Milk, sweet, to porridge, 2 gills. Milk, for drink, 2 gills. Milk, warm, 2 gills. 1 egg. Sago, arrow-root, corn-flour, 2 oz. Biscuits. Strong beef-tea. Dry tea, 2 oz., and 8 oz. sugar, for a week's supply.

RICHMOND, WHITWORTH, AND HARDWICKE HOSPITALS (DUBLIN).

LOW DIET (RICHMOND AND WHITWORTH).

BREAKFAST.—Bread, 4 oz. Tea, ¾ pint.
DINNER.—Bread, 4 oz. New milk, ¾ pint.
SUPPER.—Bread, 4 oz. Tea, ¾ pint. Whey, 1 pint.

LOW DIET (HARDWICKE).

BREAKFAST.—Bread, 4 oz. Tea, ¾ pint.
DINNER.—Bread, 4 oz. New milk, ¾ pint.
SUPPER.—Tea, ¾ pint. Whey, 1 pint.

EXTRAS ALLOWED.—1 egg. Arrow-root, ¾ pint; or beef-tea, ¾ pint, or new milk, ¾ pint, or rice milk ¾ pint. Wine, or brandy, or gin, or whiskey, or porter, ½ pint, as specially ordered.

MIDDLE DIET.

BREAKFAST.—Bread, 6 oz. Tea, ¾ pint.
DINNER.—Bread, 6 oz. Beef, boiled (exclusive of bone), ¼ lb., with broth, ¾ pint.
SUPPER.—Bread, 4 oz. Tea, ¾ pint.

EXTRAS ALLOWED.—1 egg. New milk, ¾ pint; or porter, ½ pint; or gin or wine, not exceeding 4 oz.

MUTTON DIET.

BREAKFAST.—Bread, 6 oz. Tea, ¾ pint.
DINNER.—Bread, 6 oz. Mutton, boiled (exclusive of bone), ½ lb
SUPPER.—Bread, 4 oz. Tea, ¾ pint.

EXTRAS ALLOWED.—1 egg. New milk, ¾ pint; or porter, ½ pint; or wine, not exceeding 4 oz. Fresh vegetables as ordered.

FULL DIET.

BREAKFAST.—Bread, 8 oz. Tea, ¾ pint.
DINNER.—Bread, 8 oz.; or potatoes, 1 lb. Beef, boiled (exclusive of bone), ½ lb., with broth, ¾ pint.
SUPPER.—Bread, 4 oz. Tea, ¾ pint.
EXTRAS ALLOWED.—New milk, ¾ pint; or porter, ½ pint.

Beef, with broth, to be given for dinner on five days in each week to patients on middle diet. On Wednesdays and Fridays ¾ pint of gruel to be substituted.

Potatoes, on Tuesdays, Thursdays, and Saturdays to patients on full diet, instead of bread.

Formularies.

TEA (6 pints).—Tea, 1½ oz. Sugar, 4 oz. New milk, ½ pint.

BEEF WITH BROTH (6 pints).—Beef (exclusive of bone), 4 lb. Barley, ¼ lb. Oatmeal, 2 oz. Parsley, 1 oz. Thyme, ¼ oz. Onions or leeks, ½ lb. Pepper and salt to taste.

BEEF-TEA (6 pints).—Beef (lean, without bone), 4 lb. Pepper and salt to taste.

WHEY.—New milk, 1 quart. Buttermilk, 1 pint.

GRUEL (6 pints).—Oatmeal, 12 oz. Sugar, 3 oz. Ginger to flavor. Steep the meal from night before; boil for two hours.

ARROW-ROOT (¾ pint).—Arrow-root, ½ oz. Sugar, ¼ oz. New milk, ¾ pint.

BETHLEHEM LUNATIC HOSPITAL.

BREAKFAST.—Every day—Tea, with 7 oz. of bread and butter for males, and 6 oz. for females. .

DINNER.—Every day, except Saturday—4 oz. of bread. ¾ lb. of vegetables, and 1 pint of beer, with 6 oz. for males and 5 oz. for females of boiled beef (free from bone) on Sunday; roast mutton on Monday and Thursday; boiled mutton on Tuesday and Friday; and roast beef on Wednesday. Saturday—Meat pie (16 oz. males, 14 oz. females). 4 oz. of bread. 1 oz. of cheese. Beer (males 1 pint, females ½ pint).

SUPPER. —Males, Sunday, Monday, Tuesday, Thursday, and Friday, same as at breakfast; Wednesday and Saturday, 7 oz. of bread, 2 oz of cheese, 1 pint of beer. Females, every day, same as at breakfast.

Patients in employment in the grounds, workshops, or laundry, to be allowed 4 oz. of bread, 1 oz. of cheese or ½ oz. of butter, and ½ pint of beer for luncheon; and ½ pint of beer in the afternoon.

Every patient to be allowed 1¾ oz. of tea, 8 oz. of sugar, 8 oz. of butter, and 1½ pint of milk, weekly.

On Christmas Day the dinner to be roast beef and plum pudding. On New Year's Day a mince pie to be added to the usual fare. On Good Friday a bun. On Easter and Whit Monday 6 oz. of roast veal to be allowed instead of the usual meat for the day.

The dinners to be further varied by the occasional substitution of pork and bacon, when peas and beans are in season; and also by the occasional substitution of fish, and fruit pies, when fish and fruit are plentiful and good.

The sick to be dieted at the discretion of the resident physician.

The attendants to have at all times the means of obtaining gruel for such patients as may require it.

The above to be considered maximum allowances, and all quantities unconsumed are to be taken in diminution of the next supply from the stores of the Hospital.

ST. LUKE'S HOSPITAL FOR LUNATICS.

MALE DIETARY.

BREAKFAST.—Cocoa, ½ oz. Milk, ¼ pint. Sugar, ¼ oz. Bread, 8 oz. Butter, ½ oz.

DINNER.—

Sunday.—Cooked meat, with bone, 6 oz. Potatoes, 12 oz. Bread, 6 oz. Beer, 1 pint. Pudding (farinaceous or fruit), 6 oz.

Monday.—Meat pie, with potatoes, 12 oz. Bread, 3 oz. Beer, 1 pint.

Tuesday.—Cooked meat, with bone, 8 oz. Bread, 6 oz. Beer, 1 pint.

Wednesday.—Meat pudding, 12 oz. Potatoes, 8 oz. Bread, 3 oz. Beer, 1 pint.

Thursday.—Same as Tuesday.

Friday.—Cooked meat, with bone, 8 oz. Potatoes, 12 oz. Bread, 6 oz. Beer, 1 pint.

Saturday.—Same as Tuesday and Thursday.

TEA.—Tea, ¼ oz. Sugar, ½ oz. Milk, ⅛ pint. Bread, 8 oz. Butter, ½ oz.

FEMALE DIETARY.

BREAKFAST.—Same as for males, less 2 oz. of bread.

DINNER.—

Sunday.—Same as for males, less 2 oz. of meat, 4 oz. of potatoes, and ¼ pint of beer.

Monday.—Same as for males, less 2 oz. of pie and ¼ pint of beer.

Tuesday.—Same as for males, less 2 oz. of meat and ¼ pint of beer.

Wednesday.—Same as for males, less 2 oz. of meat pudding, 2 oz. of potatoes, and ¼ pint of beer.

Thursday.—Same as Tuesday.

Friday.—Same as for males, less 2 oz. of meat, 4 oz. of potatoes, and ¼ pint of beer.

Saturday.—Same as for Tuesday and Thursday.

TEA.—Same as for males.

1 pint of beer, 8 oz. of bread, and 2 oz. of cheese, may be had for supper in place of the ordinary tea by those male patients for whom the medical officer shall think it desirable.

Patients employed in work for the hospital to be allowed 4 oz. of bread, 1 oz. of cheese, and ¼ pint of beer for lunch.

The dinners may be varied by the occasional substitution of pork, bacon, salt beef, or veal, when in season; and also the occasional substitution of fish and fruit pies, when either are plentiful and good.

Lettuce during the summer months may be substituted occasionally for other vegetables.

The sick to be dieted at the discretion of the medical officers.

The above to be considered maximum allowances; and all quantities unconsumed to be returned to the kitchen.

HANWELL LUNATIC ASYLUM.

DIET TABLE FOR PATIENTS EMPLOYED.

BREAKFAST.—
Males.—Cocoa, 1 pint. Bread, 6 oz. Butter, ½ oz.
Females.—Tea, 1 pint. Bread, 5 oz. Butter, ½ oz.

LUNCHEON.—
Males.—Bread, 3 oz. Cheese, 1 oz. Beer, ½ pint.
Females.—Bread, 3 oz. Cheese, 1 oz. Beer, ½ pint.

DINNER.—
Males—
Sunday.—Cooked meat, free from bone (roast pork, beef or mutton), 5 oz. Vegetables, 9 oz. Bread, 3 oz. Beer, ½ pint.
Monday.—Cooked meat, free from bone (boiled bacon or pickled pork), 5 oz. Vegetables, 16 oz. Bread, 3 oz. Beer, ½ pint.
Tuesday.—Cooked meat, free from bone (boiled Australian beef or mutton), 5 oz. Vegetables, 9 oz. Dumplings, 4 oz. Beer, ½ pint.
Wednesday.—Cooked meat, free from bone (meat pies), 3 oz. Pie, 4 oz. Vegetables, 12 oz. Beer, ½ pint.
Thursday.—Fish (fried or boiled, with melted butter), 10 oz. Vegetables, 9 oz. Bread, 3 oz. Beer, ½ pint.
Friday.—Cooked meat, free from bone (boiled bacon or pickled pork), 5 oz. Vegetables, 16 oz. Dumplings, 4 oz. Beer, ½ pint.
Saturday.—Cooked meat, free from bone (Irish stew), 2 oz. Stew, 16 oz. Bread, 6 oz. Beer, ½ pint.
Females—
Sunday.—Same as for males, less 1 oz. of meat and 1 oz. of vegetables.
Monday.—Same as for males, less 1 oz. of meat and 4 oz. of vegetables.
Tuesday.—Cooked meat, free from bone (boiled beef or mutton), 4 oz. Vegetables, 12 oz. Bread, 3 oz. Beer, ½ pint.
Wednesday.—Same as for males.
Thursday.—Cooked meat, free from bone (boiled Australian beef or mutton), 4 oz. Vegetables, 8 oz. Bread, 3 oz. Beer, ½ pint.
Friday.—Fish (fried or boiled, with melted butter), 8 oz. Vegetables, 8 oz. Bread, 3 oz. Beer, ½ pint.
Saturday.—Same as for males, less 2 oz. of bread.

SUPPER.—
Males.—Tea, 1 pint. Bread, 6 oz. Butter, ½ oz.
Females.—Tea, 1 pint. Bread, 5 oz. Butter, ¼ oz.

DIET FOR PATIENTS NOT EMPLOYED.

BREAKFAST.—
Males.—Cocoa, 1 pint. Bread, 6 oz. Butter, ½ oz.
Females.—Tea, 1 pint. Bread, 5 oz. Butter, ½ oz.

DINNER.—

Males—

Sunday.—Cooked meat, free from bone (roast pork, beef, or mutton), 5 oz. Vegetables, 9 oz. Bread, 3 oz. Beer, ½ pint.

Monday.—Soup, thickened with oatmeal, rice, and peas, and containing 2 oz. of meat for each patient, with a proportion of Ramornie Extract, 1 pint. Bread 6 oz. Beer, ½ pint.

Tuesday.—Cooked meat, free from bone (boiled Australian beef or mutton), 5 oz. Vegetables, 9 oz. Dumplings, 4 oz. Beer, ½ pint.

Wednesday.—Cooked meat, free from bone (meat pies), 3 oz. Pie, 4 oz. Vegetables, 12 oz. Beer, ½ pint.

Thursday.—Fish (fried or boiled, with melted butter), 10 oz. Vegetables, 9 oz. Bread, 3 oz. Beer, ½ pint.

Friday.—Cooked meat, free from bone (boiled bacon or pickled pork), 5 oz. Vegetables, 16 oz. Dumplings, 4 oz. Beer, ½ pint.

Sunday.—Cooked meat, free from bone (Irish stew), 2 oz. Stew, 16 oz. Bread, 6 oz. Beer, ½ pint.

Females—

Sunday.—Same as for males, less 1 oz. of meat and 1 oz. of vegetables.

Monday.—Same as for males, less 2 oz. of bread.

Tuesday.—Cooked meat, free from bone (boiled bacon or pickled pork), 4 oz. Vegetables, 12 oz. Bread, 3 oz. Beer, ½ pint.

Wednesday.—Same as for males.

Thursday.—Cooked meat, free from bone (boiled Australian beef or mutton), 4 oz. Vegetables, 8 oz. Bread 3 oz. Beer, ½ pint.

Friday.—Fish (fried or boiled, with melted butter), 8 oz. Vegetables, 8 oz. Bread, 3 oz. Beer, ½ pint.

Saturday.—Same as for males, less 2 oz. of bread.

SUPPER.—

Males—Tea, 1 pint. Bread, 6 oz. Butter, ½ oz.

Females—Tea, 1 pint. Bread, 5 oz. Butter, ¼ oz.

2 oz. of cheese and 1 pint of beer given to male patients for supper in lieu of 1 pint of tea and ½ oz. of butter, if requested.

Formularies.

For 1 pint of cocoa—½ oz. of cocoa, 1 oz. of treacle, and ⅛ pint of milk.

For 1 pint of tea—¼ oz. of tea, ½ oz. of sugar, and ⅛ pint of milk.

Irish stew (liquor of the meat cooked the previous day), with 2 oz. cooked Australian meat (and a proportion of Ramornie Extract), and 12 oz. of vegetables for each patient.

Currant dumplings (made with dripping or suet) are given every third Saturday, in lieu of stew, 12 oz. to the males and 11 oz. to the females. ½ pint beer at 4 p.m., and tobacco and snuff, for working patients.

25

COLNEY HATCH LUNATIC ASYLUM.

MALES.

BREAKFAST.—6 oz. of bread, and ½ oz. of butter. 1 pint of cocoa.

DINNER—

Monday.—9 oz. of pie (containing 4 oz. of meat). 9 oz. of vegetables, ½ pint of beer.

Tuesday, Thursday, Friday, and Sunday.—5 oz. of cooked meat. 9 oz. of vegetables. 4 oz. of bread. ½ pint of beer.

Wednesday.—1 pint of stew, and 6 oz. of bread, as on Saturday; or 8 oz. of fish, 9 oz. of vegetables, and 4 oz. of bread. ½ pint of beer (with either dinner).

Saturday.—1 pint of Irish stew (made with 3 oz. of meat and the liquor from meat of previous day, 12 oz. of potatoes and other vegetables, and 1 oz. dumpling). 6 oz. of bread. ½ pint of beer.

TEA OR SUPPER.—6 oz. of bread. 2 oz. of cheese or ½ oz. of butter. ½ pint of beer or 1 pint of tea.

FEMALES.

BREAKFAST.—5 oz. of bread, and ½ oz. of butter. 1 pint of tea.

DINNER.—

Monday.—9 oz. of pie (containing 4 oz. of meat). 8 oz. of vegetables. ½ pint of beer.

Tuesday, Thursday, Friday, and Sunday.—4 oz. of cooked meat. 8 oz. of vegetables. 4 oz. of bread. ½ pint of beer.

Wednesday.—1 pint of soup (made with 4 oz. of meat and the liquor from meat of previous day, peas, rice, Scotch barley, herbs, etc.), and 5 oz. of bread; or 8 oz. of fish, 8 oz. of vegetables, and 4 oz. of bread; or 12 oz. of currant dumpling. ½ pint of beer (with either dinner).

Saturday.—1 pint of Irish stew (made with 3 oz. of meat and the liquor from meat of previous day, 12 oz. of potatoes and other vegetables, and 1 oz. dumpling). 6 oz. of bread. ½ pint of beer.

TEA.—5 oz. of bread. ½ oz of butter. 1 pint of tea.

INDEX.

www.ingramcontent.com/pod-product-compliance
Lightning Source LLC
Chambersburg PA
CBHW032316280326
41932CB00009B/832